Communicating Quality 3

RCSLT's guidance on best practice in service organisation and provision

© 2006

The Royal College of Speech and
Language Therapists
2 White Hart Yard
London SE1 1NX
020 7378 1200
www.rcslt.org

First published 1991
Second edition 1996

ISBN: 0-947589-55-4

Bell

D0549966

Contents

Chapter 4 RCSLT

Chapter 5 Service Organisation

Chapter 6 Service Provision: Part 1 Care Pathway

Chapter 7 Service Provision: Part 2
Working Contexts, Tasks, Techniques and Strategies

Foreword

This is the third edition of Communicating Quality, a text that in its first edition was widely acknowledged as a seminal work on professional standards for speech and language therapists (SLTs). Its publication in 1991 marked a new era in the history of the speech and language therapy profession.

Since that time, the profession has changed its practice to reflect changes in:

- the evidence base
- national strategic direction
- legislative requirements
- technology

As part of these changes, speech and language therapy services are increasingly provided by a mix of SLTs and support practitioners working as members of multi-agency teams across a range of settings.

The future for the profession is likely to include extended scopes of practice for SLTs; an expansion in the numbers of support practitioners and an increase in partnership working with other support agencies to meet the needs of the individual with a communication or swallowing disability. The structure of this third edition of Communicating Quality has been radically changed as the result of consultation with RCSLT members and a wider group of stakeholders. The required content has been developed collaboratively over a period of twelve months. CQ3 therefore represents professional consensus opinion and reflects the profession's commitment to ongoing growth and development.

Acknowledgements

The development of this third edition of Communicating Quality has relied heavily on the extensive involvement of a large number of people. It has been a privilege to work with so many people who have been willing to contribute their time and expertise, often in the context of busy personal lives and demanding clinical and professional responsibilities, to ensure that the book was completed on time and to a high quality level.

Particular thanks are due to the people listed below who took on the lead developer role for allocated sections of CQ3. This generally involved working with a group of interested others via e-mail to agree content and wording.

The cohesion of the chapters is largely due to their hard work and shared vision of practice based on common principles.

Annie Aloysius, Helen Anderson, Ian Bell, Rebecca Bergmann, Jan Broomfield, Jayne Comins, Frances Cook, Deirdre Cotter, Hannah Crawford, Christine Currie,

Rosemary Cunningham, Calum Delaney, Ashleigh Denman, Samantha Eckman, Kamini Gadhok, Jo Graham, Kim Hartley, Celia Harding, Anne Harding-Bell, Gillian Hazell, Ruth Howes, Sue Jones, Moira Little, Neresha Maistry, Alison McCullough, Sue McGowan, Gillian McNeill, Nick Miller, Della Money, Gillian Montgomery, Jane Neil-MacLachlan, Debbie Onslow, Aileen Patterson, Sandra Polding, Lorna Povey, Christina Quinn, Victoria Ramsey, Joe Reynolds, Lynne Roberts, Margaret Rosser, Alison Stroud, Stephanie Ticehurst, Celia Todd, Wendy Wellington, Margaret White, Fiona Whyte, Georgina Willis.

Many thanks also to:

● The large number of people who formed part of the e-mail working groups and who patiently provided comments and suggestions throughout the lengthy process of revision, rewording and restructuring.

E-groups included representation from a range of stakeholder organisations including Afasic, ASLTIP, British Stammering Association, Communication Aid Centres, I CAN, RNIB, and Speakability.

● Those people who organised, ran or attended the 2004 series of meetings across the four UK countries. These early meetings formed the basis for restructuring the content and revising the format of Communicating Quality.

● The services, clinical advisors, SIGs, external stakeholders and individual members throughout the UK who took the time to comment on the first draft of CQ3 during the consultation phase in September 2005. All the feedback was carefully considered and reflected in the final version of the guidance as appropriate.

● The members of the Steering Group, especially Kamini Gadhok, Judy Lennon, Michelle Morris, Ros Rogers and Sue Roulstone for their attention to detail during the last phase of the project when deadlines were very tight.

● Pam Enderby, Alex John, Maggie Johnson and Kate Malcomess for their input to chapter nine.

● All the RCSLT HQ staff, especially Bridget Ramsay for her administrative support and Steven Harulow for his expertise around publications.

● Sarah Gentleman for proofreading.

● Annie Dilworth for preparing the index.

● Andy Smith and Denise Bell of Smith+Bell for the book design.

Special thanks to:

● The late Jayne Comins for her role in drafting out the sections on counselling and supervision.

● Sheffield Speech and Language Therapy Agency for their forbearance during my secondment to the role of CQ3 Project Manager.

● Caroline Pickstone for her unfailingly enthusiastic support during the course of the project. Caroline also shouldered some of the project manager responsibilities for a few months during 2004 at a time when I was experiencing great family stress.

Kath Williamson
CQ3 Project Manager

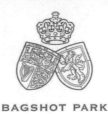

BAGSHOT PARK

It is with pleasure that I welcome the third edition of *Communicating Quality*, the professional standards document of the Royal College of Speech and Language Therapists.

Speech and language therapists provide services that are crucial to those with communication disabilities and with eating or swallowing difficulties. These services cover all ages and range from universal public health roles to targeted and specialist roles. With such a wide-ranging remit, it is important that the scope of practice of the profession and the standards of care are clearly defined and explicit. This is not only to guide speech and language therapists but also to inform the public, colleagues and users about the standards they can expect.

I congratulate members of the Royal College of Speech and Language Therapists for their diligence and creativity in producing a standards document that has been completely updated. It will be a vital tool in setting standards for the future of services for all people with communication disability.

Her Royal Highness The Countess of Wessex
Patron

Introduction

A User's Guide to Communicating Quality 3 (CQ3)

Who is CQ3 for?
CQ3 has been written with three groups in mind:
1. Members of the speech and language therapy team, including students, assistants, bilingual co-workers and SLTs who are clinicians, educators or managers
2. Commissioners and purchasers of speech and language therapy services
3. Stakeholders in speech and language therapy services, including individual users, user representatives and colleagues in other professions.

What is CQ3 for?
The text sets out to:
● Inform members of the profession and their colleagues of current guidance and standards related to the organisation, provision and development of speech and language therapy services; as well as the staff systems that underpin such provision
● Inform the process of commissioning and purchasing of speech and language therapy services

● Inform users and their representatives of the standards they can expect speech and language therapy services to meet.

What is the status of CQ3?

The content of CQ3 is for general guidance only. It does not attempt to cover every eventuality and will be subject to change over time. It is not to be relied on as legal advice. Where there are legal concerns, members are advised to seek legal assistance, initially through their employing organisation as appropriate.

However, members are advised that the guidance and standards contained within CQ3 represent current professional consensus opinion and may therefore be used in the context of disciplinary hearings to assess the reasonableness of members' actions.

What is CQ3 about?

Communicating Quality 3 sets out information, guidance and standards to support the commissioning, organisation and provision of services.

Although there is a degree of overlap between the RCSLT Clinical Guidelines, Position Papers and CQ3, the documents are complementary. CQ3 focuses on best practice in terms of service organisation and provision. The clinical guidelines and position papers focus on the details of best clinical practice with specific client groups.

RCSLT Clinical Guidelines & Position papers | Communicating Quality 3

Chapter one outlines the professional framework within which SLTs and support practitioners work. It includes a mission statement for speech and language therapy; the profession's scope of practice and the code of ethics and professional conduct.

Chapters two and three set out information in relation to the international and national contexts, whilst chapter four outlines the role of the RCSLT.

Chapter five contains guidance and standards relevant to the organisation of services, including detail on developing the workforce, use of information, risk management, public and patient involvement, resource management, staff management and partnership working.

Chapters six and seven relate to service provision, detailing guidance and standards around the notion of an individual's journey along a care pathway and within different contexts.

Chapter eight details information that will be particularly helpful for commissioners and purchasers of services. The information refers to specific client groups and is set out in the same way for each group:

● definition of group
● cross referencing with other client groups
● national guidance and sources of information
● aetiology
● incidence and prevalence
● vulnerability of individuals: risk issues
● SLT value.

Chapter nine contains information particularly aimed at service managers. It sets out information and guidance related to monitoring the quality of service provision; linking this to the processes of service improvement and development

Minimum service standards are highlighted in bold throughout the text and are summarised in Appendix 1. A list of sources of further support and information is provided in Appendix 2.

Accessibility of CQ3

The content of CQ3 forms part of the RCSLT website as well as being available in book form.

The RCSLT has taken advice from the RNIB with respect to the accessibility of this document. As a result, the chapters of this publication will be available in a large-scale format via the RCSLT website and also on request from the RCSLT headquarters.

Terminology and Abbreviations

Terminology

Individual has been used throughout the text to describe the client, patient, child or adult who may be receiving speech and language therapy

Carer has been used to refer to partner, spouse, parent, sibling, relative, friend and professional carer. This reflects the current trends in the public domain, as well as providing a more manageable, if less personal, description of those people with whom the practitioner may work.

Therapy or **intervention** have been used in preference to treatment, as these terms reflect the broader nature of speech and language therapy work with individuals and carers.

Speech and language therapist and **speech therapist** are protected professional titles under the Health Professions order 2001 and are referred to throughout the book as SLTs.

Support practitioner has been used

throughout to refer to support workers, assistants and bilingual co-workers.

Practitioner has been used to encompass both SLTs and support practitioners.

Communication disorder has been used to encompass speech, language and communication disorder

Swallowing disorder has been used instead of the term dysphagia as the term is more immediately meaningful to service users.

The term dysphagia describes eating and drinking disorders which may occur in the oral, pharyngeal and oesophageal stages of deglutition.

This therefore includes problems of positioning food in the mouth and in oral movements, including sucking, mastication and the process of swallowing.

Abbreviations

A&E	accident and emergency (department)
AAC	alternative and augmentative communication
ABI	acquired brain injury
ADD	attention deficit disorder
ADHD	attention deficit hyperactivity disorder
AfC	Agenda for Change
AHP	allied health professional
ALD	adult learning disability
AM	Assembly Member (Wales)
AOS	apraxia of speech
ARDS	acute respiratory distress syndrome
ASD	autism spectrum disorder
ASHA	American Speech-Language-Hearing Association
ASL	additional support for learning
ASLTIP	Association of Speech and Language Therapists in Independent Practice
AURE	The Alliance of UK Health Regulators on Europe
BCLP	bilateral cleft lip and palate
BME	Black and minority ethnic (groups)
CAMHS	Child and Adolescent Mental Health Services
(C)APD	(central) auditory processing disorder
CASPLA	Canadian Association of Speech-Language Pathologists and Audiologists

CCD	cognitive-communication disorder
CCI	Centre for Change and Innovation
CLD	cognitive-language disorder
CLDT	community learning difficulties team
COSHH	Control of Substances Hazardous to Health
CHP	community health partnerships
CP	cerebral palsy
CPD	continuing professional development
CPLOL	Standing Liaison Committee of Speech and Language Therapists/Logopedists in the European Union (Comité Permanent de Liaison des Orthophonistes/Logopèdes de l'Union Européenne)
CPPIH	The Commission for Patient and Public Involvement in Health
CNS	central nervous system
CNST	Clinical Negligence Scheme for Trusts
COPD	chronic obstructive pulmonary disease
CQ	Communicating Quality
CREST	The Committee for Research and Education in Speech and Language Therapy
CPR	cardiopulmonary resuscitation
CRE	Commission for Racial Equality
CSAG	Clinical Standards Advisory Group
CVA	cerebral vascular accident (stroke)
CDC	Child Development Centre
DDA	Disability Discrimination Act
DfES	Department for Education and Skills
DH	Department of Health
ECTS	European Credit Transfer System
EEA	European Economic Area
EC	European Commission
EHEA	European Higher Education Area
ELB	Education and Library Boards (Northern Ireland)
ENT	ear nose and throat
EBP	evidence-based practice
EPG	electropalatography
EPR	electronic individual record
EU	European Union
FAQs	frequently asked questions

FEES	fibreoptic endoscopy evaluation of swallowing
FETO	Fair Employment and Treatment (Northern Ireland) Order
GOR	gastro-oesophageal reflux
GP	general practitioner
HEI	higher education institution
HPC	Health Professions Council
HQ	headquarters
HR	human resources
HR&CPS	Health Records and Communication Practice Standard
HSC	Health Service Circular
HSG	Health Service Guidelines
IALP	International Association of Logopedics and Phoniatrics
ICAS	Independent Complaints Advocacy Service
ICF	International Classification of Functioning
ICIDH	International Classification of Impairment, Disability and Handicap
ICT	information communications technology
ICU	intensive care unit
IDS	International Diagnostic Standard
IDT	inter-disciplinary team
INSET	in-service training
IPR	individual performance review
IT	information technology
LEA	local education authority
LMS	local management of schools
MAT	multi-agency team
MDT	multidisciplinary team
MLA	Member of the Legislative Assembly (Northern Ireland)
MP	Member of Parliament
MSP	Member of the Scottish Parliament
MRA	Mutual Recognition Agreement
MRSA	methicillin-resistant *staphylococcus aureus*
MRI	magnetic resonance imaging
NARIC	The National Recognition Information Centre for the United Kingdom
NCSC	National Care Standards Commission
NeLH	National electronic Library for Health
NHSLA	National Health Service Litigation Authority

NHS	National Health Service
NHSSB	Northern Health and Social Services Board
NIASA	National Initiative for Autism Screening and Assessment
NICE	National Institute for Health and Clinical Excellence
NIO	Northern Ireland Office
NI	Northern Ireland
NPfIT	National Programme for Information Technology
NPSA	National Patient Safety Agency
NQP	newly-qualified practitioner
NSF	National Service Framework
NSCAG	National Specialist Commissioning Advisory Group
OCD	obsessive compulsive disorder
ODD	oppositional defiant disorder
OT	occupational therapist
PALS	Patient Advice and Liaison Services
PCP	personal care plan
PCT	primary care trust
PDP	personal development plan
PECS	picture exchange communication system
PPI	public and patient involvement
PRO	public records office
QAA	Quality Assurance Agency
QIS	Quality Improvement Scotland
R&D	research and development
RCSLT	Royal College of Speech and Language Therapists
SBH	standards for better health
SED	self-evaluation document
SEN	special educational needs
SENCOs	special educational needs coordinators
SHA	strategic health authority
SHOW	Scotland's Health on the Web
SIG	Specific Interest Group
SIGN	Scottish Intercollegiate Guidelines Network
SLCD	speech, language and communication disorders
SLD/PMLD	severe learning difficulties/profound and multiple learning difficulties
SOP	standards of proficiency
SLT	speech and language therapist
SSSC	Scottish Social Service Council

SSI	specific speech impairment
SSLI	specific speech and language impairment
TBI	traumatic brain injury
UCLP	unilateral cleft lip and palate
UNESCO	United Nations Educational, Scientific and Cultural Organisation
UNICEF	United National Children's Fund
UKCC	United Kingdom Central Council for Nursing, Midwifery and Health Visiting
UTI	urinary tract infection
VPI/VPD	velopharyngeal insufficiency/dysfunction
VOCA	voice output communication aid
WHO	World Health Organisation

See also Appendix 2 Sources of further support and information.

Chapter 1

Professional Framework

1.1 Speech and Language Therapy Mission Statement and Scope of Practice

To provide evidence-based services that anticipate and respond to the needs of individuals who experience speech, language, communication or swallowing difficulties.

Speech and language therapy works in partnership with these individuals and their families and with other professions and agencies to reduce the impact of these often isolating difficulties on people's wellbeing and their ability to participate in daily life.

1.1.1 Who are we?

Speech and language therapists (SLTs) are the lead experts regarding communication and swallowing disorders.

This does not mean that others do not work within these areas, or that others do not have many skills that may overlap with or complement those of SLTs, but that SLTs, through their pre-registration education, and later experience have greater depth and breadth of knowledge and understanding of these clinical areas and associated difficulties. This enables SLTs to lead on the assessment, differential diagnosis, intervention with and management of individuals with communication and swallowing disorders.

Where appropriate, and with the individual's agreement, the SLT will liase and work closely with other agencies and other professions, including complementary therapies.

Speech and language therapy assistants and bilingual co-practitioners are integral members of the speech and language therapy team, employed to act in a supporting role under the direction of a professionally qualified SLT.

The RCSLT is working to develop a diverse workforce that reflects the population served across the four UK countries, of England, Northern Ireland, Scotland and Wales.

1.1.2 What roles do we undertake?
In broad terms, speech and language therapy occupational roles are those of therapist, manager, researcher and educator.
Whilst an individual SLT may have a primary focus on one of these areas, each practitioner is likely to be involved in many of the following:
● health promotion work focused on identified groups or populations
● prevention work focused on identified groups or populations
● assessment and differential diagnosis of speech, language, communication and swallowing disorders
● intervention focused on the individual with communication and/or eating and drinking difficulties
● individual 1:1 therapy
● group therapy
● advising and counselling carers
● advocacy
● consultancy (eg expert medico-legal practitioner; second opinions)
● professional advice
● learning and education
● training and assessment of speech and language therapy students and speech and language therapy support practitioners
● training of volunteers and other members of the team
● teaching
● lecturing
● peer review
● peer support including formalised support of newly-qualified therapists
● supervision, audit and performance management
● service management
● research
● quality assurance
● working within a team.
SLTs need to maintain a clear sense of their personal scope of practice and competence.
SLTs need to remain clear when it is appropriate to refer on; to seek further advice or to seek training in order to maintain or extend their competence.

Extended roles

The *National Health Service (NHS) Plan (England)* in 2000 formally introduced the idea that registered staff, including SLTs, could formally broaden or add to their scope of practice. This involves taking on additional roles (eg consultancy, developing practice, prescribing medication, undertaking invasive procedures) in relation to identified individual groups that might previously have been undertaken by other professional groups.

1.1.3 Who do we work with?

● Children (from neonates through to school age), adolescents and adults with special needs in communication, communication disability and/or swallowing disorders associated with:
● diagnosed impairments, genetic and medical conditions
● trauma
● developmental delays
● mental health problems
● learning disability.
● Children (from neonates through to school age), adolescents and adults with special needs in the following areas:
● speech
● voice
● fluency
● language
● psychologically based communication disorders
● social skills
● problem solving
● literacy
● swallowing functions
● alternative and augmentative communication (AAC).
● Parents and families, caregivers, communication partners, friends and colleagues of people with communication and swallowing disorders.
● Employers.
● General public/community.
● Volunteers.
● Other professionals including:
● allied health professionals
● doctors, medical and surgical consultants, general practitioners (GPs)
● social workers

- early years practitioners
- teachers
- therapy assistants
- interpreters
- nurses
- psychologists.
- Speech and language therapy students.
- Speech and language therapy colleagues.

1.1.4 Where do we work?
- Education:
- local education authority (LEA) nurseries and schools (mainstream and special)
- language and communication units and colleges of further education
- independent nurseries and schools
- playgroups
- government funded initiatives (eg education action zone projects).
- Health and social care:
- hospitals, day hospitals and hospices
- specialist centres: child development centres, rehabilitation centres, specialist joint consultative clinics
- primary care: community clinics, community day centres
- supported living homes
- intermediate care
- mental health services
- initiatives in areas of social deprivation (eg Sure Start).
- Legal system:
- penal system/prisons
- court tribunals
- adult and child protection.
- Voluntary/charitable organisations.
- Independent practice.

1.1.5 What are the health, educational and psycho-social benefits that speech and language therapy can contribute to?
- improvement in general health and wellbeing
- increased independence
- improved participation in family, social, occupational and educational activities

- improved social and family relationships
- reduction in the negative effects of communication disability and the harm or distress this may cause to the individual and others
- reduced risk of surgical intervention and poor nutrition in the case of individuals with swallowing disorders
- reduced health risks and length of hospital stay through the prevention of respiratory problems associated with swallowing difficulties
- reduced risk of surgical intervention by maintaining healthy voice mechanisms
- reduced risk of educational failure
- reduced risk of social isolation
- prevention of certain speech, language and communication disorders.

1.1.6 What are the outcomes of speech and language therapy that will contribute to these health, educational and pyscho-social benefits?

- diagnosis of communication and/or swallowing disorders
- maintenance of optimal communication and/or swallowing abilities
- improvement in the speech, language, communication abilities of individuals
- improved use of existing function
- reduction of communication anxiety and avoidance
- provision and use of AAC where oral communication is limited or precluded by a physical condition
- improvement in interaction and effective social communication
- increased awareness of others about communication and/or swallowing disorders, intervention and management
- improved communication environment
- greater opportunities for communication
- improvement in the individual's understanding of the nature and implications of a communication and/or swallowing disorder.

1.1.7 How are speech and language therapy services provided?

- All intervention is delivered on the basis of ongoing assessment and review of progress with the individual (and/or carer as appropriate) as measured against targeted outcomes.

● Various approaches or models of working have been developed to meet the needs of individuals and context.

● The following are key principles guiding the provision of services:

● the rights, wishes and dignities of each individual and their carers are respected at all time

● effective intervention is based on a holistic understanding of the individual, including their social, cultural, economic, political and linguistic context

● the safety of the individual is paramount

● speech and language therapy intervention aims to be efficient and effective ie best results against targeted outcomes within given resources.

● Speech and language therapy services may operate at three levels:

● the level of the person (working with individuals)

● the level of their environment (working with people, processes or settings)

● the level of the wider community (influencing attitude, culture or practice).

● The form of intervention will vary according to the changing needs of the individual and contexts.

● Speech and language therapy works to encourage individual autonomy and to discourage dependency on the therapist.

● Intervention aims are relevant, achievable and likely to have the greatest impact on daily life.

● People with speech, language, communication or swallowing disorders have a right of equal access to services regardless of age, time post-onset, severity of disorder, geographical location, economic status, linguistic and cultural background.

● Services are provided in settings that will most readily facilitate the development of communicative function.

● The SLT works as an active member of the team to provide coordinated services.

● Speech and language therapy services are planned and developed with reference to current evidence-based practice, research findings, user perspective and expert opinion.

1.2 Regulation of the Profession

In October 2000 speech and language therapy became a state regulated profession, regulated by the Health Professions Council (HPC).

This means that anyone who wishes to practise in the UK as an SLT must be registered with the HPC. No SLT is entitled to use the title or allowed to work in the UK without HPC registration.

Registered practitioners are accountable to the HPC and to the RCSLT in terms of standards of practice and individual care.

Further information on the HPC is in chapter four, RCSLT.

At present, speech and language therapy support practitioners are not subject to regulation, although this is likely to change during the next few years (DH, 2004).

1.3 Role of the RCSLT

The Royal College of Speech and Language Therapists (RCSLT) is a membership organisation providing and promoting:
● support and professional leadership for members, including the setting of standards
● strategic direction for the profession
● consistent, effective and accurate professional representation to external bodies and the government
● heightened public awareness of the medical, social and emotional effects of communication, eating, drinking and swallowing difficulties
● heightened awareness of the contribution of speech and language therapy with the public, government, other professions and the media.
For further information see chapter four, RCSLT.

1.4 Role of the ASLTIP

The Association of Speech and Language Therapists in Independent Practice (ASLTIP) has two main functions:
● to provide information on independent speech and language therapists throughout the United Kingdom
● to support therapists in independent practice.
All ASLTIP therapists are certified members of the RCSLT (Cert.MRCSLT) and registered with the HPC.
For further information visit: www.helpwithtalking.com

1.5 Professional Indemnity Insurance

The RCSLT provides an insurance policy that indemnifies all its practising SLT members in the UK, Channel Islands and the Isle of Man. This covers proven liability arising from alleged professional negligence, breach of professional conduct and damage to property. The policy covers the legal liability for injury to an individual occurring during a community visit and also covers members who see individuals in their own home.

It is essential that the RCSLT is **informed immediately** of any incident that may give rise to a claim. No liability should be admitted and no correspondence entered into without reference to the RCSLT. Members are liable for the first part of any claim, at present £250.

Speech and language therapy support practitioners are not covered by professional indemnity insurance in their own right, but are covered for claims brought against them whilst carrying out duties under the supervision of an SLT.

1.6 Code of Ethics and Professional Conduct

The RCSLT code of ethics is grounded in the broad ethical principles of healthcare, these being:

- **Respect for autonomy** (self determination of individuals and therapists). Enabling individuals to make reasoned and informed choices.
- **Beneficence** (the imperative to do good). There will be some benefit to the individual.
- **Non-maleficence** (the imperative to avoid doing harm).
- **Distributive justice** (the notion that individuals in similar positions should be treated in a similar manner).

Beyond these principles, the RCSLT code of ethics espouses:

- the values of personal and professional integrity
- a commitment to competent and effective practice
- care for the individual who is the focus of practice
- inclusion
- team working.

Practising SLTs will:

- hold an appropriate professional qualification
- be registered with the HPC.

All practising SLTs are bound by the HPC standards of conduct, performance and ethics, visit: www.hpc-uk.org

This provides the starting point for the RCSLT standards of ethical conduct and performance, which will apply to all members of the RCSLT, *including all support practitioners.*

The RCSLT endorses the HPC position in stating that the paramount concern of RCSLT members must be the wellbeing of individuals for whom a speech and language therapy duty of care exists.

The RCSLT therefore requires its members to be competent and to maintain the highest ethical standards in the performance of their duties. Every member is personally accountable for their conduct and performance.

RCSLT members must:

- act in the best interests of individuals using speech and language therapy services
- respect the confidentiality of individuals using speech and language therapy services
- maintain high standards of personal conduct
- report any important relevant information about personal conduct, competence or health to their employers, the RCSLT and the HPC
- be engaged in a process of keeping personal professional knowledge and skills up to date
- act within the limits of personal knowledge, skills and experience
- maintain proper and effective communication with individual service users, carers and other members of the team
- effectively supervise delegated tasks
- get informed consent to work with an individual (except in an emergency)
- keep accurate records in relation to individuals using speech and language therapy services
- deal fairly and safely with the risks of infection
- limit work or stop practising if personal performance or judgement is affected by health issues
- carry out all duties in a professional and ethical way
- behave with integrity and honesty
- follow HPC guidelines when advertising SLT services
- make sure that personal behaviour does not damage the speech and language therapy profession's reputation.

In addition to the HPC standards listed above, in relation to individuals using speech and language therapy services, RCSLT members must:

- recognise the ethical dimension that exists within every clinical decision taken
- respect the needs and opinions of the individuals to whom a duty of care is owed

- ensure that the wellbeing of individuals is not compromised by any action or omission on the part of the SLT
- respect the legal, social and moral norms of the society and the communities in which they work
- strive to maintain objectivity in all their judgements
- avoid activities which may give rise to a conflict of interest, and to make explicit to all concerned any potential conflicts of interest
- disregard prospects of professional advancement or personal gain when making clinical or professional decisions
- decline gifts or hospitality from individuals which could be construed as inducements to gain preferential therapy
- refrain from guaranteeing the results of therapy and from making false or exaggerated claims when promoting services
- agree fees in advance in accordance with RCSLT recommended norms and only charge for professional services rendered
- in association with the RCSLT, educate and inform the public regarding communication disability, ensuring the accuracy of such information
- retain the strictest confidentiality of information including that acquired in the course of non-clinical duties, except in the following cases:
- where there is valid written consent by the individual or the individual's authorised representative
- where necessarily imparted to a close carer in the individual's best interests when, due to the nature of the individual's impairment, it is not possible for consent to be gained
- where there is a wider ethical or legal duty to disclose information
- where required by the order of a court.
- help protect the individual from the consequences of the disclosure of confidential information
- refrain from discrimination on the basis of age, cultural background, gender language, race, religion, or any other consideration. Selection for therapy should only be made on the basis of relevant individual information and accepted standards of best practice
- abstain from undertaking unnecessary therapy, or prolonging therapy unnecessarily, by continually monitoring and evaluating therapy effectiveness
- make onward referrals of individuals as appropriate
- not enter into inappropriate or disruptive personal relationships with individuals

● inform individuals of the nature and likely course of proposed intervention and of the status of those involved in their care

● gain valid consent for intervention from the individual and/or carers, as appropriate, and respect the individual's autonomy to give and withdraw consent at any time. Consent must not be assumed except in emergency situations (*see HPC guidance*), and should be in writing for research purposes, or when videotaping

● ensure familiarity with national guidelines and relevant legislation and ensure that these are observed by all staff for whom the RCSLT member has responsibility.

In relation to involvement in research and development, RCSLT members must:

● conduct all research within an ethical framework and obtain approval for research projects, from the appropriate Ethics Committees

● ensure that the presentation and reporting of research results protects the anonymity of subjects

● engage in audit and research using agreed and well-structured methodology.

See chapter 9, Service Monitoring, Improvement, Evaluation and Development

In relation to students RCSLT members must:

● facilitate the development and education of students

● share information, knowledge and skills to an appropriate level with students

● ensure adequate support and supervision for students, delegating to them only such duties as fall within their competence, and to accept full responsibility for their actions.

See RCSLT Position Paper *The National Standards for Practice-based Learning*, 2006 at: www.rcslt.org

In relation to colleagues RCSLT members must:

● share information, knowledge and skills to an appropriate level with fellow professionals and support practitioners

● ensure adequate support and supervision of speech and language therapy support staff, delegating to them only such duties as fall within their competence, and to accept responsibility for their actions

● facilitate the development and education of colleagues as appropriate

● refrain from collaboration in therapy with practitioners who are not

appropriately qualified for the tasks they are undertaking
- maintain liaison with professional colleagues in cases of concurrent therapy
- refrain from disparaging the competence or character of colleagues
- make concerns regarding professional competence of colleagues known to the appropriate employing, professional, statutory and/or regulatory body.

See Intercollegiate position paper on *Supervision, Accountability and Delegation of Activities to Support Workers*, 2006, at: www.rcslt.org

In relation to an employer RCSLT members must:
- work to the highest level of their ability within an agreed job description
- work within their employer's quality assurance frameworks, policies and procedures
- endeavour to satisfy the requirements of the employer except when:
- this conflicts with the best interests of the individual
- the employer gives false information or issues misleading statements
- the directions of the employer place the SLT in significant physical or psychological danger
- the directions of the employer conflict with agreed professional standards.

It is in the best interest of individuals that RCSLT members exercise independent professional judgement at all times.

For further information on ethics see the UK Clinical Ethics Network at: www.ethics-network.org.uk

1.7 Working within a Legal Framework

1.7.1 Principles

In order to meet the needs of all service users regardless of race, religion or gender, it is incumbent upon all therapists to take action to address inequalities in access to services and to adapt and develop service models as appropriate.

It is imperative that SLTs are aware of their responsibilities within current legislative frameworks and that individuals recognise their personal and professional duty in complying within their statutory obligations.

The levels of responsibility/accountability can be defined as follows:

1.7.2 Organisational responsibility

Each organisation is accountable for ensuring compliance with the implementation of its local strategies and policies at national and regional levels. Regional government may have existing structures and organisations in place.

For example, the Commission for Racial Equality (CRE) can take action and has a role to play in the monitoring of the Race Relations (Amendment) Act (2000) in England.

1.7.3 Service level responsibility

Each head of service or professional lead has a responsibility to ensure that they and their staff are informed as to how their organisation is responding to national/regional legislation. This will require a knowledge of:

● Which legislation is being implemented through local strategy and policy and how this is being achieved.
● What the gaps are.
● What actions are required to ensure full service compliance.
● What response will be required from the organisation.

It is important that service leads recognise that legislation can and should be used to strengthen the case for improving local service delivery by driving forward service developments which reflect national and regional policies.

For example, the Race Relations (Amendment) Act includes a duty to promote race equality. This duty provides service managers with a legislative framework within which to develop a business case to develop speech and language therapy services to ensure that they are able to meet the linguistic, cultural and religious needs of people from black and minority ethnic (BME) communities. The RCSLT Bilingualism Specific Interest Group (SIG) has guidance to support managers.

Service managers need to ensure that their policies meet the required legislative requirements. Service managers are urged to identify the leads in their organisation in order to facilitate them in this task.

Service managers have a duty to highlight any policies that fail to meet the requirements due to organisational or service constraints. The issues should be raised with senior managers through appropriate communication lines to ensure that their organisation has ownership and responsibility for service improvement.

It is recommended that service managers resource existing examples of good practice. It may be helpful to identify a 'buddy' service that has experience in order to help support this process.

Demographic information, prevalence and incidence data, assessment of need, along with the legislative frameworks and any policy directives should all be used to inform service improvement and business plans.

See chapter 3, UK Political Context and chapter 8 Service Provision: Part 3, Working With Specific Client Groups.

1.7.4 Personal responsibility

● All members have a responsibility to ensure that policies and practice that fall within their personal scope of practice are in line with legislation. This responsibility includes raising any concerns along with potential solutions to address these issues.

● With the advent of clinical governance, health professionals are being increasingly called upon to examine the ethics that lie behind all practice decisions.

● Increasingly, processes related to ethical decision-making are being undertaken in the public arena and are therefore subject to public scrutiny. For example, as evidence grows regarding cost-effective care, health managers are expected to be able to justify the management of scarce resources. There is increasing debate about national evidence-based recommendations, such as those produced by the National Institute of Clinical Excellence (NICE), that limit treatment for individuals, in order to shift resources to healthcare areas which will benefit the majority.

● SLTs are required to consider all aspects of professional decisions, actions and omissions in relation to individual safety, practice efficiency and practice effectiveness and should be able to justify these decisions to individual individuals and the general public.

● All decisions should therefore clearly reflect policy direction at each level to ensure that service delivery is not found in breach of ethical or moral guidelines.

Table 1 (below) sets out the types of accountability that all practitioners need to be aware of.

1.7.5 Individual consent to care

Individuals have a fundamental legal and ethical right to determine

Table 1: Types of accountability for practitioners

Individual accountability	Accountability to whom?	For what?	
a) **Contractual accountability**	Employer (organisation or individual)	Efficiency Effectiveness Safety and wellbeing of individual	
b) **Professional accountability**	HPC professional conduct committee	Efficiency Effectiveness Safety and wellbeing of individual	
c) **Societal accountability**	Public	Effectiveness Safety and wellbeing of individual	
	Individual/individual	Effectiveness Safety and wellbeing of individual	

Requirements: fiscal and quality standards to be adhered to	Monitored and assured through…	Enforced by…
• Employment law • Contract of employment • Local standards of practice • National Service Frameworks (NSFs) • Service-level agreements	• Individual Performance review (IPR) • Supervision/peer review • Individual feedback • Audit • Reporting systems • Outcome measures	• Civil courts and • Industrial tribunals
• HPC and RCSLT codes of conduct • Standards of proficiency • RCSLT guidance (CQ, clinical guidelines and position papers) • Ethical research guidelines • Duty of care	• HPC registration process • RCSLT continuing professional development (CPD) process • IPR • Outcome measures • Supervision/ peer review • Individual feedback	• HPC
Criminal law	• Individual report • Supervision/peer review	• Criminal courts
• Civil law (for negligence, trespass and other civil wrongs) • Duty of care	• Individual report • Supervision/ peer review	• Civil courts

what happens to their own bodies. Valid consent to treatment is therefore absolutely central in all forms of healthcare, providing personal care to undertaking major surgery. Seeking consent is also a matter of common courtesy between health professionals and individuals.
See Consent Key Document, *Reference Guide to Consent for Examination for Treatment*, at: www.dh.gov.uk/consent

In order for consent to be valid, the individual needs to be:
● competent to take the decision
● have received sufficient information to take the decision
● not be under any pressure from any other source at the time.
Therapists are required to seek the consent of an individual, obtaining either written or verbal consent from the individual or their carer prior to service involvement.
As consent is an ongoing process, rather than a one-off decision, therapists are also required to ensure that an individual/carer continues to give consent throughout the process of service involvement.
Services will need to consider, in relation to each client group, at what points in an individual's journey through the service it may be appropriate to seek further consent and how this might be documented.

Capacity to consent

A key principle of law is that every adult is assumed to have the capacity to make his or her own decisions unless it is proved otherwise. Some people may need help or support to be able to understand the decision they are being asked to make and then to communicate that choice, but the need for help and support does not remove their right to make their own decisions.
Where there is doubt about an individual's capacity, a doctor's assessment may be requested.
In broad terms, the individual:
● must be able to understand the nature and effect of making or not making the proposed decision
● must be able to retain the information
● must be able to exercise choice.
Legally, in England, Northern Ireland and Wales, no person can give or withhold consent to healthcare and treatment on behalf of another adult. However, for individuals who lack capacity to consent for themselves, health professionals are generally allowed to provide

treatment without consent if it is considered to be clinically necessary and in the best interests of the individual. (Mental Capacity Act, 2005). In Scotland, a proxy decision maker who has the power to give consent on behalf of the person may be appointed. (Adults with Incapacity [Scotland] Act, 2000).

Working with children and young people – the legal position

Consent for assessment and intervention of children under the age of 16 will normally be sought from the parent/guardian.

However, children under the age of 16 can give consent providing that:

● the practitioner raises the issue of their involvement with the parent/guardian and documents their response, and
● the child has sufficient maturity to understand the nature, purpose and likely outcome of the assessment or intervention.

Efforts should be made to encourage the child that his/her parent/guardian should be informed (except in circumstances where it is clearly not in the child's interest to do so) – (NHS Scotland, 2004).

When services are provided in an educational setting, the headteacher cannot give consent for a child to be seen. This must come from a person with parental responsibility:

● one of the child's parents
● legally appointed guardian
● a person in whose favour the court has made a residence order concerning the child
● a local authority designated in a care order in respect of the child
● a local authority or other authorised person who holds an emergency protection order in respect of the child.

Foster parents do not automatically have full parental responsibility and clarity on this issue should be sought from those concerned (Children Act, 1989).

Generally speaking, consent given by one person with parental responsibility is valid, even if another person with parental responsibility withholds consent.

Young people of 16 and over are able to give their own consent for assessment and intervention, but this does not change the position of parental responsibility. This means that two forms of consent are possible between the ages of 16-18 (Family Law Reform Act, 1969). Wherever a young person aged 16-18 has sufficient understanding of what treatment is being proposed, that young person may consent to a therapist assessing and intervening. The therapist must be satisfied that any such young person has sufficient understanding of what this involves. A full record should be made of the factors taken into account by the therapist in the making of her/his assessment of the young person's capacity to give a valid consent.

Parental consent should always be obtained where the young person of 16-18 does not have sufficient understanding.

Standards and guidance

● Each service/practice should have a clear policy relating to individual consent. NHS organisations will have detailed guidelines on consent and speech and language therapy department policies and procedures should be in line with this guidance.

● Consent may be implied or expressed. In many cases, individuals do not explicitly give express consent but their agreement may be implied by compliant action, eg keeping an appointment. Express consent is given when an individual confirms their agreement to treatment in clear and explicit terms whether orally or in writing. Written consent formalises the process and should be linked to procedure and applied consistently.

● Where therapists are practising in environments where consent cannot be assumed, carer consent must be obtained to see the child, eg screening in nurseries/schools.

● It is recommended that written consent is obtained for:
● individual participation in teaching exercises
● intervention involving working with a student
● individual participation in research projects
● photographic or audiovisual recordings
● use of invasive procedures.

● Consent should be routinely recorded in case notes.

● Individuals should be fully informed about proposed intervention and consent should be gained for all care. It is good practice to provide a written information leaflet explaining any procedures/interventions.

● The most important element of consent is the duty to ensure that individuals understand the nature and purpose of the proposed intervention, together with the expected outcome. SLTs should ensure that information about consent, and the way in which consent is requested, is provided in the most appropriate and accessible format for the individual/s concerned.

● Where intervention options exist, the therapist must advise the individual of her/his recommendations together with the reasons for selecting a particular course of action. Sufficient information must always be given by the therapist to ensure that the individual understands the nature and consequences of each option. This is to enable the individual to take a decision based on that information. The therapist should assume that all individuals wish to be well-informed.

An individual's rights in accepting or refusing aspects of assessment and intervention

● An individual has the right under common law to give or withdraw consent prior to examination or intervention.

● Care must be taken in respect of the individual's wishes. This is particularly relevant where individuals may be involved in student training and/or research. An explanation should be given of the need for practical experience and/or research, and agreement obtained before proceeding. It should be made clear that an individual may refuse to agree without adversely affecting his/her care.

● SLTs must ensure that where an individual does not accept any aspect of assessment or intervention, the therapist should respect that decision and withdraw, recording the situation in the case notes.

Key documents

Legal frameworks to ensure that people who lack capacity are protected:

● Adults with Incapacity (Scotland) Act, 2000: www.scotland.gov.uk/topics/justice

● The Mental Capacity Act, 2005: www.dca.gov.uk/menincap/bill-summary.htm#keyprinciples

● The code of practice related to the Mental Capacity Act (2005) outlines how capacity is assessed and by whom: www.dca.gov.uk/menincap/mcbdraftcode.pdf

● The Department of Constitutional Affairs has produced a guide for professionals in relation to the Mental Capacity Act: www.dca.gov.uk/family/mi/index.htm

● Two sets of documents written from different perspectives for the public and professionals can be accessed at: www.dh.gov.uk/PolicyAndGuidance/HealthAndSocialCareTopics/Consent/Consent GeneralInformation/fs/en

● Consent – what you have a right to expect. Guidance for adults, children and young people, people with learning disabilities, parents and carers

● Seeking consent from children, older people, people in prison, people with learning disabilities. Guidance for therapists.

● The DH website has consent forms for particular groups, including children and young people, older people and people with learning disabilities: www.dh.gov.uk/consentforms. It also has consent forms in various formats, which cater for people from different linguistic backgrounds.

● Human Rights Act, 1998 (Adults).

● Children Act, 1989 (Children).

1.7.6 Confidentiality

What is confidentiality?

Confidentiality may be defined as maintaining security of information obtained from an individual in the privileged circumstances of a professional relationship.

This includes non-health information, for example, name, address and details of financial or domestic circumstances.

Principles around maintaining confidentiality

● Individuals have a right to expect that information given in confidence will be used only for the purpose for which it is given and will not be released to others without permission.

● Whenever possible, consent should be sought to sharing of information that is personal to an individual.

● There are limits to confidentiality and circumstances may arise where a health professional may be bound to breach it.

Breaching confidentiality

A breach of confidence is unethical, unprofessional and in some cases, unlawful.

However, it should be remembered that a breach of confidence cannot occur where prior permission to disclose has been sought and obtained from the individual or carer.

Standards and guidance around confidentiality

● Practitioners should retain the strictest confidentiality of information,

including that acquired in the course of non-clinical duties, except in the following cases:
● where there is valid written consent by the individual or the individual's authorised representative
● where necessarily imparted to a close carer in the individual's best interests when, due to the nature of the individual's impairment, it is not possible for consent to be gained
● where there is a wider ethical or legal duty to disclose information
● where required by the order of a court
● if information is requested by another professional authorised to receive that information, who also owes the individual a duty of care.
In each of these situations, only as much information as is necessary for the purpose should be released.
● In the context of developing integrated care pathways and inter-agency working, there is an increasing need to share information on individuals. Services are encouraged to develop shared protocols around what, when and how information will be shared.

Consent to disclosure of information

● There may be occasions when a carer or individual requests that information is not passed on. On these occasions, the practitioner must indicate that, although every effort will be made to maintain confidentiality, it can never be guaranteed: the information may need to be shared with others on a need-to-know basis.
● When an individual consents to disclosure of information, the practitioner should ensure that they understand what will be disclosed, the reasons for disclosure and the likely consequences.
● Individuals should be informed whenever information about them is likely to be disclosed to others involved in their care and be given the opportunity to withhold permission.
● In a situation where permission has not been sought or obtained, but disclosure of information about a individual by a professional is under consideration, the professional must ask the following questions of herself/himself:
● Was I categorically asked not to disclose?
● Will withholding information affect the wellbeing of the individual?
● Is the disclosure relevant?
If the answers to the above are positive, then maintaining confidentiality may actually militate against the individual.

If a decision is taken to disclose confidential information, the practitioner must be prepared to explain and justify their decision. The individual should be informed of the decision.

See the NHS Confidentiality Code of Practice: www.dh.gov.uk

Guidelines for observing individual confidentiality when obtaining support and in supervision

● Confidential information from the individual can be discussed in supervision. If it is to be discussed with colleagues, permission must be obtained from the individual.

● Support or opinions can be obtained from colleagues, providing the individual cannot be identified. Individuals should be told that you may wish to discuss their case with a colleague, but that any information disclosed is confidential to the department. A pre-appointment leaflet or charter could also explain this.

● Notes should be clear but brief if an individual gives details of their personal life and emotional state.

● Providing anonymity is kept, separate notes may be made for supervision. These may include the subjective experiences of the SLT and are for the SLT's own learning objectives. They are therefore not the case notes of the individual, nor should they become case notes.

More information can be accessed on the DH's website, visit: www.dh.gov.uk

1.7.7 Duty of care

The information in this section is based on the work of K Malcomess, 2005.

The concept of duty of care sits in common law and is defined as "doing what is reasonable" ie the care that would be given by a reasonable person in the same position.

The standard by which practitioners are judged is that expected from their position, standing and declared competence. The higher the standard claimed, the higher the expectation of competence.

The definition of what is reasonable is that which a "respectable body of opinion within the profession" would confirm to be so.

From a professional point of view, the duty of a therapist is determined by the stage of therapeutic involvement the individual is at along the timeline from pre-referral to post-discharge. It is critical for a therapist to understand each stage of duty and the implications of opening a duty of care to an individual.

Table 2 (below) outlines in brief the duty at each stage of therapeutic involvement.

It is important to note that professional duty of care to an individual does not open until the practitioner has decided and agreed to intervene. By accepting a referral, the practitioner opens a duty to assess and it is only once they have assessed the individual's clinical risk that the decision about whether to open a duty of care should be made. Duty to assess is not equivalent to duty of care and therapists should take care to keep their individual and referrer well informed of what their duty is at each stage of therapeutic involvement and when they are moving to another stage.

Once a therapist has opened a duty of care, the extent of that duty will rely heavily on the clinical risk for the individual. It is the role of all therapists to identify whether the general risk faced by an individual (ie foreseeable harm) constitutes a clinical risk and, therefore, whether a duty of care applies, ie should it be managed or addressed by this practitioner?

The only person who can identify a speech and language therapy clinical risk is an SLT. An individual may present as being at general risk as a result of a speech, language, communication or swallowing difficulty, but this does not automatically indicate that a speech and language therapy **clinical** risk exists. Whether or not an individual can be helped by speech and language therapy will determine the existence of a clinical risk.

Another important characteristic of duty of care is that therapists are autonomous and fully responsible for their clinical decisions. As such, therapists should always take care to record the reason for their clinical judgements in order to support a view on what was reasonable at the time. The test of what is reasonable, relates both to the stage of therapeutic involvement the therapist is involved at, as well as to the seniority and professional standing of the practitioner offering the care; that is, a junior therapist will not be expected to have the same accuracy of judgement as a senior one. However, even a junior therapist cannot plead higher order, as acting on the instructions of a senior therapist or manager when the therapist's judgement contradicts these instructions, is not considered reasonable.

However, the introduction of clinical governance structures within the

Table 2: Professional duty at each of the six

Stage of therapeutic involvement	Duty	Specific duties at this stage include:	
Service Levels 1 and 2: Focus on general risk of the population; how to do the most good and least harm for the most people	To the **population**	• health promotion/prevention • education of referrers, general public and other agencies about access, risk and scope of practice • informing commissioners about population risks • support for self-help and support for other professionals working with individuals	
Service Level 2 **REFERRAL:** Focus is on deciding whether or not to accept the referral	To the **referrer**	• to process the referral in a timely way • to have clear referral criteria based on risk • to communicate the decision (acceptance/non-acceptance) to the referrer • to communicate the length of wait expected to the referrer, who holds on to the duty of care	
Service Level 3 **ASSESSMENT:** Focus is on whether there is a duty of care	To **assess**	• to identify the nature and impact of the presenting difficulties • to identify general risks • to predict whether the individual will benefit from intervention (clinical risk) • to identify the risks of intervening/not intervening	

stages of therapeutic involvement

Stage of therapeutic involvement	Duty	Specific duties at this stage include:
Service Level 3 **INTERVENTION:** Focus is on discharging duty of care by reducing clinical risk or identifying that individual cannot be helped	Duty of **care** to the individual	• to identify the individual's goals and desired outcomes • to inform the individual of and negotiate the likely outcomes of care • to evidence effectiveness and negotiate any further input • to prepare the individual and carers for discharge
Service Level 3 **DISCHARGE/ TRANSFER TO SPECIALIST SERVICE OR SELF-MANAGED CARE:** Focus is on handing over the management of any residual or future risks	Duty to **individual/ referrer/ receiving service**	• to hand back or hand over management of residual risk effectively • to inform individual of re-referral routes and reasons • to identify possible future risks and ways of managing these
POST-DISCHARGE, SELF-MANAGED CARE: Focus is on reviewing effectiveness and adjusting policies	Duty to the **public**	• to evaluate clinical effectiveness and cost-effectiveness of care offered • to identify an changes in policy required based on effectiveness • support for self-help and support for other professionals working with individuals • health promotion/prevention

NHS (DH, 1998) means that therapists employed within the NHS can pass a decision up through the clinical governance mechanisms of their organisation. In this way the organisation can agree to take on that risk on their behalf as long as they have clearly articulated the risks of following a particular instruction. It is recommended that this is done in writing.

In essence, the therapist has the duty to do good and not harm and, as such, the degree to which harm is foreseeable determines the extent of the duty of care. Should harm occur to a individual whilst a therapist has an open duty to that individual, the test of whether they have breeched their duty of care will relate closely to whether the harm was foreseeable and the therapist took reasonable steps to avoid/reduce the harm to the individual.

If the therapist has breached their duty of care, they can then be judged to be negligent. Three dimensions must be present to prove negligence. They are:

- the therapist must have an open duty of care
- there must be a breach of that duty, either by act or omission
- there must be resultant harm directly from the breach of duty of care.

For example, negligence could be proved where:

- intervention should only have been undertaken by someone more highly experienced or with specialist expertise
- onward referral should have been made and such referral was not made, and harm resulted.

1.7.8 Delegation

The information in this section is based on the Intercollegiate Position Paper *Supervision, Accountability and Delegation of Activities to Support Workers*, 2006.

When delegating work to others, registered practitioners have a legal responsibility to have determined the knowledge and skill level required to perform the tasks within the work area. The registered practitioner retains accountability for the delegation and the support practitioner is accountable for accepting the delegated task and for his/her actions in carrying out the task. This is providing that the support practitioner has the skills, knowledge and judgement to perform the assignment, the delegation of task falls within the guidelines and protocols of the workplace, and the level of supervision and feedback is appropriate.

What is delegation?

In this context, delegation is the process by which a registered practitioner can allocate work to a support practitioner who is deemed competent to undertake that task. This practitioner then carries the responsibility for that task.

There is a distinction between delegation, and assignment. In the former case the registered practitioner retains accountability for the outcome of the activity. In the latter case both the responsibility and accountability for an activity pass from one individual to the other.

Choosing tasks or roles to be undertaken by support staff is a complex professional activity; it depends on the registered practitioner's professional opinion. For any particular task, there are no general rules. Additionally it is important to consider the competence of the support practitioner in relation to the activity to be delegated.

Principles of delegation

The registered therapist must ensure that delegation is appropriate. The following principles should apply:

● The primary motivation for delegation is to serve the interests of the individual.

● The registered therapist undertakes appropriate assessment, planning, implementation and evaluation of the delegated role.

● The person to whom the task is delegated must have the appropriate role, level of experience and competence to carry it out.

● Registered therapists must not delegate tasks and responsibilities to colleagues that are beyond their level of skill and experience.

● The support practitioner should undertake training to ensure competence in carrying out any tasks required. This training should be provided by the employer.

● The task to be delegated is discussed and if both the therapist and support practitioner feel confident, the support practitioner can then carry out the delegated work/task.

● The level of supervision and feedback provided is appropriate to the task being delegated. This will be based on the recorded knowledge and competence of the support practitioner, the needs of the individual, the service setting and the tasks assigned.

● Regular supervision time is agreed and adhered to.

● In multi-professional settings, supervision arrangements will vary and depend on the number of disciplines in the team and the line management structures.

● The organisational structure has well defined lines of accountability and support practitioners are clear about their own accountability.

● The support practitioner shares responsibility for raising any issues in supervision and may initiate discussion or request additional information and/or support.

● The support practitioner will be expected to make decisions within the context of a set of goals/care plan which have been negotiated with the individual and the healthcare team.

● The support practitioner must be aware of the extent of his/her expertise at all times and seek support from available sources, when appropriate.

● Documentation is completed by the appropriate person and within employers' protocols and professional standards.

For further information see :

Intercollegiate Position Paper, *Supervision, Accountability and Delegation of Activities to Support Workers*, 2006: www.rcslt.org

RCSLT Competencies Project: Support Practitioners Framework, 2002: www.rcslt.org

RCSLT Standards for Working with Support Practitioners, 2003

Chapter 5, Service Organisation.

1.8 Competent Practice

Practice as an holistic concept

Professional practice draws on and consists of a set of fluid and changing ideas, knowledge, understandings, theories and frameworks, skills, values and attitudes which interrelate with each other and are integrated in a personal and unique way by each therapist. The context of work is equally complex, existing as it does, within the arena of social engagement and an ever-changing set of priorities, structures and systems.

Therapy is about making sound judgments and decisions through the application of principles and frameworks.

Thus, professional practice, whilst open to a degree of functional analysis and articulation, will always remain more than the sum of its parts.

The fundamental requirement of therapists is that they should act from a position of commitment and care about the work they are engaged in. Flowing from this comes a desire to continually improve the quality of individual practice through a process of critical reflection and the

Figure 1

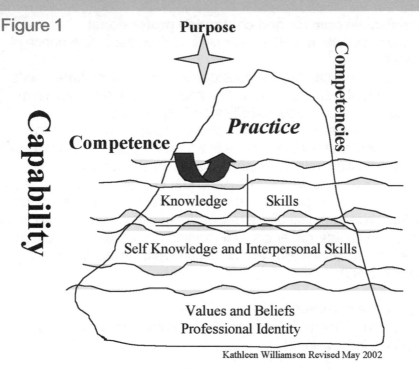

Kathleen Williamson Revised May 2002

integration of evidence from the "outsider knowledge base". Quality of professional practice will be achieved and improved on primarily by individual professionals working with integrity in a critically reflective way. Further, professional autonomy is increased through greater understanding of the decision-making process (RCSLT, 2001).

What is competence?

Put at its simplest, competence is an individual's ability to effectively apply all their knowledge, understanding, skills and values within their designated scope of practice. It is witnessed by:
● the effective performance of the specific role and its related responsibilities
● an individual's critical reflection on their practice.

See figure 1

Capability sits beyond competence. It relates to an individual's full range of potentials that may go beyond current role and responsibilities.
Competencies (singular **competency**) are statements about what needs to be carried out within the workplace and therefore form part of how practice can be described.

Critical reflective practice and continuing professional development activities (CPD) underpin and drive the maintenance of competence.

Individuals and services need to consider both their **immediate** needs (related to current responsibilities and competence) and **longer-term** needs (related to future responsibilities and capability).

"In view of the diversity of individuals and unpredictability of health issues that might present themselves in any given practice, it is evident that clinical practitioners and supporting staff must have a wide and constantly updated knowledge base, and that they are required to keep abreast of latest developments and emerging trends. They also require an excellent understanding of the rest of the healthcare system so that individuals can be referred and supplementary services can be ordered as appropriate". (National Primary Care and Trust Development Programme, 2002).

A structure for competencies

A cross section of the model reveals hidden complexities in relation to competencies (see figure 2).

Figure 2

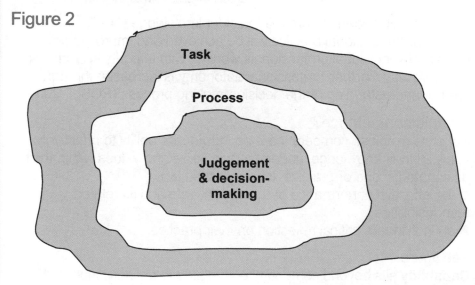

Task

The most visible and obvious aspect of practice relates to task, ie what is done.

Process

A further aspect of practice relates to process, ie *how* the tasks are being carried out.

Judgement and decision-making

The least visible aspect, and one that lies at the heart of practice, is that of professional judgement and decision-making.

Judgement and decision-making, based on a constant process of clinical and ethical reasoning, emerges as the least visible yet most important aspect of practice.

Professional issues do not present as given problems ready to be solved. Instead, the problems need to be framed through the process of *judgement* (Schon, 1983).

Framing involves selecting and prioritising the aspects that are felt to be relevant to the situation. As the process is therefore inevitably based on personal values, theories of practice and certain assumptions that are likely to be operating at a subconscious level, *judgement* emerges as the fundamental aspect of practice and one that carries with it the highest level of professional responsibility.

The process of confronting professional experience and uncovering the values and assumptions that surround practice is key to professional competence and professional development.

1.9 Decision-making

Professional action can never be pinned down and prescribed in absolute terms beforehand. Professional practice is far greater than the ability to deliver a service through a pre-determined care plan or pathway. A therapist is constantly facing unique situations and practice dilemmas not just in relation to individual individuals, but in relation to managing caseload demands and all the unexpected happenings that characterise practice.

Decision-making builds on the process of framing and results in the therapist determining the best course of action at any one time given the particular set of circumstances. A competent therapist therefore needs to have high level reasoning skills in order to work with the many relevant factors and perspectives involved when identifying the best possible option.

In the public sector, the political and moral imperative for transparency of decision-making, about clinical care and allocation of resources, has never been higher. The demand for evidence-based practice is reflected

Figure 3

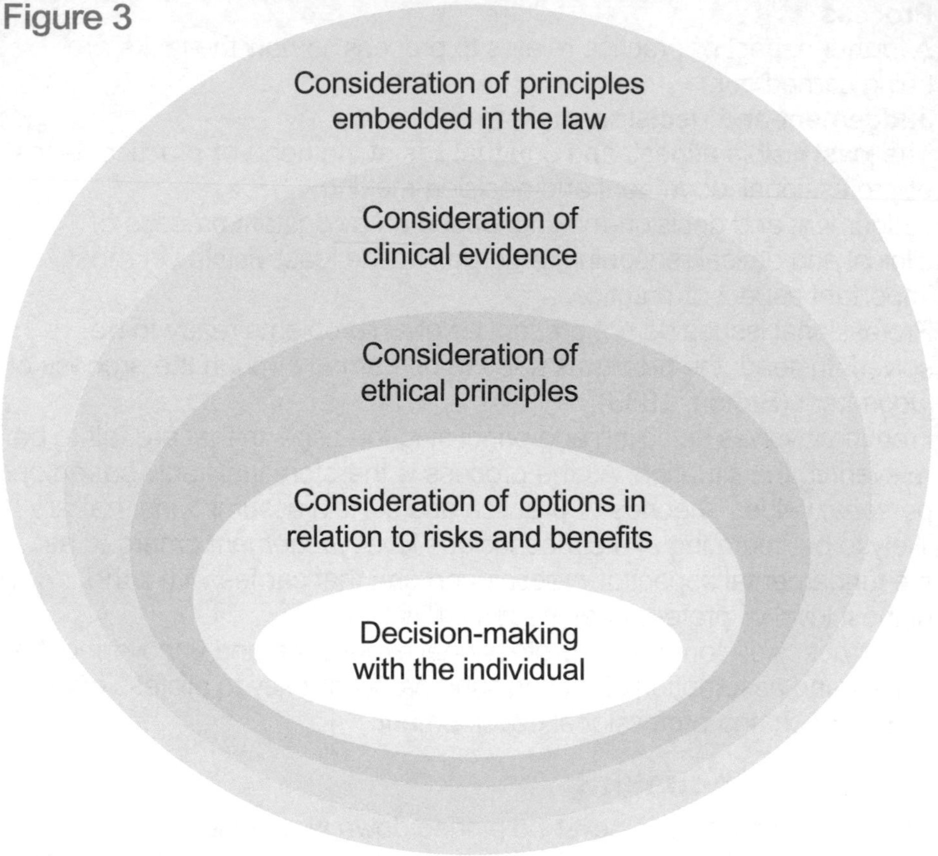

Consideration of principles
embedded in the law

Consideration of
clinical evidence

Consideration of
ethical principles

Consideration of options in
relation to risks and benefits

Decision-making
with the individual

in professional regulation and accountability structures, with
professional re-registration relying more and more on an ability to
demonstrate reflective decision-making.

Practitioners should recognise that every practice decision, whether
relating to an aspect of service provision or to an intervention with an
individual, involves legal, ethical and clinical reasoning (Figure 3).
Ethical reasoning and ethical decision-making are closely related to
clinical reasoning and clinical decision-making. They are also closely
related to legal reasoning and legal decision-making.

However, each has a different set of guiding principles and it is possible
therefore, as a result of ethical reasoning to come to a different decision
from one which may result exclusively from clinical or legal reasoning.
Any professional decision-making process should take account of:

1) Reasoning from a legal perspective:

Involving principles that are embedded in the law.
Examples of this are:
● Respect for other individuals (Human Rights Act, 1998; The Children Act, 2004).
● Protection of vulnerable individuals (Care Standards Act, 2000; The Children Act, 2004; Protection of Children (Scotland) Act, 2003).
● Confidentiality (Data Protection Act, 1998, Freedom of Information Act, 2000, Prevention of Terrorism Act, 1989, Computer Misuse Act, 1990).
● Need for consent (Mental Health Act, 1983; Human Rights Act, 1998; The Children Act, 2004; Family Law Reform Act, 1969; Adults with Incapacity (Scotland) Act, 2002).
● Providing quality services (Health and Personal Social Services Act (Northern Ireland) 2003; Health Act, 1999).
● Promotion of equality (Disability Discrimination Act, 1995, Section 21; Race Relations (Amendment) Act 2000, Special Educational Needs & Disability Act, 2001).
The Acts referenced above are not exhaustive, but are examples of where principles are embedded in the law. Where an Act is applicable to only one of the four UK countries, equivalent legislation is to be found in relation to the relevant country.
For further details see section 1.7, Working within a Legal Framework.
Also see information related to legal acts within the four UK countries, in Chapter 3, UK Political Context.

2) Reasoning from a clinical perspective:

Involving consideration of professional evidence at various levels (personal expertise, peer opinion, professional consensus opinion, published evidence) in relation to dimensions such as:
● best practice (methods, timing etc)
● predicted outcomes
● degree of certainty
● risks of intervention
● risks of non intervention.
See also sections on Service Organisation and Service Provision in chapters 5,6,7 and 8, RCSLT Clinical Guidelines, 2005 and RCSLT position papers.

3) Reasoning from an ethical perspective:
Involving consideration of broad ethical principles (Beauchamp and Childress, 2001):
- respect for autonomy
- beneficence
- non-maleficence
- justice.

See also section 1.6 on Code of Ethics and Professional Conduct.

4) Consideration of options:
Involving a comparison of the risks and benefits of each of the possible options, both for the individual and, as appropriate, for the wider community. See also 5.4.3 on Workload Management and 5.6.1 on Risk Management

5) Decision-making with the individual:
Involving a balancing of various factors, including consideration of:
- The wishes of the individual. (The individual may be an individual, an at-risk group or a commissioner).
- The needs and interests of the individual, the organisation and society.
- The course of action which will minimise risk and maximise good.
- What is reasonable and possible.

Complexity of decision-making
Decision-making is becoming more complex for a number of reasons:
- Advances in practice knowledge and technology.
- The influence of mass media making practice knowledge public property.
- Increased scrutiny of practice.
- Move to team decision-making.
- Financial and resource constraints.

This, coupled with an increased emphasis on holding professionals accountable for their acts and omissions, means that practitioners and managers must be prepared to make their reasoning processes explicit. Some practice decisions have become embedded in custom and practice in the form of policies and procedures (for example, discharging individuals on the basis of non-attendance). The RCSLT recommends that these decisions should be revisited by managers or lead-therapists as part of a service review.

Practitioners also have a responsibility to challenge policies where they feel these are not in the best interests of individuals.

References

Beauchamp, TL & Childress, JF. *Principles of Biomedical Ethics*, 5th edition. Oxford University Press, 2001.

Department of Health. *The NHS Confidentiality Code of Practice*, 2003. www.dh.gov.uk

Department of Health. *The NHS Plan: A plan for investment, a plan for reform*, 2000. www.dh.gov.uk

Department of Health. *Reference guide to consent for examination or treatment*, 2001. www.dh.gov.uk

Department of Health. *Regulation of Health care support Staff in England and Wales*, 2004. www.dh.gov.uk

Intercollegiate Position Paper on *Supervision, Accountability and Delegation of Activities to Support Workers*, 2006.

Malcomess, K. The Care Aims Model in Anderson C, van der Gaag A (eds) *Speech and Language Therapy: Issues in Professional Practice*. Whurr Publishers, 2005; pp43-71.

NHS Modernisation Agency. *National Primary Care and Trust Development Programme*, 2002. www.natpact.nhs.uk

NHS Scotland. *Fraser guidelines, teenagers, consent and confidentiality*, 2004. www.show.scot.nhs.uk

Taylor-Goh, S. *RCSLT Clinical Guidelines*. RCSLT, 2005. www.rcslt.org

RCSLT. *Competencies Project: Support Practitioner Framework*, 2002. www.rcslt.org

RCSLT. *Model of Professional Practice and Professional Competencies*, 2001.

RCSLT. *Position Paper – The National Standards for Practice-based Learning*, 2006

Schon, DA. *The Reflective Practitioner: How Professionals Think in Action*. Basic Books, 1983.

Scottish Executive Health Department and Social Work Services Inspectorate. *Regulation of Health and Social Care Support Staff in Scotland*, 2004. www.scotland.gov.uk

Williamson, K. *Capable, confident and competent*, RCSLT Bulletin, 592,12-13.

Acts of Parliament

All available at: www.opsi.gov.uk

Adults with Incapacity (Scotland) Act 2000

Care Standards Act 2000

The Children Act 1989

The Children Act 2004

Computer Misuse Act 1990

Data Protection Act 1998

Disability Discrimination Act 1995

Family Law Reform Act 1969

Freedom of Information Act 2000

Health Act 1999

Health and Personal Social Services Act (Northern Ireland) 2001

Human Rights Act 1998

Mental Capacity Act 2005

Mental Health Act 1983

Prevention of Terrorism Act 2005

Protection of Children (Scotland) Act 2003

Race Relations (Amendment) Act 2000

Special Educational Needs and Disability Act 2001

Chapter 2
International Context

2.1 Introduction

Healthcare systems are commonly organised at the level of the nation-state, and many professional networks and organisations follow this same pattern. However, international dimensions of health and professional organisation are becoming more important, and it is necessary to consider them as a part of the overall context within which our profession works. International networks have for many years been important in the development of the scientific knowledge base of the profession. With an increase in globalisation and professional mobility, an interest in professional and educational issues has also increased. This has resulted in greater international collaboration between professional associations.

Within Europe, the European Union (EU) has increasing influence on the status of employed and independent practitioners within professions, and its Bologna Agreement aims to increase the alignment of higher education systems across Europe that may influence the development of the profession in the future. The RCSLT adopts a proactive role in participating in and influencing these international and European initiatives, and international involvement forms part of the RCSLT's strategic aims, see: www.rcslt.org/about/strategicplan

2.2 International Influences on the Profession

World Health Organisation

The World Health Organisation (WHO) is another major influence on many aspects of healthcare. Its family of International Classifications provides universal terminology for descriptions of conditions, health outcomes and interventions.

The major revision of the International Classification of Functioning, Disability and Health (ICF), 2001, has moved away from being a "consequences of disease" classification (as in the 1980 version) to become a "components of health" classification. Within a social model framework, this takes into account the social aspects of disability and has gone some way to provide a tool for SLTs to communicate with colleagues about communication disability and healthcare across the world.

However, many issues still remain a challenge in providing common terminologies and taxonomies for speech and language therapy, not just across languages and cultures but even within and across English speaking countries. More information on the WHO and its publications can be found at: www.who.int/en

Free movement of European nationals

A Directive of the European Parliament and of the Council on the Recognition of Professional Qualifications was adopted in June 2005 (COD) 2002/0061 (presented by the Commission pursuant to Article 250 (2) of the EC Treaty). The Directive aims to simplify existing rules on the mutual recognition of professional qualifications by consolidating existing sectoral and general systems Directives under one umbrella piece of legislation.

The basic principle behind these Directives is: if you are qualified to practise a profession in your home country, you are qualified to practise the same profession in any other EU country. You are entitled to recognition to work in another EU member state under the Directive if your professional qualifications (education and professional experience) enable you to work in your home EU member state. Requirements are placed on both the individual seeking to work in another member state and on the host state responsible for processing the individual applications.

SLTs should note that the legislation acknowledges that professionals treating patients have to meet appropriate and consistent standards, including language competence. The Directive states that applicants should have the necessary knowledge of the language of the host country. This allows member states to check the applicant's language skills before granting the authorisation to practise. The host member state has the right to request that an applicant undertakes "compensation measures" which can be additional tests or courses, to ensure that he/she has the knowledge and skills necessary to practise his/her profession in the host member state.

Health professionals must ensure that EU initiatives to facilitate the free movement of European Economic Area (EEA) migrants are coupled with arrangements guaranteeing the systematic exchange of fitness to practise information among all member states, in order that public protection is not compromised.

SLTs who want further information about the implementation of the

Directive and the employment of European trained SLTs, or who wish to seek employment in another European country may find the following sources of information useful:

www.cplol.org

CPLOL is the **Standing Liaison Committee of Speech and Language Therapists and Logopedists in the EU** and provides details of education for SLTs and professional practice in European countries and useful contact addresses.

www.naric.org.uk

The National Recognition Information Centre for the United Kingdom (UK NARIC) is the national agency under contract to the Department for Education and Skills (DfES) and is the official source of information and advice on the comparability of international qualifications from over 180 countries worldwide to those in the UK.

www.aure.org.uk

The Alliance of UK Health Regulators on Europe (AURE), includes the Health Professions Council (HPC), and campaigns on behalf of UK regulators for standards in Europe.

The Bologna Process

The Bologna Process is an EU reform process that aims to establish a European Higher Education Area (EHEA) by 2010. It follows on from the Bologna Declaration of 19 June 1999, signed by the education ministers in 29 European countries, including the UK. By 2005, 40 countries agreed to harmonise their systems of higher education to facilitate academic and professional recognition and allow greater mobility of students, teachers and researchers. The aim of the process is to make the higher education systems in Europe voluntarily converge towards a more transparent system. The links between research and education are seen to benefit from synthesis between the EHEA and the European Research Area. The different national systems are to cooperate with regard to quality assurance, degrees should be easily readable and comparable and to this end higher education should adopt:

● A common framework based on two cycles: undergraduate degree/bachelor level (at least three years study), and postgraduate master level (conditional upon successful completion of first cycle) leading up to a doctorate. Most UK speech and language therapy qualification programmes fit this model for education. The issue, however, is whether the professional qualification is achieved at bachelor's level or masters or even doctorate level, with there being a strong view within Europe that the professional qualification should be at postgraduate level, and in some countries this is already the case.

● A system of accumulation and transfer of credits based on an European Credit Transfer System. This is already used successfully under the EU Socrates-Erasmus training programme to quantify study and allow mobility of students as well as provide a means of comparing one programme of study with another.

● A commitment to lifelong learning.

The progress of the Bologna Process across Europe is being regularly monitored and meetings of ministers set targets for achievement of each part of the process. They have laid emphasis on the need to make the EHEA attractive to the rest of the world. It is therefore incumbent upon existing and new programmes of study in the UK to comply with the Bologna Process and to ensure appropriate quality assurance measures are in place, not only at institutional and national level, but that they meet European standards.

2.3 Speech and Language Therapy Practice in other Countries

Practice and service provision can vary quite legitimately between different places within the UK and between different countries. There has always been a debate about the limits of the profession and its scope within the UK, and some of the activity on the international level is to do with this debate.

There are different views about what types of practitioner should be accepted as fitting any given definition of the speech and language therapy profession, and how far they should be accepted as fit to practise in a country other than the one where they trained. It cannot be taken for granted in every case that someone who calls themselves an SLT is officially qualified to be one.

Consequently assessing the equivalence of individual practitioners is a complex process. Questions can also arise in considering what type of recognition particular organisations might be accorded within international forums such as CPLOL. The different titles for professionals used in different languages further illustrate this complexity, as can be seen in the list within the CPLOL statutes. For more information, visit: www.cplol.org

2.4 International Speech and Language Therapy Professional Bodies

The speech and language therapy profession has developed in a variety of ways in the countries where it is practised, and the history and national context of the country involved has a big impact on the shape of the profession and its networks today.

For example, in countries like Belgium and Switzerland, there are separate associations covering the linguistic communities within the population. Within other countries, there are separate speech and language therapy professional organisations, that may be in competition with each other.

In some countries, a professional speech and language therapy organisation has a role both in setting professional standards, and in negotiating with governments and employers on employment conditions and pay.

Professional associations can have varying levels of influence or control over the education of SLTs. Some countries have a body focusing on communication disorders, but may include a range of other professionals as members, not purely SLTs.

SLTs within other countries may work more in independent and private practice, or be reimbursed by state health insurance systems. All these factors have a big impact on how professional bodies are set up, how they operate, and how they deal with international matters and international networks.

2.5 International Bodies concerned with Communication Disorders and Professional Matters

CPLOL

The Standing Liaison Committee of Speech and Language Therapists and Logopedists in the EU is generally known by its French abbreviation, CPLOL, which stands for "le Comité Permanent de Liaison des Orthophonistes et Logopèdes de l'Union Européenne". It was created in 1988, when the French professional association, la Fédération Nationale des Orthophonistes invited professional bodies in the EU (then the European Economic Community) countries to meet and work together, in response to the actions of the European authorities in laying down new requirements for professional training and regulation.

The then College of Speech Therapists (CST) was a founder member of the Committee. CPLOL has monitored the actions of the EU, and worked to influence the EU on speech and language therapy issues. Members have been particularly concerned about the free movement of workers and the recognition of qualifications, as well as working to ensure that the language competencies required for speech and language therapy practice could not be undermined. The Committee has also worked on a range of projects related to professional training and standards of practice, sharing experience, resources and materials. Particularly for smaller countries and newer professional associations, CPLOL has offered important networking and support. CPLOL has regularly run scientific conferences and maintains a major interest in speech and language therapy education.

For details of current and past projects, visit: www.cplol.org

IALP

The International Association of Logopedics and Phoniatrics (IALP) was founded in 1924. It has a worldwide membership of over 50 national societies from 38 countries, and more than 400 individual members. It aims to help clinicians around the world to improve the treatment of people with communication disorders.

IALP holds scientific congresses and publishes the journal *Folia Phoniatrica* six times a year. It has informative status with world bodies including the United Nations Children's Fund, the United Nations Educational, Scientific, and Cultural Organisation and the WHO.

Membership of IALP is not restricted to SLTs or to speech and language therapy organisations, and some member bodies are multidisciplinary organisations in clinical fields such as voice disorders. The RCSLT is a corporate member of IALP.

For more details, visit: www.ialp.info

2.6 Other Professional and Service User Associations

In addition to the national associations and international bodies concerned with the practice and practitioners of speech and language therapy, there are also national and international associations and networks that cater for the professional, academic and individual or carer interests within different client groups serviced by SLTs. Links to many of these are on the RCSLT website, visit: www.rcslt.org/resources/links/

2.7 Broadening of the European Union and its Implications for Speech and Language Therapy

The EU continues to expand, and in May 2004 its 15 members received 10 new member states into the Union, including countries from the former Eastern block and Cyprus and Malta. It is likely to expand still further in the future. The countries within the EU have a variety of speech and language therapy professional systems, and these are of particular interest to CPLOL as the European umbrella body for speech and language therapy.

The expansion of the EU does not change the freedom of movement for qualified workers as described above, and also in the sections below. There is so far no indication of a large influx of qualified SLTs to the UK from other countries (either existing or new EU members), looking for employment or self-employment.

There are, however, more requests for clinical placements in UK services, even though the profession in the UK has at times had difficulty providing enough placements for home students. There has always been a regular exchange of SLTs to and from the Republic of Ireland, both for training and for employment, arising out of long-standing links and contacts between the speech and language therapy professions in the two countries.

2.8 International Practice Standards

There is some variation of standards for clinical practice across different countries. These have arisen as a consequence of historical differences in the ways the professions have evolved in these countries in relation to other services, and of the differing cultural, social and legal contexts. However there are also some broad similarities, particularly where SLTs approach their practice within a strong ethical framework, and are viewed as autonomous practitioners by the society within which they work.

Greater alignment of standards is emerging as professional associations have given attention to the movement of SLTs between countries and the consequent increasing internationalisation of their workforce.

2.9 UK SLTs Working Abroad

Many UK trained SLTs have worked abroad in the past. SLTs who are interested in this should note however that, with increasing regulation of health professionals, this can be a complicated matter. It may take some time to complete the official procedures in order to obtain official authorisation to practise in a foreign country and the systems change frequently. It is therefore important to start the research and information-gathering needed in good time, and certainly well before leaving the UK. The RCSLT provides detailed information on working overseas, visit: www.rcslt.org/cpd/internationalworking

2.10 Overseas SLTs Working in the UK

Many SLTs who have qualified outside the UK are able to practise within the UK. The specific requirements will depend on where the applicant was educated, and if they can meet the professional and English-language requirements laid down by the HPC. Again, the situation changes from time to time and more up-to-date information is available from the RCSLT and the HPC.

2.11 The Mutual Recognition of Credentials Agreement

A Mutual Recognition of Credentials Agreement (MRCA) was signed on 31 August 2004 and came into effect on 1 January 2005. The MRCA provides for the mutual recognition of professional certification between the four speech and language therapy/pathology associations in America (the American Speech–Language–Hearing Association), Australia (Speech Pathology Australia), Canada (the Canadian Association of Speech–Language Pathologists and Audiologists) and the UK (the RCSLT).

These associations established that the professional knowledge and competencies of their respective practitioners were substantially equivalent and that it was therefore possible for certified members of one association to become recognised by the other associations. The MRCA is not one of reciprocal recognition, in that each association requires certain conditions to be met before granting certification to practise in each country. It also does not extend to provincial, state or country licensing/registration, which is the responsibility of the respective licensing or registration authorities. The MRCA only applies to the certified practitioners of the respective associations.

In seeking common understandings of the practice of speech–language pathologists and of the means by which the associations maintain practitioner competence and safeguard the interests of clients, it was recognised that responsibility for ethical practice is assumed individually by autonomous practitioners, and collectively by autonomous associations.

The associations also recognised that similar competency outcomes can be achieved through different educational and professional practices. The associations exercise a fundamental role in monitoring the standards of education and practice, and practitioners collaborate by complying with these standards. Thus the MRCA rests on the reliance by each of the associations on the integrity of the systems and procedures of the other associations for ensuring a level of competence of practitioners substantially equivalent to that of their own certified members.

The associations agreed that many benefits exist to the international community in establishing a transparent, robust, and professionally and ethically sound basis for the mutual recognition of credentials of speech–language therapist/pathologists. These are:

● Assisting the academic community, continuing education providers, industry, regulatory authorities and the public by identifying common standards of clinical competence.

● Facilitating the ongoing exchange of knowledge as it relates to research, continuing professional development, emerging technologies and other aspects of professional practice.

● Promoting greater international understanding of the role of speech–language therapists/pathologists.

● Responding to governmental interests to reduce trade barriers.

● Streamlining the mutual recognition process for individuals who are certified by the signatory associations and improving mobility for employment abroad.

● Providing a process for the inclusion of other countries interested in the mutual recognition of qualifications and credentials for speech–language therapists/pathologists.

The MRCA has facilitated an exchange of knowledge and understanding between the associations that has permitted a deeper appreciation of their respective standards and procedures and of the principles underlying these. This has contributed to the continuing development of standards within the associations and to the intent to maintain this understanding through the monitoring of the MRCA. Just as the negotiation of the MRCA was approached in a spirit of fostering understanding and inclusion, the associations are also committed to exploring ways of broadening this inclusion and understanding to other associations. The associations believe that the principles upon which the current MRCA is based provide viable guidelines and mechanisms for achieving this.

2.12 Conclusion

The world is more global and international than ever before. International developments and influences will become increasingly important in the future for the profession and for health and education systems more generally.

Individual SLTs are increasingly interested in travel and in working abroad and, at a corporate level, there are more reasons to develop the international profile and involvement of speech and language therapy. The transformation of communications systems and easier travel will have longer-term consequences that may not yet be obvious. These are already reflected in the international strategy being developed by the RCSLT, and in the increasing contact between professional bodies as described above.

As a profession concerned with communication, it is important that SLTs play an active part in building the profession around the world and developing networks to support better care for individuals.

Chapter 3
UK Political Context

3.1 What is Government?

All governments in the UK divide into two parts:

a) The Executive, made up of ministers (elected politicians), their deputies or juniors and the civil service, eg Department of Health (DH). The Executive or cabinet is also sometimes called "the government". In Scotland the generic term for Ministers plus the civil service is "the Executive".

b) Parliament or Assembly – made up of elected politicians who are not Ministers. In the UK Parliament or Westminster there are Members of Parliament (MPs); in Scotland there are Members of the Scottish Parliament (MSPs); in Wales, Assembly Members (AMs); and in Northern Ireland, Members of the Legislative Assembly (Northern Ireland) (MLAs).

3.1.1 The UK Executive

The UK Executive, or government, is the institution that runs the country. It formulates policy and introduces legislation in Parliament.

3.1.2 The UK Parliament

The United Kingdom Parliament today comprises members from England, Northern Ireland, Scotland and Wales. There are two-chambers: the House of Lords (the upper house) and the House of Commons (the lower house). The legislative process involves both Houses of Parliament and the Monarch.

The main functions of Parliament are to:

● make UK law (other than that dealt with by devolved governments) by voting to accept or reject proposals for law (sometimes called Bills or White Papers) emanating from the Executive or from individual MPs (a Private Members Bill). Once accepted and given "Royal Assent" by the Queen, a Bill becomes an Act

● approve, including voting for taxation, the means of carrying on the work of government

● scrutinise government policy and administration, including proposals for expenditure

● debate the major issues of the day

● protect the public and safeguard the rights of individuals

● examine European proposals before they become law

●hear appeals in the House of Lords, the highest Court of Appeal in Britain.

UK Parliament and Government Departments

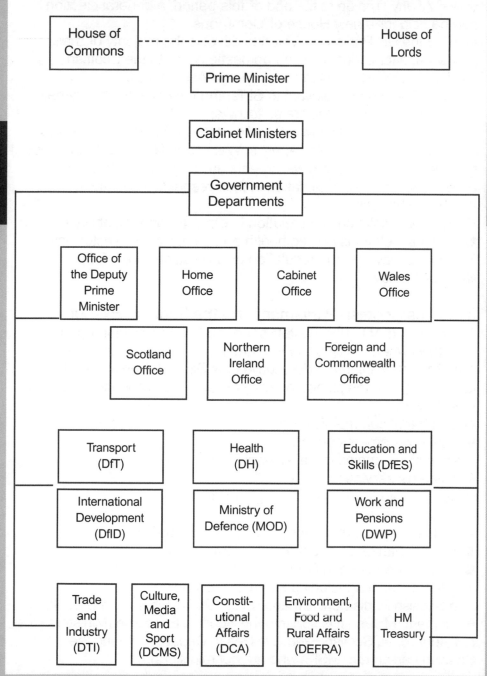

An Executive and Parliament can be in place for a maximum of five years. At any time up to the end of this period, a general election can be held for a new House of Commons.

In 1998 the UK Parliament voted to devolve the majority of their powers and functions covering domestic policy to the Scottish Parliament, Welsh and Northern Ireland Assemblies.

The policies and law relevant to SLTs and their clients, that remain the remit of Westminster, are as follows;

● All English domestic law and policy, eg health, education, social work, etc. These laws also apply in Wales and Northern Ireland but the respective devolved governments are empowered to produce orders affecting implementation in their respective countries.

● Tax and benefits.

● Equality legislation, ie in relation to ethnicity, gender, ability etc.

● Industrial relations law, eg health and safety, public sector pay, Trade union laws, some regulation of professions, (ie HPC).

● European law.

3.1.3 The Scottish Parliament and the Scottish Executive

The Scotland Act (1998) established the Scottish Parliament on 1 July 1999 when the Scottish Parliament assumed its full powers. The Scottish Parliament (Executive plus Scottish Parliament) has jurisdiction over the following policy areas of relevance to SLTs and their clients:

● health and community care
● local government/councils
● education – mainstream, special
● children's services
● lifelong learning – including higher education
● rural development
● justice – including protection of vulnerable people
● implementation of equal opportunities legislation
● public expenditure in Scotland
● voluntary sector including some direct funding.

The Scottish Parliament is made up of 129 Members of the Scottish Parliament (MSPs). It is split into the Scottish Executive (Ministers plus civil service, eg Scotish Executive Health Department) and the Scottish Parliament (MSPs who are not ministers).

The Scottish Executive

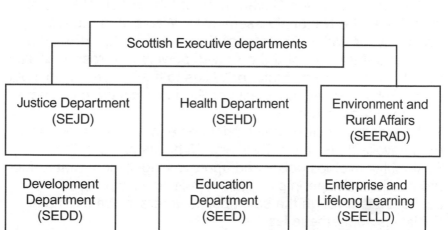

First Minister

Deputy First Minister

Scottish Executive ministers

- Minister for Communities
- Minister for Education and Young People
- Minister for Enterprise and Lifelong Learning
- Minister for Environment and Rural Development
- Minister for Finance and Public Services
- Minister for Health and Community Care
- Minister for Parliamentary Business
- Minister for Justice
- Minister for Tourism Culture and Sport
- Minister for Transport

Scottish Executive departments

- Justice Department (SEJD)
- Health Department (SEHD)
- Environment and Rural Affairs (SEERAD)
- Development Department (SEDD)
- Education Department (SEED)
- Enterprise and Lifelong Learning (SEELLD)

Ministers in the Executive are accountable to the Scottish Parliament. The Scottish Parliament has statutory committees matching the portfolios of Ministers, eg Scottish Parliament Health and Community Care Committee, Education Committee, Communities Committee, Equal Opportunities Committee, etc. These committees are made up of MSPs from all political parties.

The Scottish Parliament:
● makes Scottish law and approves policies by voting to accept or reject proposals for law or policies (Bills) emanating from the Executive, from individual MSPs (Private Members' Bills) or from Scottish Parliament committees. Once accepted and given "Royal Assent" by the Queen, a Bill becomes an Act
● scrutinises, votes on and eventually approves the budget for expenditure proposed by the Executive
● may vote to approve or reject UK-wide legislation – such a vote sends a "signal" to Westminster but has no influence in statute
● debates the major issues of the day.

For further information see the Scottish Executive website and the Scottish Parliament website: www.scottish.parliament.uk

3.1.4 The National Assembly for Wales and Welsh Assembly Government

Parliament passed the Government of Wales Act, 1998, that established the National Assembly for Wales, and the National Assembly for Wales (Transfer of Functions) Order, 1999, that enabled the transfer of the devolved powers and responsibilities from the Secretary of State for Wales to the Assembly on 1 July 1999. Subsequently many acts of Parliament have given new powers to the Assembly.

The Assembly decides on its priorities and allocates the funds made available from the Treasury. Within its powers, the Assembly develops policy and approves legislation, that reflect the needs of the people of Wales. Politicians, who are accountable through the ballot box to voters in Wales, make decisions about these issues.

The National Assembly for Wales consists of 60 AMs. It has

The National Assembly for Wales

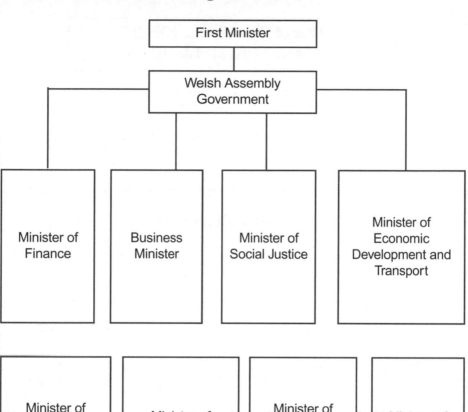

First Minister

Welsh Assembly Government

Minister of Finance

Business Minister

Minister of Social Justice

Minister of Economic Development and Transport

Minister of Education and Life long Learning

Minister of Health and Social Care

Minister of Culture, Welsh Language and Sport

Minister of Planning and Countryside

delegated many of its powers to the First Minister, who, in turn, has delegated to the cabinet ministers – the Welsh Assembly Government.

Wales remains part of the UK and the Secretary of State for Wales and MPs from Welsh constituencies continue to have seats in Westminster. Laws passed by Parliament in Westminster still apply to Wales.

For more information, visit: www.wales.gov.uk

The Northern Ireland Assembly

```
┌─────────────────────────────────────┐
│   Office of First Minister (OFM)     │
│  and Deputy First Minister (DFM)     │
└─────────────────────────────────────┘
              │
   ┌─────────────────────────────┐
   │   NI Executive (Ministers)   │
   └─────────────────────────────┘
              │
   ┌─────────────────────────────┐
   │   NI Executive Departments   │
   └─────────────────────────────┘
```

Regional Development	Enterprise, Trade and Investment	Agriculture and Rural Development

Culture, Arts and Leisure	Environment	Education	Employment and Learning

Finance and Personnel	Health, Social Services and Public Safety	Social Development

3.1.5 The Northern Ireland Office and the Assembly

The role of the Northern Ireland Office (NIO) is to support the Secretary of State for Northern Ireland in securing a lasting peace, based on the Good Friday Agreement. When power has been devolved to the Northern Ireland Executive, the Secretary of State retains responsibility for constitutional and security issues as they relate to Northern Ireland, in particular law and order, political affairs, policing and criminal justice. Victims issues are handled by the NIO's Victims Liaison Unit and the NIO also has responsibility for matters relating to the licensing and legislation concerning firearms and explosives.

The Northern Ireland Assembly was established in December 1999 as part of the Belfast Agreement and meets in Parliament Buildings. The Assembly is the prime source of authority for all devolved responsibilities and has full legislative and executive authority. During devolution, economic and social matters are the responsibility of the Northern Ireland Executive.

The Executive's main function is to plan each year, and review as necessary, a programme of government with an agreed budget. This is subject to approval by the Assembly, after scrutiny in Assembly committees, on a cross-community basis. The Assembly has ten statutory committees. Membership of committees is in broad proportion to party strengths in the Assembly to ensure that the opportunity of committee places is available to all members. Each committee has a scrutiny, policy development and consultation role in relation to its department and a role in the initiation of legislation. For more information visit: www.niassembly.gov.uk and www.nio.gov.uk

3.2 Legislation Relevant to the Profession

3.2.1 UK wide

All available to view or download from: www.opsi.gov.uk.

Disability Discrimination Act, 1995 (Section 21)

This section gives material and publications about the implementation of Section 21 of the Disability Discrimination Act, which is the section of the Act with implications for health service provision, practice, policies and procedures.

The Race Relations (Amendment) Act, 2000

The Race Relations Act (2000) provides new laws for race equality. It strengthens the Race Relations Act (1976). The 2000 Act outlaws race discrimination (direct, indirect and victimisation) in all public authority functions not already covered by the 1976 Act.

It outlaws race discrimination in the terms and conditions that apply to public appointments. It also places a general duty on listed public authorities to be proactive in promoting race equality. This will require them to work to avoid unlawful discrimination before it occurs and to promote equality of opportunity and good relations between persons of different racial groups.

Disability Discrimination Act, 2005

Places a duty (Disability Equality Duty) on public bodies to carry out their functions with "due regard" to the need to eliminate discrimination against and harassment of disabled people; promote greater equality for disabled people; promote positive attitudes to disabled people, and encourage disabled people to participate in public life. It comes into affect from 4 December 2006. Associated codes of practice and guidance is published or to be published by the Disability Rights Commission, visit: www.drc.org.uk

Data Protection Act, 1998

The Data Protection Act (1998) seeks to strike a balance between the rights of individuals and the sometimes competing interests of those with legitimate reasons for using personal information.

The Data Protection Act gives individuals certain rights regarding information held about them. It places obligations on those who process information (data controllers) while giving rights to those who are the subject of that data (data subjects). Personal information covers both facts and opinions about the individual. Visit: www.informationcommissioner.gov.uk

See also chapter 5, Service Organisation, section 5.5 Use of Information.

3.2.2 England

Care Standards Act, 2000

The Care Standards Act (2000) established a major regulatory framework for social care to ensure high standards of care and will improve the protection of vulnerable people. Its implementation led to the establishment of the independent National Care Standards Commission (NCSC). The DH standards and regulations in regard to the Act can be found at: www.dh.gov.uk/publications

Health Act, 1999
An Act to amend the law about the National Health Service (NHS). It makes provision in relation to arrangements and payments between health service bodies and local authorities with respect to health and health-related functions.

NHS Reform and Health Care Professions Act, 2002
This Act received Royal Assent on 25 June 2002. This Act contains an updated version of guidance issued to primary care trusts (PCTs) and strategic health authorities (SHAs) and can be used as a reference for major legislative and organisational changes resulting from the passage of this Act.

Mental Capacity Act, 2005
The Act provides a statutory framework to protect vulnerable people, carers and professionals. It makes it clear who can take decisions in which situations and how they should go about this. The Act starts from the fundamental viewpoint that a person has capacity and that all practical steps must be taken to help the person make a decision.

Mental Health Act, 1983
The Mental Health Act (1983) makes provision for the compulsory detention and treatment in hospital of those with mental disorders.

Education Act, 2002
The Education Act (2002) received Royal Assent in July 2002. The Act implements the legislative commitments set out in the White Paper *Schools – Achieving Success*. It is a substantial and important piece of legislation, intended to raise standards, promote innovation in schools and reform education law.
Visit: www.dfes.gov.uk/educationact2002

Special Educational Needs and Disability Act, 2001
This Act strengthens the right to a mainstream education for pupils

with special educational needs (SEN), where parents want it and where it is compatible with the efficient education of other children. It requires local education authorities (LEAs), schools, colleges, universities and providers of adult education not to discriminate against disabled people in their access to education, for reasons relating to their disability. It requires LEAs and schools to plan to increase progressively, and over time, access to schools by disabled pupils and prospective pupils. Visit: www.dfes.gov.uk

The Children Act, 2004
This Act provides a legislative spine for the wider strategy for improving children's lives. This covers the universal services that every child accesses, and more targeted services for those with additional needs. Its overall aim is to encourage integrated planning, commissioning and delivery of services as well as improve multi-disciplinary working, remove duplication, increase accountability and improve the coordination of individual and joint inspections in local authorities. The legislation is enabling rather than prescriptive and provides local authorities with a considerable amount of flexibility in the way they implement its provisions. Visit: www.dfes.gov.uk/publications/childrenactreport

The Children Act, 1989
The Children Act (1989) covers the following: reforms the law relating to children; makes provision for local authority services for children in need and others; amends the law with respect to children's homes, community home, voluntary homes and voluntary organisations; makes provision with respect to fostering, childminding and day care for young children and adoption, and for connected purposes. Visit: www.dfes.gov.uk/publications/childrenactreport

Freedom of Information Act, 2000
This Act gives the right to access information held by public authorities including: central government; local authorities; NHS services; schools; police. Visit: www.informationcommissioner.gov.uk See chapter 5, Service Organisation, section 5.5 Use of Information.

The Care Standards Act, 2000

The Care Standards Act (2000) changed the regulatory framework covering regulated care providers. Under the Act, the National Care Standards Commission (NCSC) becomes responsible for regulating care standards. This Act explains how care service providers should transfer their registration or licences to the NCSC, as specified by the Act's Transitional Provisions Order. The transfer arrangements cover residential care homes, nursing homes, children's and nurse agencies. The Act introduced new registration categories and requires a number of previously exempt services, such as boarding schools, to be registered. It sets out detailed guidance in these areas and also includes a timetable for data transfer and sample data transfer documentation.

3.2.3 Scotland

Useful websites

www.scotland.gov.uk – information on all Scottish Executive departments and contacts, including health, education, communities (covering equal opportunities) and justice. It provides several useful links to government bodies.

www.show.scot.nhs.uk – "Scottish Health on the Web" (SHOW) contains Scottish Executive documents and policies, plus a lot more.

www.scottish.parliament.uk – information on the Scottish Parliament; details the progress of bills, debates, motions and petitions; and lists all MSPs with their contact details.

Anyone can register on any of these websites to get regular updates. All public libraries in Scotland should provide access to legislation and/or policies, as can your MSP (see the Scottish Parliament website for contact details of your local MSP).

Regulation of Care (Scotland) Act, 2001

This Act set up the:

a) Scottish Commission for the Regulation of Care (Care Commission), which sets national care standards. It uses these standards to regulate and inspect the following care services in Scotland:

- care homes
- school care accommodation
- independent healthcare services

- nurse agencies
- childcare agencies
- secure accommodation services
- offender accommodation services
- adoption and fostering services
- adult placement services
- childminding
- day care of children – including nurseries
- housing support services.

Information on the Commission and national care standards are available at: www.scotland.gov.uk

b) Scottish Social Services Council (SSSC) which deals with regulation and training of social service workers, including social workers and care assistant.

More information is available at: www.sssc.uk.com

Community Care and Health (Scotland) Act, 2002
This Act:
- provides for expansion of access to direct payments for non-residential service users, giving people the ability to purchase their own services
- enables expansion of joint resourcing and management of services relevant to health and community care between NHS Scotland and local authorities, ie the Joint Future Agenda.

More information is available at: www.scotland.gov.uk

National Health Service Reform (Scotland) Act, 2004
This Act:
- establishes Community Health Partnerships (CHPs) including statutory right of AHPs to have representatives on CHP lead committees. Contact the RCSLT Scotland Office for more information on CHPs and what they mean for SLTs
- places a duty on Health Boards and Special Health Boards to involve the public in the planning, development and operation of health services
- places a duty on the Health Boards to take action to promote health improvement
- provides for the governance of NHS staff (ie family friendly policies, etc)

● provides for the promotion of equal opportunities in the NHS.
More information is available at: www.scottish.parliament.uk and
www.scotland.gov.uk

Education (Additional Support for Learning) (Scotland) Act, 2004

The Education (Additional Support For Learning) (Scotland) Act
2004 came into effect in November 2005, and establishes a new
framework for supporting children and young people with additional
support needs.
The Act establishes:
● the concept of "additional support needs" which is much wider
and more encompassing than "special educational needs"
● new duties on education authorities and others. Education
authorities are required to identify and make adequate and efficient
provision for the additional support needs of children and young
people
● more rights for parents – parents can request an education
authority to establish whether their child has additional support
needs and whether they require a coordinated support plan
● new dispute resolution arrangements for parents, in addition to
mediation
● a new Code of Practice that sets out how the new system will
operate, entitled *Supporting Children's Learning,* 2005
● better planning and preparation for transition to post-school life
● removal of the current Record of Needs and the introduction
of the new Coordinated Support Plan for those who need it.
A Coordinated Support Plan must be prepared for those with
enduring complex or multiple needs that require support from
outwith education services.
● The act obliges "other agencies" including health to "help" the
education authority fulfil its duties within certain timescales set by
regulations – to be issued (and alterable) by ministers. Definitions
of "help" have been agreed by the AHP Action Group and are
available from the Scottish Executive Additional Support Needs
Division
A summary of the Act is available at: www.scotland.gov.uk/Topics
/Education/School-Education
More information is also available at the Enquire website, designed

specifically for parents and guardians of children with additional support needs, visit: www.childreninscotland.org.uk/enquire/
A multi-agency training pack on the implementation of the Codes and leaflets about the role of AHPs including a specific leaflet for SLTs is also available from the Scottish Executive website.

Education (Disability Strategies and Pupils' Educational Records) (Scotland) Act, 2002

The Act requires education authorities to:
● prepare accessibility strategies to improve access to education for pupils with disabilities
● review and implement these strategies.
More information is available at: www.scottish.parliament.uk and www.scotland.gov.uk

The Standards in Scotland's Schools etc Act, 2000

This Act places a duty on education authorities to improve the quality of school education and to ensure education is directed to the development of the personality, talents and mental and physical abilities of the child or young person to their fullest potential. In carrying out their duties, an education authority must have due regard, so far as is reasonably practicable, to the views (if there is a wish to express them) of the child or young person, in decisions that significantly affect that child or young person, taking account of the child or young person's age and maturity.
More information is available at: www.scottish.parliament.uk

Protection of Children (Scotland) Act, 2003

An Act establishing a list of individuals whom they consider to be unsuitable to work with children and prohibiting these individuals from doing certain work relating to children. The list must be checked by prospective employers and added to by employers at time of identification.
More information is available at: www.scottish.parliament.uk and www.scotland.gov.uk

Children (Scotland) Act, 1995

This Westminster Act covers:
● parental responsibilities and parental rights

- promotion of children's welfare by local authorities and by children's hearings, etc
- support for children and their families.

More information on the Act can be found at: www.scotland.gov.uk

Adults with Incapacity (Scotland) Act, 2000

This Act makes provision in relation to the property, financial affairs and personal welfare (including healthcare) of adults who are incapable by reason of mental disorder or inability to communicate. Part V of the Act (revised late 2005/early 2006) refers to medical treatment and consent to treat.

The extensive roles and responsibilities of SLTs in respect of this Act and its associated Codes of Practice are available from the RCSLT Scotland Office. An RCSLT Adults with Incapacity Network in Scotland also provides support to SLTs.

The Act was slightly amended in 2005 (as part of the Smoking, Health and Social Care [Scotland] Act) to extend the range of professionals who can issue certificates of incapacity (in lieu of direct consent by the adult) and to extend the time that a certificate can apply to up to three years.

More information is available at: www.scotland.gov.uk

Mental Health (Care and Treatment) (Scotland) Act, 2003

The 2003 Act replaces the 1984 Act. It establishes new arrangements for the detention, care and treatment of persons who have a mental disorder.

This comprehensive Act covers:
- the welfare of the child in mental health services
- equal opportunities
- Mental Welfare Commission
- medical examinations
- provision of services for people under 18 and mothers
- emergency detention
- Compulsory Treatment Orders and Care Plans
- assessment of needs in the community
- safeguards regarding consent to medical treatment by those who are "incapable"
- treatments given over time
- patient representation

- advocacy
- provision of information to patients
- provision of information to patients with communication difficulties.

More information, including easy to read guides and guidance notes to be published, is available from:
www.scotland.gov.uk/Topics/Health/health/MentalHealth/mhlaw/home

Joint Inspection of Children's Services and Inspection of Social Work Services (Scotland) Bill, 2005

This Bill gives authority for multiple agency inspections and gives these agencies the legal powers to access and share information jointly – including health records and speech and language therapy records for the purposes of child protection. These bodies will be required to ensure that the joint handling and sharing of any sensitive information is carried out in full compliance with legal obligations set out in the Human Rights Act 1998 and the Data Protection Act 1998. The Bill will be supported by robust protocols that enable information to be provided and ensure the necessary confidentiality.
See: www.scottish.parliament.uk

3.2.4 Wales

Health (Wales) Act, 2003

An Act to make provision about Community Health Councils in Wales; to establish and make provision about the Wales Centre for Health and to make provision for the establishment of, and otherwise about, Health Professions Wales.

Children's Commissioner for Wales Act, 2001

This Act implements the policy of the Government and the National Assembly for Wales on establishing a Children's Commissioner for Wales with a wide-ranging scope, which encompasses all children in Wales and different sectors and services.
For more information visit: www.wales.gov.uk

3.2.5 Northern Ireland

Useful websites

www.niassembly.gov.uk – includes Bills before Assembly.

www.parliament.uk – includes details of Bills currently before Parliament.

www.opsi.gov.uk – includes the text as passed of General Acts from 1988, Local Acts from 1991, Statutory Instruments from 1987, all Statutory Rules from 1997 and a large number from 1981 to 1986. Also all Acts of the Assembly.

www.bailii.org – includes text of Statutes Revised Northern Ireland. Also UK Statutes from 1996.

www.opsi.gov.uk/legislation/northern ireland/ni-acts.htm – information on Northern Ireland Acts and Orders.

The Mental Health (Northern Ireland) Order, 1986

This is the principal Act governing the treatment of people with mental health problems in Northern Ireland. The Order covers all aspects of compulsory admission and subsequent treatment. Besides these emergency procedures, there are other sections of the Act under which a person can be detained in hospital without their consent.

In October 2002, the Department of Health, Social Service and Public Safety initiated a major, wide-ranging and independent review of the law, policy and provision affecting people with mental health needs or a learning disability in Northern Ireland.

Visit: www.opsi.gov.uk

The Health and Personal Social Services (Quality, Improvement and Regulation) (Northern Ireland) Order, 2003

This Order creates an independent body, the Northern Ireland Health and Personal Social Services Regulation and Improvement Authority, and introduces a number of measures to address quality issues and procedures within health and personal social services in Northern Ireland.

Visit: www.opsi.gov.uk

The Commissioner for Children and Young People (Northern Ireland) Order, 2003

The principal aim of the Commissioner in exercising his functions under this Order, is to safeguard and promote the rights and best interests of children and young persons. In determining whether and, if so, how to exercise his functions under this Order in relation to any

particular child or young person the Commissioner's paramount consideration shall be the rights of the child or young person and/or the regard in particular to the ascertainable wishes and feelings of the child or young person (considered in light of age and understanding)
Visit: ww.opsi.gov.uk

The Equality (Disability, etc) (Northern Ireland) Order, 2000

The Disability Discrimination Act is the main anti-discrimination legislation for disabled people in the UK. However, the European Convention on Human Rights may help fill in some gaps. The Convention was brought into UK law by the Human Rights Act (1998), and thus differs from most international conventions in the relative ease with which individuals can rely on their rights under it.
Visit: www.equalityni.org

Health and Safety at Work (Amendment) (Northern Ireland) Order, 1998

The Health and Safety at Work (Amendment) (NI) Order (1998) imposes duties on employers and employees in all aspects of health and safety in the workplace. This legislation, together with the Management of Health and Safety at Work Regulations (NI) (1992) and other relevant laws applicable to this workplace, must be adhered to at all times.
Visit: www.niassembly.gov.uk/

The Fair Employment and Treatment (Northern Ireland) Order, 1998

The Fair Employment and Treatment (Northern Ireland) Order (1998) makes it unlawful to discriminate against someone on the ground of religious belief or political opinion. This includes a person's supposed religious belief or political opinion and the absence of any religious belief or political opinion.
The Order defines three types of unlawful discrimination:
● Direct discrimination – where a person, on grounds of religious belief or political opinion, is treated less favourably than others are, or would be, treated in the same or similar circumstances.
● Indirect discrimination – occurring where a provision, criterion or practice, although applied equally to all, would put persons of a

particular religion or belief at a particular disadvantage compared with other persons unless that provision, criterion or practice is objectively justified by a legitimate aim.

● Victimisation – treating someone less favourably than others because they have, for example, complained of alleged discrimination or have assisted someone else to do so.
Visit: www.ofmdfmni.gov.uk

The Access to Health Records (Northern Ireland) Order, 1993

This gives individuals certain rights regarding information held about them. It places obligations on those who process information (data controllers) while giving rights to those who are the subject of that data (data subjects). Personal information covers both facts and opinions about the individual.
Visit: www.opsi.gov.uk/legislation/northernireland/acts/
See chapter 5, Service Organisation, section 5.5 Use of Information.

Health and Personal Social Services Act (Northern Ireland), 2001

This Act amends the law about the national health service regarding provision in relation to arrangements and payments between health service bodies and local authorities with respect to health and health-related functions. It confers powers to regulate any professions concerned (wholly or partly) with the physical or mental health of individuals. In particular this act introduced the concept of primary care trusts.
Visit: www.opsi.gov.uk/legislation/northernireland/acts

Personal Social Services (Preserved Rights) Act (Northern Ireland), 2002

This Act introduces new arrangements for funding and managing the care of people with social security "preserved rights". Previously, anyone who could find a place in an independent sector residential care home could have that place funded by social security, subject only to a means test. From April 1993, this changed and, before anyone is admitted to a care home paid for from public funds, assessment under a Health and Social Services Trust's care

management procedures is mandatory. This ensures those admitted to homes actually need that level of care, and to help maintain people in their own home with appropriate support where that is a feasible alternative.
Visit: www.opsi.gov.uk/legislation/northernireland/acts

Special Educational Needs and Disability (Northern Ireland) Order, 2005

The Special Educational Needs and Disability (Northern Ireland) Order (2005) came into operation on 1 September 2005.The law increases the rights of children with special educational needs (SEN) to attend mainstream schools and introduces disability discrimination laws for the whole education system in Northern Ireland for the first time. Further information on the SEN aspects of the law is available from the local Education and Library Board (ELB) SEN advice service, or from the Department of Education. For further information on disability discrimination visit: www.deni.gov.uk

The Education and Libraries (Northern Ireland) Order, 2003

One of the main purposes of this Order is to provide the Department of Education with an enabling power to introduce a single common formula for the calculation of school budgets for all schools funded under Local Management of Schools (LMS) arrangements *(Articles 3-9)*. The Order also contains a range of other provisions on education matters, which introduce technical or minor amendments to existing legislation. These provisions can be grouped under the following generic headings:
● best value in the delivery of ELB services *(Articles 13-16)*
● improve the operation of certain elements of the education system for the benefit of pupils/parents/ELBs/department *(Articles 20, 21, 23-27, 31 and 37)*
● provide for the greater delegation of authority from the Department to ELBs *(Articles 29, 30 and 32)*
● strengthen elements of children's rights *(Articles 17-19, 34 and 36)*
● access to the special education system for pupils from outside Northern Ireland *(Article 22)*.
Visit: ww.deni.gov.uk

3.3 Government Strategy across the UK

3.3.1 What is strategy?
A strategy is a long-term plan of action spanning normally five to 10 years. It generally starts with a vision (a definition of where the organisation wants to be in 10 years time). The vision is often broken into several "themes". Under each theme there are common aims, which may, or may not, be further broken into objectives the organisation is going to implement to achieve their vision. Aims and objectives can be spelled out in detail but they always represent the overarching work plan for the whole organisation in the medium to long term.

3.3.2 NHS and social care strategies
NHS Scotland – *Our National Health: A Plan for Action, A Plan for Change*, 1999, www.show.scot.nhs.uk
NHS England – *The NHS Plan: A Plan for Investment, A Plan for Reform,* 2000 – www.dh.gov.uk
NHS Wales – *Improving Health in Wales: A Plan for the NHS with its partners,* 2001 – www.wales.gov.uk
NHSSS Northern Ireland – *Investing for Health,* 2002 – wwwinvestingforhealthni.gov.uk

Common themes
● **Public health agenda and reducing health inequalities**
Governments across the UK are demanding and supporting:
a) the development of attitudes and services which promote healthy lifestyle choices for all communities (particularly those who historically reflect above average mortality and morbidity such as the unemployed, older people, people with disabilities and black and ethnic minority communities)
b) improving the life circumstances of the whole community. Health is no longer seen as the preserve of those working in the health service. Prevention of ill health and promotion of good health is the responsibility of every individual and every public, private and voluntary sector worker and organisation should promote this. Policies contributing to this agenda include:
● equity of access

- patient information – to improve access to services
- healthy lifestyles in respect of diet, smoking, alcohol, exercise, stress management, health at work, etc
- improving life circumstances such as housing, transport, environments, employment
- good mental health initiatives
- Sure Start/parenting skills
- social inclusion.

● The service quality agenda, service structures and relationships

Governments across the UK have established organisations that set standards of practice for all levels of service provision. The standards increase the accountability of services to the public they serve and to increase the parity of services across the country in relation to all care groups.

Accountability drives efficiency and effectiveness in service provision including the streamlining of decision-making structures.

Accountability has also driven a change in what influences services, how they are planned, how they are delivered (and by whom) and where and how innovation is encouraged and supported. In all four countries, health services are statutorily required to listen to patients and work in close partnership with local authorities (education, social work), the voluntary sector and the independent or private sector.

Policies contributing to this agenda include:
- setting national standards – NICE, SIGN, Quality Improvement Scotland (QIS) guidelines, standards etc
- regulation of staff – HPC, etc
- service inspections, audits and reviews
- informatics
- performance related funding for services
- streamlining bureaucracy and speeding up decision-making
- improving and integrating planning and decision-making leading to integrated services, joint management and pooled budgets (children's trusts, foundation hospitals, community health partnerships, etc)
- listening and responding to individuals and communities – patient and public involvement
- empowering change from the ground up – encouraging staff to problem solve, devolving planning and funds "down" the structure,

made safe by the requirement to work within standards
● patient centred services.

● Services redesigned around an easily accessible, speedier, smoother patient journey

All four governments take the patient-centred approach to service change – focussing on the perspective of the patient and carers, prioritising what they prioritise and changing in order to create the services that patients would create if they were running the health service themselves. This is a change in perspective from preceding decades when services appeared more focused on the needs of the bureaucracy and those providing the services.

This change of perspective drives service redesign. Service redesign from the perspective of the patient starts with examination of the patient's pathway or patient's journey – the good, efficient, economic and effective parts and the slow, overly expensive parts that have little or no positive outcomes for patients. Having examined the patient's journey every step along the way (as defined by the evidence available), circumstances are altered, as necessary, with a view to making the whole journey a better overall experience for the patient. Service redesign also aims to make effective use of the NHS's most valuable (and expensive) asset – staff. Service redesign is about creating services that match every patient's needs and expectations and that gets the optimum output from the collective knowledge, skills, experience and work time of every member of the healthcare team.

Policies contributing to this agenda include:
● achieving better, fairer access to services and more flexible services (in terms of where, when, how and who delivers them)
● increasing patient choice
● reducing waiting times
● improving communication and breaking down barriers between acute and community services, different staff groups, etc
● increasing skill mix within teams
● competencies frameworks, knowledge and skills frameworks
● extending roles within multidisciplinary and uni-disciplinary teams
● workforce planning
● continuing professional development (CPD)
● sharing good practice and guidelines on good practice
● joint case records

Chapter 3

- informatics
- change and innovation/modernisation.

● Public and patient involvement

All four governments are addressing the balance of power within the health service, redistributing it away from traditionally powerful groups (generally large groups of providers, such as doctors and nurses or managers and accountants) towards those who have traditionally been absent from any decision-making and/or fund holding bodies – particularly patients and the public. As with service redesign, a change in the distribution of power within the health service is extremely challenging. The NHS Plan for Scotland recognises this, "More than any other area, change here depends on a wholesale shift in the culture of the NHS. That will take more than words in a Plan; it will take commitment and involvement from staff at all levels." (NHS Scotland, 1999).

Policies contributing to this agenda include:
- giving patients a stronger voice – a seat or seats on boards
- changing the make up of boards, trusts and other bodies and structures to reflect the multi-disciplinary and multi-agency service provision on the ground, eg AHP Advisory Forums, etc
- patient focused, public involvement strategies
- patient involvement in service evaluation, reviews and planning at an individual and organisational level
- communication, information and consultation mechanisms and strategies
- working with professional bodies but also hearing the independent voice
- patient advocacy services.

● Priority care groups (as at 2005)

- cancer
- heart disease (and sometimes stroke)
- mental health
- children (and sometimes young people)
- older people
- chronic illness
- unplanned (emergency) care
- learning disabled/special needs.

All four governments have the same priorities in terms of health service provision and development. These priorities are determined by health statistics, including inequalities between, for example, high and low-income communities. Within each board or authority expenditure on these policies should reflect the local assessed need. However, services falling outside these priorities still need funding, policy initiatives and encouragement.

Policies contributing to this agenda include:

- National Service Frameworks
- stroke, cancer, mental health strategies, etc
- older people strategies
- learning disability frameworks.

● Partnership working between government, employers, trade unions and managers' organisations

All four governments – and by extension NHS managers – are naturally keen to engage with, and have the support of, those who will deliver the change agenda for them. Accountability to tax payers and a moral obligation to the wellbeing of the public drives them to get the most out of staff – accounting for over 80% of the NHS budget. Similarly the vast majority of staff are keen to contribute their skills, knowledge and experience and energy to the benefit of patients but they also naturally want to be recognised, respected, valued and fairly rewarded for that contribution.

Healthcare provision is, without exception, focused on interaction between people acting in the roles of provider or patient. To provide a health service, government and employers require enough staff to match as closely as possible the needs of patients. Training, recruiting and retaining is central to health service provision and as demographic and technical changes increase the numbers of patients, the case for action is becoming increasingly more urgent. All four governments have strategies to address the supply side of the health service – its work force.

Policies contributing to this agenda include:

- work force planning
- working in partnership with trade unions – involving staff in service planning, evaluation, review and change
- family friendly policies, flexible working, etc
- pay and conditions – Agenda for Change, including knowledge and skills framework directly linking contribution to pay, health and safety etc
- equality and diversity strategies
- innovation awards and schemes

- careers opportunities/pathways
- changes in education and routes to entry to professions
- regulation of staff.

● Supporting service change

All four governments recognise that change requires movement through a process and that changing an organisation as big as the NHS requires change agents and development of a "can do" attitude throughout the organisation. To this end, all four governments have put developments in place to push and pull the NHS towards change. Policies contributing to this agenda include:

- leadership development
- management development
- organisation development
- service redesign
- best practice
- research and development.

3.3.3 Children's services/education strategy

The **Every Child Matters: Change for Children** programme, whilst England based, encapsulates key policy direction that is echoed in Scotland, Wales and Northern Ireland. The move towards integrating children's services is a common strategy across the UK.
Visit: www.everychildmatters.gov.uk

The common themes which emerge across the UK include:

● Commissioning of integrated services

Commissioners will take overarching policy leadership for children's service across the traditional boundaries of health, education and social care. These posts have been established in England, Wales, Scotland and Northern Ireland.

Local services will see the appointment of Directors of Children's Services or, in Wales, Lead Chief Officers for Children, whose role will be to ensure that services are redesigned to meet the needs of all children, including those who are vulnerable and/or have additional specialist needs, as locally and flexibly as possible.

● Integrated delivery of services around the child and their family.

This includes the development of Sure Start programmes, Early Support Programmes and the development of Children's Centres and Children's Trusts or their equivalent.

● **Multi Agency working** focused on five outcomes for children:

i. Be healthy

ii. Stay safe

iii. Enjoy and achieve

iv. Make a positive contribution

v. Achieve economic well-being.

www.everychildmatters.gov.uk

● **Inclusion** of children with special (or additional) needs in mainstream settings and the need for specialist services to be delivered flexibly in order to enable inclusion

● **Reduction of inequalities** due to disadvantage of whatever sort

● **Development of primary care services**

● **Increased emphasis on health promotion**

● **The redesign of professional roles** focusing on the competencies required to deliver new integrated services.

For further information on providing speech and language therapy within integrated children's services see: RCSLT Position Paper, *Supporting children with speech, language and communication needs within integrated children's services,* 2006. Available at: www.rcslt.org

For further information on the commissioning of children's services see: The Commissioner for Children and Young People (Northern Ireland) Order 2003 www.nics.gov.uk/press/ofmdfm/030626a-ofmdfm.htm
For Scotland's Children: Better Integrated Children's Services, 2001 www.scotland.gov.uk/library3/education/fcsr-00.asp
Children First programme in Wales, 2004. www.wales.gov.uk/subichildrenfirst/documents/circulars/circ8-e.htm

For further information on early intervention initiatives visit:
www.earlysupport.org.uk
www.scotland.gov.uk/Topics/People/Young-People/children-families
www.scotland.gov.uk/library5/education/sure_start_mapping.pdf
www.wales.gov.uk/subichildren/content/circulars/start/start-e.htm
www.wales.gov.uk/subichildren/content/entitlement/early-entitlement-2004-e.pdf

For further information on the development of Children's Trusts or their equivalent see:
www.surestart.gov.uk/_doc/0-1D9968.pdf

Chapter 3

www.earlysupport.org.uk/pilot2/index.htm
www.allchildrenni.gov.uk
www.nics.gov.uk/press/hss/041216a-hss.htm

For further information on inclusion see:
Removing Barriers to Achievement, DfES, 2004
www.standards.dfes.gov.uk/literacy/publications/inclusion/883963
Special Educational Needs and Disability Order 2005
www.opsi.gov.uk/si/si2005/20051117.htm
The Education (Additional Support for Learning) (Scotland) Act 2004
www.opsi.gov.uk/legislation/scotland/acts2004/20040004.htm
Shaping the Future for Special Education – An Action Programme for
Wales www.wales.gov.uk/subieducationtraining/content/special/
spcled_cnts_e.htm

For further information on health promotion see:
Health for All Children www.health-for-all-children.co.uk

For further information on the redesign of professional roles see:
Children's Workforce Strategy, 2005 www.everychildmatters.gov.uk/
deliveringservices/workforcereform/
Common Core of Skills and Knowledge for a Children's Workforce
www.dfes.gov.uk/commoncore/docs/5610_COMMON_CORE.pdf

References

Department of Health. *The NHS Plan: A plan for investment, a plan for reform*, 2000. www.dh.gov.uk
Gascoigne, M. *Supporting children with speech, language and communication needs within integrated children's services – position paper*, RCSLT, 2005. www.rcslt.org/news/childrens_services
NHSScotland. *Our National Health: A plan for action, a plan for change*, 1999. www.show.scot.nhs.uk
NHSSS Northern Ireland. *Investing for Health*, 2002.
www.investingforhealthni.gov.uk
NHS Wales. *Improving Health in Wales: A plan for the NHS with its partners*, 2001. www.wales.gov.uk

Acts of Parliament
All available at: www.opsi.gov.uk

The Access to Health Records (Northern Ireland) Order 1993
Adults with Incapacity (Scotland) Act 2000
The Care Standards Act 2000
The Children Act 1989
Children (Scotland) Act 1995
The Children Act 2004
Children's Commissioner for Wales Act 2001
The Commissioner for Children and Young People (Northern Ireland) Order 2003
Community Care and Health (Scotland) Act 2002
Data Protection Act 1998
Disability Discrimination Act 1995
Disability Discrimination Act 2005
Education Act 2002
Education (Additional Support for Learning) (Scotland) Act 2004
The Education and Libraries (Northern Ireland) Order 2003
Education (Disability Strategies and Pupils' Educational Records) (Scotland) Act 2002
The Equality (Disability, etc.) (Northern Ireland) Order 2000
The Fair Employment and Treatment (Northern Ireland) Order 1998
Freedom of Information Act 2000
Health Act 1999
The Health and Personal Social Services (Quality, Improvement and Regulation) (Northern Ireland) Order 2003
Health and Personal Social Services Act (Northern Ireland) 2001
Health and Safety at Work (Amendment) (Northern Ireland) Order 1998
Health (Wales) Act 2003
Human Rights Act 1998
Joint Inspection of Children's Services and Inspection of Social Work Services (Scotland) Bill 2005
NHS Reform and Health Care Professions Act 2002
National Health Service Reform (Scotland) Act 2004
Mental Capacity Act 2005
Mental Health Act 1983
Mental Health (Care and Treatment) (Scotland) Act 2003
Mental Health (Northern Ireland) Order 1998
Personal Social Services (Preserved Rights) Act (Northern Ireland) 2002

Protection of Children (Scotland) Act 2003
Race Relations (Amendment) Act 2000
Regulation of Care (Scotland) Act 2001
Special Educational Needs and Disability Act 2001
The Special Educational Needs and Disability (Northern Ireland)
Order 2005
The Standards in Scotland's Schools etc Act 2000

Chapter 4
RSCLT

4.1 The RCSLT's Role

4.1.1 Mission statement

The RCSLT is the professional body for SLTs and support practitioners. The RCSLT provides leadership so that issues concerning the profession are reflected in public policy and people with communication, eating, drinking or swallowing difficulties receive optimum care.

The RCSLT will provide and improve services to its membership and lead an inclusive profession whose members deliver quality services to meet diverse needs.

4.1.2 Key purposes of the RCSLT

External focus

● To increase public, professional and government awareness of the health, educational and psychosocial impact of communication and swallowing disorders on the lives of individuals.

● To ensure that the profession is consistently, effectively and accurately represented to external bodies and the government.

● To increase public, professional and government awareness of the contribution of the speech and language therapy profession.

Internal focus

● To define the strategic direction of the profession.

● To provide guidance, standards and professional leadership for RCSLT members.

● To provide support for the professional development of RCSLT members.

● To develop diversity within the profession.

● To increase the level of membership involvement in the work of RCSLT.

4.1.3 Relationship with the Health Professions Council

In October 2000, the speech and language therapy profession became regulated by the Health Professions Council (HPC). This means that anyone wishing to practise in the UK must apply to be registered with this body.

Students from programmes approved by the HPC should apply for registration on graduation. They will not be allowed to work in the UK without HPC registration.

As part of its remit to protect the public, the HPC has three main functions:

● To ensure that pre-registration programmes in speech and language therapy are appropriate and of a satisfactory quality.

● To approve the qualifications of overseas educated SLTs working in the UK.

● To regulate the profession and to investigate complaints and take appropriate disciplinary action where necessary.

There are a number of sanctions available to the HPC if allegations are proved against an SLT:

i. Strike-off register

ii. Suspend registration for up to a year

iii. Impose conditions of practice

iv. Caution the person concerned

v. Conditions iii and iv will require the registrant to comply with certain requirements in order to continue to practise.

The RCSLT has produced advice sheets for these therapists, their managers and prospective mentors. The RCSLT has a process for managing members who are given a sanction by the HPC. There is also a RCSLT complaints process for RCSLT members who are not registered with the HPC.

By 2009, all SLTs will have to provide evidence of continuing professional development (CPD) in order to re-register with the HPC. For the HPC renewal in 2009, SLTs will be expected to provide evidence of, and reflect on, the CPD they have undertaken in 2007 and 2008. The RCSLT has developed an online CPD diary and toolkit to support this process.

4.1.4 Professional indemnity insurance

The RCSLT provides an insurance policy that indemnifies all its practising members in the UK, Channel Islands and the Isle of Man. This covers proven liability arising from alleged professional negligence, breach of professional conduct and damage to property. The policy covers the legal liability for injury to a client occurring during a community visit and also covers members who see individuals in their own home.

It is essential that RCSLT is informed immediately of any incident that may give rise to a claim, no liability should be admitted and no correspondence entered into without reference to the RCSLT. Members are liable for the first part of any claim, at present £250.

4.1.5 Diversity

It is the policy of the RCSLT that:

● The diversity of the clients served by the profession should be represented within the speech and language therapy workforce.
● Every effort should be made to ensure that all members of the community who need speech and language therapy services have equal access to them.

The RSCLT has produced guidelines to help services to develop their diversity strategy. The RCSLT is currently developing standards to support the recruitment and development of bilingual co-workers.

4.2 RCSLT Structure

4.2.1 Membership and categories

Certified membership equates to full, practising members who have agreed to meet the standards on professional conduct and CPD. All practising UK therapists must comply with this, and therapists working overseas can choose whether or not it is appropriate for them to do so.

Certified members:

Practising members (includes UK and overseas members who have agreed to meet the standards on professional conduct and CPD). MRA members (members entering the UK under the mutual recognition agreement [MRA] scheme).

Non-certified members:

● Practising overseas members (overseas members who have not agreed to meet the standards on CPD).
● Practising members new to the RCSLT.
● Newly-qualified practitioners.
● Returners to practice.
● Therapists working for a charity overseas (have the option to

become certified if they comply with conduct and CPD standards).
- Non practising.
- Retired (over 59 years old and non-practising).
- Speech and language therapy assistants, technical instructors, bilingual co-workers.
- Student members (those enrolled on a recognised course of study in the UK leading to a qualification in speech and language therapy).
- *Bulletin* subscribers (associated professionals, non UK-based therapists not registered with HPC).

4.2.2 Governance

Council
Council's role is to define the strategic direction of the profession and provide professional leadership to implement this strategy. Council is comprised of a number of trustees. It consists of the chair and deputy chair of the RCSLT, the chairs of each board, the country councillors and lay representation. All council members' duties are carried out on a voluntary basis.

Following a reorganisation and the introduction of a new staff structure, the following boards were approved in December 2005:

Professional Standards and Development Board: to oversee the strategic management and policy development of pre- and post-registration training, CPD and the needs of the speech and language therapy workforce.

Membership and Communications Board: to oversee the strategic management and policy development regarding membership, communications, publications, marketing and events.

Policy and Partnerships Board: to follow the strategic direction defined by Council, to govern the influencing and lobbying function of the RCSLT to the UK and devolved country governments and to promote and oversee policy and partnership functions.

Finance and Organisational Resources Board: to provide and develop corporate leadership and implement strategic objectives within the areas of finance, performance and contracts, human resources, IT and health and safety.

"Task and Finish" groups: any board may establish time-limited specialist groups to complete clearly defined pieces of work.

4.2.2 RCSLT governance structure

```
┌─────────────────────────────────┐
│            RCSLT HQ             │
│ To operationalise the strategy  │
│ of Council and boards and ensure│
│ corporate management of HQ      │
└─────────────────────────────────┘
                │
                ▼
┌─────────────────────────────────┐
│            COUNCIL              │
│ To define the strategic         │
│ direction for the profession    │
│ and provide professional        │
│ leadership to implement this    │
│ strategy. All boards and        │
│ committees report to Council    │
└─────────────────────────────────┘
```

Secretariat

| Policy and Partnerships Board | Membership and Communications Board | Professional Standards and Development Board | Finance and Organisational Resources Board |

Task and Finish groups

| Specialist Interest Groups | Specialist advisors | Local groups |

4.2.3 Headquarters structure

The RCSLT employs a small number of staff to operationalise the strategy of Council and its boards and ensure corporate management. Staff are organised into four functions under the Chief Executive Officer:

Customer Relations: membership, publications, communications, events and marketing.

Policy and Partnership: policy formulation, promotion and advice. This includes policy officers working in Wales, Scotland, England and Northern Ireland.

Professional Development: professional training and development, professional guidance and standards, research and development.

Performance and Contracts: performance management and contract processes (finance, human resources, information technology and administration) across all functions.

4.2.4 Professional networks

The RCSLT works with a range of professional networks to support its membership. This includes the regional managers groups, Specific Interest Groups (SIGs) and advisor networks and the Adult Learning Disability Network. The RCSLT also links with:

CREST: The Committee for Research and Education in Speech and Language Therapy

ASLTIP: The Association of SLTs in Independent Practice

CPLOL: The Standing Liaison Committee of Speech and Language Therapists/Logopedists in the European Union (known by it's French acronym, le Comité Permanent de Liaison des Othophonistes/Logopèdes de l'Union Européenne) is the organisation for professional speech and language therapy bodies in Europe. It aims to give support, to develop professional consensus and to unify standards and strategies in Europe.

4.3 RCSLT Processes

Becoming a councillor or board member: Vacancies on Council and the boards are advertised in *Bulletin*. Nominations are matched against clear criteria. The initial term of office is two years, and this may be renewed for a further two years. The chair is elected for a four-year period, two years for a deputy chair and two for a chair.

Similarly, the Honorary Treasurer is elected for a four-year period with two years acting as deputy.

Contacting boards and Council: Issues that need to be raised at a board or Council should be directed towards the appropriate country councillor or country policy officer. They ensure that the matter is brought to the attention of the relevant board and that decisions and actions are communicated to the membership.

Influencing what is happening in the profession: The RCLST consists of its members, who all have a responsibility for shaping the future of the profession. This may be through serving on a board, contributing to policy development, providing feedback or promoting the implementation of policies and guidelines.

Requesting a position paper: If a member feels that a position paper or policy statement is needed in a particular area, this is communicated through their country councillor, country policy officer or to the chair of the appropriate board. Following debate and investigation, Council decides the level of priority within its existing work programme and, if appropriate, commissions the work from a board.

4.4 RCSLT Functions

4.4.1 Membership and communication

Membership and information services: Providing information about membership, careers advice and signposting to other organisations. Holds a database of RCSLT specialist advisors and SIGs.

Specialist advisors: Acknowledged experts in their specific field who have gone through a nomination and approval process. As well as offering advice to individual members they contribute to responses to government papers and the development of RCSLT policy.

Specific Interest Groups (SIGs): These are groups of practitioners who organise meetings and study days that focus on a specific area of speech and language therapy practice. As well as providing support to members, these groups may also contribute to the development of RCSLT policy.

Publications: The RCSLT produces a wide range of publications for membership and to promote the profession to the general public.

Many of these are available as files that can be downloaded from the website (visit: www.rcslt.org) or can be purchased from the RCSLT headquarters. Publications include:

● a monthly **Bulletin** featuring clinical and professional news and articles

● a fortnightly **Bulletin Supplement** containing job vacancies and information on courses, meetings and conferences

● the **International Journal of Language and Communication Disorders**: a bi-monthly peer reviewed journal on the latest speech and language research

● **leaflets**: on RCSLT policies and guidance

In addition, the RCSLT produces a wide range of tools to support professional practice. There is a mechanism in place to ensure that these tools (outlined below) are reviewed and revised on a regular basis.

● **RCSLT Clinical Guidelines:** These were published in book form in 2004, and are also available on the RCSLT website. The guidelines are a set of recommendations developed from the clinical research evidence base in order to support the use of research findings within practice. They were developed in consultation with a large number of SLTs working with different client groups. As well as a core guideline, the following specific areas are covered:

aphasia	dysfluency
autistic spectrum disorders	dysphagia
cleft palate	head and neck cancer
deafness	pre-school children
dysarthria	school-age children
mental health	voice disorders

● **Position papers:** There are a number of areas where the evidence base is insufficient for the development of guidelines. In this case the RSCLT have worked with specialists in the profession to provide a position paper. Currently position papers exist for:

● adults with learning disabilities

● dementia

● clinical placements

● supporting children with speech, language and communication needs.

The RCSLT has also produced policy statements on endoscopy and Fibreoptic Endoscopic Evaluation of Swallowing (FEES).

● **Communicating Quality:** Contains information, guidance and professional standards which define the parameters for the provision and the development of speech and language therapy services across a range of areas.

● **Clinical competencies frameworks** (SLTs and support practitioners): The competency statements allow practitioners to identify their strengths and weaknesses and define their development needs. The framework relates to three layers of professional practice:

● task (what is done)
● process (how tasks are carried out)
● professional judgement and decision making (the why of practice).

● **RCSLT *Reference Framework: Underpinning Competence to Practise* (2003):** contains information about the knowledge and skills required to work with particular client groups.

● **CPD toolkit:** contains guidance to support members in meeting the CPD requirements of the RCSLT and the HPC.

4.4.2 Policy and partnership

The RCSLT:

● raises the profile of the speech and language therapy profession through contacts with the media, government, parliamentary bodies, statutory and voluntary organisations and service user groups. This involves:

● Lobbying governments and contributing to local and national policies.
● Issuing press releases presenting RCSLT views on relevant issues.
● Providing information and supporting initiatives to promote speech and language therapy services to the general public.
● Providing comments to the media from informed and specialist SLTs.

● influences the development and implementation of policy affecting the profession

● represents the profession at the highest levels

● provides consultancy and lobbying to the government and commissioning authorities

● contributes to the development of multi-professional guidelines through organisations such as the National Institute for Health and

Clinical Excellence (NICE), the Scottish Intercollegiate Guidelines Network (SIGN) and the National Patient Safety Agency (NPSA). The team includes policy officers representing and working in England, Northern Ireland, Scotland and Wales.

4.4.3 Workforce planning and career pathways

Bringing people in to the profession:
The RCSLT produces careers materials and information for potential speech and language therapy students. The RCSLT is involved with the Allied Health Professions (AHP) *New Generations* project which aims to change perceptions and raise awareness of AHP career options for seven to nineteen year olds, particularly within demographic groups that are currently under represented.

Newly-Qualified Practitioners (NQP) transition: The *NQP Competency Framework* was published in 2005. This is a tool for the NQP and his/her manager to support the transition to full RCSLT membership.

Recruitment and retention: In 2005 the RCSLT initiated a project to support workforce planning and commissioning of speech and language therapy. The outcome will be a toolkit to help managers to analyse activities being carried out in the service.

Return to practice: The RCSLT has developed a *Returners Pack,* 2005 and a *Return to Practice* course to ensure that SLTs returning to the profession following a career break will be able to fulfil the HPC requirements.

Skill mix: The RCSLT supports the development and implementation of policy, standards and tools related to skill mix within the workplace. For example, see the *RCSLT Support Practitioner Framework* and published *Standards for Working with Support Practitioners*, available at: www.rcslt.org A collaborative AHP statement supporting the development of foundation degrees aimed at support workers has been issued and guidance will be produced for members on the new National/Scottish Vocational Qualification in allied health professions support.

Managers: The RCSLT provides support to managers through regional managers groups and networks. These groups contribute to the work of RCSLT in a number of ways. For example, see the *Information Pack for New SLT Managers*, 2005 at: www.rcslt.org

Extended scope practitioners: The RCSLT is involved in

developing position papers to support SLTs working in new areas, for example, see the paper on the *Fibreoptic Endoscopic Evaluation of Swallowing (FEES): The role of speech and language therapy*, at: www.rcslt.org

4.4.4 Research and development
The RCSLT:
● raises awareness and supports the development of the research capacity of the profession
● influences the research agenda by building partnerships with others in the statutory and voluntary sectors
● influences workforce planning to inform research roles and develop leaders.
See *Approaching Research in Speech and Language Therapy* (2003), at: www.rcslt.org. An e-mail network exists for those interested in research. RCSLT grants are available to support members who wish to undertake research. The RCSLT is setting up a new professional development unit that will review the grants process and identify how the RCSLT can support research and development as part of CPD and career pathways.

4.4.5 Education and training
Pre-registration education is now regulated by the HPC. The RCSLT continues to work with educational establishments to ensure that their programmes meet the needs of the profession. The RCSLT has developed a position paper on pre-registration education and training, curriculum guidelines and standards for practice-based learning. The RCSLT also provides representation to higher education institutes quality assurance events to act as a "critical friend" to the course.
The RCSLT holds an annual meeting with admissions tutors and links with the Committee for Research and Education in Speech and Language Therapy (CREST).
Post-registration education: The RCSLT has a range of initiatives to support post-registration education. There is a distance learning *Return to Practise* course developed and accredited by the RCSLT and franchised to a number of universities. The RCSLT registers and runs a range of short courses and has developed tools to support CPD. These will ensure that RCSLT members will meet the criteria

and have collected the appropriate evidence needed for re-registration with the HPC.

4.4.6 Employment
The RCSLT does not deal directly with issues relating individual pay and conditions of employment as it is not a trade union. Trade union matters are dealt with by the union representing the profession, currently Amicus (2006).

However, the RCSLT will become involved if issues are likely to have an impact on the profession. For example, the RCSLT worked with Amicus to produce profile guidance for the speech and language therapy profession as part of the Agenda for Change (AfC) process and lobbied at a national level.

References
All available at www.rcslt.org

Taylor-Goh, S. *RCSLT Clinical Guidelines*, RCSLT, 2005.

RCSLT. *Approaching Research in Speech and Language Therapy*, 2003.

RCSLT. *Fibreoptic Endoscopic Evaluation of Swallowing (FEES): The role of speech and language therapy – policy statement*, 2005.

RCSLT. *Information Pack for New SLT Managers*, 2005.

RCSLT. *Newly-qualified Practitioners Competency Framework to Guide Transition to full RCSLT Membership,* 2005.

RCSLT. *Reference Framework: Underpinning Competence to Practise,* 2003.

RCSLT. *Returners Pack,* 2005.

RCSLT. *Standards for Working with Speech and Language Therapy Support Practitioners*, 2003

RCSLT. *Competencies Project: Support Practitioner Framework*, 2002.

Chapter 5
Service Organisation

This chapter contains guidelines and signposting pertaining to different areas of service organisation. However, practitioners will also need to refer to their organisation's local polices and procedures.

5.1 Definition of Health

"Being confident and positive and able to cope with the ups and downs of life" is how good health is defined by the Secretary of State for Health in *Our Healthier Nation*, (DH, 1998).
Health is therefore seen as a resource for everyday life. It is a positive concept emphasising social and personal resources, as well as physical and mental capability. It is not simply defined by an absence of disease or infirmity.

5.1.1 Responsibility for health
The concept of health as the responsibility of the individual, as well

as of society or government, has been increasingly emphasised in government strategy documents from as far back as *Prevention and health, everybody's business: A reassessment of public and personal health* (1976).

5.1.2 Framework for health

The World Health Organisation's (WHO) International Classification of Functioning, Disability and Health (ICF) 2000 provides a common framework for describing the health of an individual. The dimensions used for this description are:
- body functions and structure
- activities
- participation

In addition, a fourth dimension of environmental factors is included. This allows for the description of factors within the environment that interact with the three dimensions above, either as barriers or facilitators at an individual, service and/or organisational level.

5.2 Range of Speech and Language Therapy Services

In line with this definition and framework of health, speech and language therapy works with referred individuals or targeted at-risk groups to:
- provide information on the promotion of health, particularly in relation to communication and swallowing
- provide information on existing or anticipated risks in relation to communication and swallowing
- assess the nature of any speech, language, communication or swallowing difficulty
- assess how involvement in everyday activities is being compromised
- assess what environmental facilitators or barriers exist
- assess the capacity for change at an individual or environmental level.

Based on needs that are identified jointly by the individual and professional, intervention is likely to include work to improve or maintain individuals' functional ability; to reduce the health, educational and psychosocial risks faced by individuals and to ensure that communication and swallowing disorders do not preclude opportunities for self-determination, fulfilment and participation in community life.

People with speech, language, communication and/or swallowing disorders can expect services that will:

● be accountable to the service commissioners, the public, service users and carers
● be responsive to identified needs
● offer choices that promote independence
● be accessible, so that non-discriminatory help is available when and where needed
● be well coordinated between all staff and agencies
● be clear and open about what therapy options are available
● offer appropriate and effective care
● promote the safety of individuals and staff
● empower and support staff members
● involve service users in planning and delivery of care
● provide continuity of care for as long as necessary.

Minimum standards for service organisation and provision

Minimum service standards are included at appropriate points within this text. A full summary is available in Appendix 1.

Service standard 1: The service audits its performance against the RCSLT minimum service standards as part of a regular process of service review.

Service standard 2: Policies are reviewed at least every three years.

5.3 Developing the Workforce

5.3.1 Recruitment

All practising SLTs must be registered with the HPC.

Service standard 3: The service has a system for monitoring SLT's HPC registration status.

Services may also require therapists to be certified members of the RCSLT.

It is recommended that independent practitioners are members of the ASLTIP.

Support practitioners are currently (2005) not subject to regulation, but may be at some point in the future.

All staff should be subject to police checking as part of the recruitment process.

There are national policy initiatives within the NHS on recruitment, retention and return to practise. Further information is available on the Department of Health's website.

Robust recruitment is crucial for the delivery of an effective service. Each employing organisation will have a recruitment policy that aims to guide managers through the recruitment process by advising of legislation, good practice and creativity within recruitment and selection.

Employing organisations should provide training for managers regarding the recruitment and selection process. This should include equal opportunities. Staff involved in recruitment must understand the areas where discrimination may occur. They should take positive action to recruit the best candidate thereby giving individuals the opportunity to demonstrate their abilities regardless of their race, sex, religion/belief, age, disability, marital status or sexual orientation.

Managers should be aware of current human resources policies covering issues such as flexible working arrangements, family friendly policies, career breaks, childcare, etc.

For further guidance around recruitment and selection, see the RCSLT's *Information Pack for New SLT Managers 2005* available at: www.rcslt.org

5.3.2 Retention

All staff should develop their professional and personal skills. An effective way of doing this is to broaden experience across a number of organisations. Consequently it is never possible to retain all staff. However it is important to consider why staff decide to leave a post and to ensure that it is not due to any avoidable shortcomings.

Service standard 4: Exit interviews are conducted with all staff who leave the service.

5.3.3 Staff supervision and support

The following areas should be addressed to ensure that staff feel valued and supported:

Terms and conditions of service
Service standard 5: All staff have a clear and up-to-date contract of employment.
This includes locums and staff on fixed short-term contracts. University staff should have an honorary contract for clinical work.
Service standard 6: All staff have a clear and up-to-date job description.
● Job descriptions should be kept in personal files.
● Staff should be familiar with the content.
● Job descriptions should be subject to annual review.
● Where a sole practitioner service is delivered, there should be a description of the parameters of the service, including what is not offered.

From 1 October 2004, the Whitley terms and conditions of employment were replaced by the new NHS pay system, *Agenda for Change*. This mechanism was jointly agreed by the Department of Health and the trade unions. As a consequence there is now one set of terms and conditions for all directly employed NHS staff, except doctors and dentists and the most senior managers at, or just below, board level. These new conditions include the number of hours worked in a full-time week and the number of annual leave days. Further information is available on the Department of Health website, under the Agenda for Change section at:
www.dh.gov.uk/PolicyAndGuidance

Staff who were employed on a local trust contract prior to 1 October 2004, ie contracts not based on the national Whitley terms, were given the choice whether or not to move onto the new pay system.

SLTs both within and outside the NHS should be clear about their terms and conditions of service at the time of their employment. SLTs are advised to take full advice from their trade union in respect of terms and conditions of employment.

Monitoring of staff absence
Service standard 7: The service has a system for monitoring staff absence.
● There should be a clear policy in place for the notification and monitoring of staff absence.
● Staff should be familiar with the procedure.

- Records should be kept.
- There should be a process to support return to work in the case of extended absence for whatever reason.
- There should be a process of review of the information, and action planned if required.

Induction training

Carefully planned induction programmes should include input from both the employer organisation and the local team/service.

Service standard 8: The service provides a planned orientation, induction and support programme for all new staff, including locum staff, and returners.

The programme of support will include:

- preparation for roles and responsibilities
- familiarisation with policies and procedures
- explanation regarding emergency procedures
- information regarding health and safety, including risk
- mentoring/supervision/support mechanisms
- identification of personal development needs.

Records of the induction process should be kept, signed and dated by the staff member and manager.

A range of written policies and procedures in relation to clinical and organisational processes should be readily available for staff. These are likely to be developed locally and may apply to a range of services beyond speech and language therapy.

During their first year or so of practice, newly qualified practitioners consolidate their previous knowledge and apply their learning to clinical practice. This period of development, prior to full certified membership of the RCSLT, is subject to additional support and supervision. The focus of this is guided by a set of competencies laid out in the RCSLT's *Newly-qualified Practitioner Competency Framework*, available at: www.rcslt.org.

Supervision

A key factor in delivering a quality speech and language therapy service is supervision. Supervision refers to a formal arrangement which enables an SLT or support practitioner to discuss their work regularly with someone who is experienced and qualified.

Two forms of supervision are recommended:

● **line management**
● **clinical supervision.**

Managers need to ensure that the system of management and supervision used in their department is understood by all staff and that it is offered on a regular basis with adequate time made available and necessary recording and follow-up actions taking place.

The management and supervision processes should allow the supervisee the opportunity to consider their strengths and needs. The process may involve case review, either on a random or case selection basis.

The management and supervision sessions should provide information and data that contributes to the formal performance review, while dealing with day-to-day challenges in a positive way.

Service standard 9: There is an up-to-date organisation and service profile showing clear lines of responsibility and accountability within the organisation.

Line management aims to:

● enable the practitioner to fulfil their person specification and job description

● provide information for carrying out individual performance reviews

● encourage and support practitioners in meeting objectives set during the formal appraisal

● give advice on managing caseloads and any problems that may cause problems in the day-to-day functioning of the service

● ensure that the practitioner is aware of the professional standards and codes of conduct expected of them, and to facilitate their adherence to such professional standards

● discuss professional development needs in relation to service delivery

● assist the practitioner in relating practice to theory and theory to practice thereby promoting CPD.

It is essential that the practitioner's manager is trained in appraisal and performance review skills as well as being able to deal with difficult situations that could result in disciplinary action. This is in order to prevent possible abuse of these procedures.

In instances where significant difficulties are encountered in achieving acceptable standards of conduct or performance, and where opportunities have been offered to help the practitioner overcome any difficulties, the manager needs to know his/her level of authority for using the disciplinary procedure.

The manager and practitioner should consider all possible avenues for resolving difficulties that may arise before resorting to disciplinary procedures.

Service standard 10: All staff have an annual performance review supported by a systematic approach to training and development including a PDP and appropriate CPD opportunities.

Service standard 11: The service has a system for reviewing the requirements of a post in terms of knowledge and skills.

Where specialist skills are required, training should be provided.

Service standard 12: The service has agreed mechanisms in place to support practitioners working within external agencies.

These mechanisms might include service level agreements and regular joint planning meetings.

Independent SLTs and line management

Normally independent SLTs are not required to take part in job description reviews, an appraisal process, performance reviews, or caseload prioritisation, and therefore are exempt from line management. However, the system of annual certification with the RCSLT and the two-yearly HPC registration, encourages all SLTs to reflect on their professional development.

Clinical (non-managerial) supervision provides an opportunity for practitioners to obtain case supervision outside the line management structure.

It is a formal arrangement where SLTs can discuss their interventions, including the feelings that are engendered.

There are a range of clinical supervision models, including collegial supervision, co-supervision, peer supervision, telephone supervision and group supervision.

However, clinical supervision is commonly carried out by a peer, or in situations where the practitioner has a predominantly counselling role, from a psychiatrist/psychotherapist who can enable the SLT to explore the psychodynamics of the therapeutic relationship.

Clinical supervision aims to:

● Create a learning environment which promotes critical reflective practice.

● Help the practitioner overcome some of the considerable demands created by the nature of the work, by helping to develop an understanding of the interactive processes in relationships with individuals.

● Help the practitioner deal with difficulties such as establishing a therapeutic alliance, over-involvement with individuals and professional boundary issues. The supervisor aims to help the practitioner understand the dynamics of the therapeutic relationship.

● Reinforce and offer feedback on effective clinical skills as well as enabling the supervisee to talk about areas of their work that are thought to be ineffective.

● Assist in the management of issues arising out of the location of delivery and the SLT's confidence in managing complex inter-disciplinary situations.

● Provide a supportive role to help prevent crises or disillusionment arising.

● Enable the practitioner to be challenged by their clinical experiences and to be able to question their practice in a safe and confidential environment.

Service standard 13: The service has an up-to-date policy and system of clinical supervision for all clinical staff.

Having chosen a supervisory model, for example group or individual supervision, a supervision contract should be made and agreed between both parties and, if appropriate, the manager.

The contract should include the frequency and length of meetings and should have a confidentiality clause. It is advisable that a clause should state that, if a difficulty cannot be overcome within the supervisory relationship, the supervisor or supervisee can take the difficulty to the manager. It is good practice to discuss this in the first supervision session. The supervisor's role and responsibilities to the supervisee will be clearly negotiated.

Service standard 14: SLTs access an appropriate form of clinical supervision at least once every 12 weeks.

For therapists with a predominantly counselling role, one and a half hours per month is an appropriate level of supervision, but this may need to be increased depending on the caseload.

The supervisor must ensure that they are sufficiently experienced, competent and appropriately trained to provide individual or group supervision as appropriate.

Training for supervision

It is recommended that SLTs who offer managerial or clinical supervision should receive training. The following organisations are possible sources for training:

- the RCSLT
- the ASLTIP
- individual trusts
- the British Association of Psychotherapists
- psychotherapy organisations, such as member organisations of the British Confederation of Psychotherapists
- Oxford and Cherwell College.

For guidance on observing individual confidentiality when obtaining support and in supervision, see Chapter 1, Professional Framework section 1.7.6 Confidentiality.

Support

The RCSLT recognises that SLTs require easy access to support networks both from within and outside the profession and that the SLT should recognise when they need to access support. Good clinical practice relies upon therapists' recognition of the limits of expertise and their ability to secure clinical support in the provision of their services. Managers and practitioners at all levels of expertise require support in order to exchange information and share expertise to help raise the quality of services provided.

Practitioners may require extra specialist support and training when starting a new specialism, for example through buddying or formalised external supervision.

Professional support should be available through:

- the management structure of the employing authority
- colleagues within and/or outside the service
- RCSLT SIGs, managers and ASLTIP groups.

The RCSLT acknowledges the potential for pressures arising from professional practice where the unique relationship with the individual is paramount.

The RCSLT suggests that adequate provision of support leads to reduced stress levels and the enhanced ability to "manage" distressing or complex situations. This is especially important for newly-qualified therapists and those who may find themselves working in isolation.

The RCSLT recommends that, wherever possible, joint initiatives and close collaboration should be a normal part of service delivery in order to prevent isolation and resulting difficulties.

It is important for SLTs working in a service structure to be confident in their manager's ability to offer responsive and sensitive support in times of difficulty.

The speech and language therapy manager recognises that their commitment to staff will at times extend to facilitating personal support. It is likely that the support will be more appropriately offered outside of the management line. However, the SLT may need help in accessing appropriate support, for example, from the occupational health department, staff counsellors, employee assistance programmes or assertiveness training courses.

In situations where especially high levels of stress are likely, owing to the nature of the SLT's caseload or work environment, it is important to encourage group support to provide mutual support and promote problem solving.

In summary: The RCSLT recognises that SLTs may require support throughout their career and urges employing authorities, speech and language therapy managers and fellow clinicians to deal sensitively with these needs as they arise.

Service standard 15: The service has a system for accessing clinical advice or second opinions.

There should be a policy on staff seeking advice or second opinions from senior staff or external agencies, detailing opportunities for joint working, guidance or support.

Policy relating to staff health and safety issues

The service makes the health and safety of staff a priority. For more information see section 5.6.4 Health and Safety at Work.

5.3.4 Competence

What is competence?

Put at its simplest, competence is an individual's ability to effectively apply all their knowledge, understandings, skills and values within their designated scope of practice.

It is witnessed by:
● the effective performance of the specific role and its related
responsibilities
● an individual's critical reflection on their practice.
For further exploration of competence, see Chapter 1 on
Professional Framework.

SLT competence
SLTs are accountable to the HPC and the RCSLT in terms of their
personal standards of practice and care for individuals.
SLTs need to maintain a clear sense of their personal scope of
practice and competence. This includes knowing when it is
appropriate to refer on; to seek further advice or to seek training in
order to maintain or extend their competence.
When identifying their personal scope of practice, SLTs may wish to
start with a consideration of their practice roles (in broad terms,
those of therapist, manager, researcher and educator).
Each role may then be described in the form of competencies.
For information on competencies see:
● NHS KSF
● RCSLT Clinical Competency Framework
● RCSLT Manager Competencies
● AHP Ten Key Roles for AHPs.

RCSLT six outcomes model of competence
The six outcomes model was piloted as part of a national Allied
Health Professional (AHP) project carried out during 2003.
Within this model SLTs show that they:
● understand, work within and respond appropriately to the limits of
professional practice
● demonstrate effectiveness in practice
● practise within the profession's moral and ethical framework
● think critically about personal practice and its context
● deal appropriately with the new and non-routine
● communicate and collaborate effectively.
In 2004–2005, the model was incorporated into the RCSLT
professional log on a pilot basis as part of RCSLT membership
requirements. Feedback from the membership at the end of the year
led to a decision to stop using the six outcomes.

However, the outcomes remain valid ways of expressing key dimensions of practice and members may wish to incorporate these notions into their philosophy of practice.

Newly-qualified practitioners

Under current arrangements newly-qualified practitioners (NQPs) are entered into the supervised category of RCSLT membership when they graduate from a qualifying course accredited by the HPC and recognised by the RCSLT.

On joining the professional body, NQPs are issued with a certificate of RCSLT membership. These entrants to the profession are expected to complete approximately one year in a clinical setting under supervision before being accepted as an autonomous clinician and given full RCSLT membership.

This time frame is given as a guide and may vary according to the individual. However, it is unlikely that an SLT will have met the requirements in less than twelve months, but they should have done so within two years.

Service standard 16: The service uses the competency based framework to structure the learning of the newly qualified practitioner during the initial twelve month period and as evidence of readiness to transfer to full RCSLT membership.

A Speech and Language Therapy Competency Framework to Guide Transition to Full RCSLT Membership for Newly-qualified Practitioners (2005) is available at:

www.rcslt.org/resources/newlyqualifiedpractitioner

The framework encompasses eight dimensions of competence that an SLT is expected to develop during the first twelve to eighteen months of practice:

● communication
● personal and people development
● health, safety and security
● service improvement
● quality
● equality and diversity
● assessment and care planning to meet health and wellbeing needs
● health and wellbeing needs intervention.

These headings link directly with the core dimensions and others listed in the NHS KSF to reflect current thinking within the NHS.

The competencies set out within each dimension of competence are broad and can be added to if there are particular local requirements. The framework contains suggestions as to the type of evidence that may be provided to indicate competence across the eight dimensions. This is not intended to be prescriptive. Evidence can be collated throughout the year and gathered in a variety of ways, eg through discussion, professional portfolio, observation, case note checks, presentations, etc.

This transitional supervised period of working helps NQPs to:
● develop a detailed knowledge of a particular working context and its impact on practice
● build up a bank of supervised cases in relevant areas of case work to support future independent clinical judgments and decisions
● reinforce certain key aspects of autonomous professional practice.

It is not recommended that a newly-qualified practitioner works as a locum during the transitional period or that an NQP works in independent practice, except where this is as a member of a large independent practice able to provide the required level of support and supervision.

The detailed programme of support for the NQP is a matter for local decision. However, the RCSLT recommends that the following types and levels of support should be in place:
● a work place mentor or buddy to assist each NQP in learning about everyday work place practice and procedures
● regular line management supervisory meetings (weekly during the first three months and monthly thereafter) to assess progress and to identify further development needs. The manager will also be expected to support the NQP in finding appropriate ways in meeting those development needs
● attendance at clinical meetings to develop an understanding of current clinical issues and debates
● opportunities to access specialist advice to support clinical judgment and decision making
● a clinical supervisor to support development of critical reflective practice.

Any performance or capability issues should be addressed immediately they become apparent through a programme of opportunities and additional support to meet the NQP's needs.

Transfer of NQPs to full RCSLT membership

Before recommending the NQP for transfer to full RCSLT membership, the manager should be satisfied that the NQP is competent and ready to work autonomously, ie is performing consistently to the required standards. The main responsibility for producing evidence lies with the NQP.

The form for transfer to full membership should be submitted fully completed to the RCSLT and can be submitted any time during the year. Most NQPs will therefore qualify in year one; submit a form in year two and appear on the full membership section in the spring of year three. A few will transfer during the following year.

Transfer forms will be scrutinised by the RCSLT but any disputes should be resolved locally. The transfer form must be completed correctly and in full and signed by the manager/supervisor therapist. Receipt of the completed form by the RCSLT will trigger removal of the NQP from the supervised section of membership.

The transfer form will be retained in the individual member's file in the registered office of the RCSLT.

Guidance on any aspect of the above procedure can be provided by the RCSLT.

Information about the framework is also included in the RCSLT's *Starting your career as a speech and language therapist: An essential guide,* 2004 available at: www.rcslt.org/resources/publications

Returners to practice

Since 2001, the regulation of health professionals has changed and there are now rules in place for SLTs returning to practise.

The rules have been designed to ensure that all health professionals are practising in an up-to-date way and are aware of the changes that have taken place whilst they have not been working.

All SLTs are required by law to register with the HPC in order to practise in the UK. The HPC requires individuals to ensure that their knowledge and skills are up to date and that the HPC's standards of proficiency (SOPs) are met. More information is available on the HPC's website at: www.hpc-uk.org

The RCSLT provides guidance and support for speech and language therapy returners. It includes information on finding a clinical placement and guidance on registering with HPC. SLTs who have been out of practice for more than two years should apply to become a returner member of RCSLT. This status is held for a year prior to being transferred on to the full membership list again.

The RCSLT's *Returners Pack* is available on the RCSLT website. The RCSLT also has a distance-learning course for SLTs who have been out of practice for more than two years. This course is to help SLTs meet the HPC requirements for additional study. The course is designed in units and there are nine units, each requiring approximately 10 hours of study time.

Each unit has specific aims, learning outcomes, reading material and self-assessment questions that must be answered in order to complete the unit. The self-assessment questions are submitted to the RCSLT as evidence of completion of each unit. The RCSLT then issues a certificate of completion to the SLT.

This course does not cover all areas of clinical practice. It is designed to bring individuals up to date with key areas of professional practice, legislation and new developments.

Once the course has been completed, individuals may need to undertake courses on specific clinical areas to update knowledge and skills still further. The RCSLT can provide a list of short courses currently available through its own programme and other programmes based in universities and voluntary sector organisations throughout the UK.

Support Practitioners

Speech and language therapy support practitioners are integral members of the speech and language therapy team, employed to act in a supporting role under the direction of a professionally-qualified SLT. **Support practitioners need to maintain a clear sense of their personal scope of practice and competence. This includes knowing when it is appropriate to seek advice or training in order to maintain or extend their competence.**

At present, speech and language therapy support practitioners are not subject to regulation, although this is likely to change during the next few years.

For information on support practitioner competencies see:

● *NHS KSF*

● *RCSLT support practitioner core clinical competencies (2002).* This looks at competency levels for a newly appointed support practitioner, established support practitioner and advanced support practitioner. It contains a useful exploration of the terms support, supervision and direction, as well as identifying what support practitioners are not expected to do. Available at: www.rcslt.org

Manager competence

Managers need to maintain a clear sense of their personal scope of practice and competence. They have a responsibility to ensure they develop and sustain their management and leadership skills and to seek advice as appropriate.

They should ensure that staff are provided with an opportunity to do likewise.

The RCSLT information pack for new speech and language therapy managers includes a model of competencies for speech and language therapy managers, available at: www.rcslt.org

The model covers the following areas:

- organisation
- leadership
- operational management
- resource management
- health and safety
- collaborative/partnership working
- influencing policies
- people management
- clinical effectiveness
- patient and public involvement.

5.3.5 Learning organisation

The delivery of high quality healthcare services is integral to clinical governance. In order to adhere to the clinical governance agenda, organisations, (eg trusts, local education authorities, voluntary organisations, etc) need to demonstrate they are learning organisations. Learning organisations have responsibilities as illustrated in the following examples.

The management board of the organisation is responsible for:

- promoting clinical governance as integral to its work
- promoting a supportive learning culture
- ensuring adequate resources are available to deliver the clinical governance agenda

- the overall accountability for clinical governance.

Managers are responsible for:
- supporting individuals (appraisal, service development, supervision, direction, leadership) to provide evidence-informed care
- ensuring accountability arrangements and systems are in place within their services
- promoting a culture that supports improvement and learning.

Individual practitioners are responsible for:
- ensuring the provision of high quality services
- being evidence-aware
- professional accountability and self regulation
- commitment to appraisal and CPD
- accessing learning opportunities
- input to appraisal process
- clinical audit and risk management
- sharing good practice.

Information and guidance on clinical governance is available on the NHS Clinical Governance Support Team's website at: www.cgsupport.nhs.uk

Service standard 17: The service supports the monitoring of clinical practice through managerial and clinical supervision, staff development review and personal development plans.

Learning culture

Service standard 18: The service has an up-to-date policy for dealing with staff concerns about clinical care, including a confidential procedure for staff to follow.

Staff should be aware of their responsibility to report concerns and action should be taken to investigate any concerns.

Service standard 19: As appropriate, service managers are involved in influencing and defining the objectives of the wider organisation.

Service standard 20: All staff have the opportunity to participate in the planning, decision making and formulating of policies which affect service provision.

Involvement may occur for example through staff meetings, membership of committees or individual responsibilities.

It is essential that managers ask staff for their views and listen to and take on board their comments. The NHS undertakes staff surveys on an annual basis. However service specific surveys may be necessary to obtain more detailed information.

Service standard 21: The service has up-to-date administrative policies that relate to speech and language therapy working practices and are written by, or in consultation with, a registered SLT.

Service standard 22: The RCSLT's professional standards and guidelines inform the development of policy and practice.

In support of this, copies of the RCSLT standards and guidelines should be readily available in each clinical setting.

5.3.6 Evidence-based practice: research utilisation

The evidence base for intervention has grown considerably over recent years and continues to do so, although there is a need for much more research in some areas. Research and evaluation play an essential role in ensuring quality in healthcare.

It is essential that professionals contribute to the development of the evidence base in diverse ways including generating research questions, critical reflective practice and evaluation.

Service standard 23: The service has a strategic and systematic approach within each clinical team to establish an evidence-based resource as the basis for provision of clinical care, organisation of services and service development.

The RCSLT recognises that increasing the use of evidence-based or evidence-informed practice requires changes at the level of the individual practitioner and at the level of the organisation.

Individual practitioners need:
● a positive attitude towards research findings
● to know where to find the evidence
● access to people working in the same field, eg peers and advisers, to help filter and analyse evidence
● access to specialist people and other resources
● baseline competencies in researching skills for using electronic databases
● baseline competencies in critical appraisal of published research
● knowledge of levels of evidence
● knowledge of research designs, especially what design is appropriate for which types of questions and what its limitations are.

More information is available on the Critical Appraisal Skills Programme website at: www.phru.nhs.uk/casp/casp.htm
● baseline competencies in measuring clinical practice, ie designing, implementing and analysing clinical audits
● baseline competencies in implementing clinical change.
See also Chapter 9, Service Monitoring, Improvement, Evaluation and Development section 9.1.4. Service Monitoring and Improvement

Services need to provide:

A research culture
● protected time in line with local organisational policy and active management support
● active encouragement to staff to read relevant literature regularly and to use library resources as part of professional duties. The professional development plan (PDP) process is core to this

Learning and development opportunities
Opportunities for education and updating learning in the accessing and use of:
● electronic library resources, especially subject-based researching and the saving of search terms
● critical reading of research literature
● methodology and application of evidence-based practice (EBP).

Structure and systems
● a robust means of peer support/clinical supervision, in which facilitators/supervisors are evidence-aware and encourage appropriate discussion of evidence
● designated members of staff who are able to provide specific support for EBP/audit/research
● active encouragement of "journal club" activities
● a system of ensuring SLTs are properly trained to evaluate research
● a system for checking that therapists use evidence-based information, (eg as part of CPD/annual appraisal interview and/or other associated meetings. For example SLTs have their notes audited and decision making is looked at as part of that process)

● a strategic and systematic approach within each clinical team to establish an evidence-based resource as the basis for service planning and to ensure efficient use of staff time, (eg to reduce duplication of searching for research evidence, etc)

● designated people with responsibility to access and evaluate research findings in relation to a particular clinical area and with responsibility to skill up the rest of the clinical team

● collaborative networks with higher education institutions (HEIs)/research teams

● contacts for additional assistance with all the above when required.

Resources

These can include:

● departmental library resources, having access to books, journals and magazines, with remote access/borrowing particularly for services in rural/sparsely populated areas and supported by the facility to access to university/post-graduate medical or other relevant tertiary library resources

● appropriate information and communications technology (ICT) support and internet access so therapists can access clinical guidelines, electronic libraries such as e-library (Scotland) and the NHS's National electronic Library for Health (NeLH) with local/national subscriptions to relevant full-text journals.

5.3.7 Audit

Audit is a way of measuring and assuring service quality. Audit results are used to support the processes of service improvement and development.

Audit is covered more comprehensively in Chapter 9, Service Monitoring, Improvement, Evaluation and Development; section 9.1.4.

Service standard 24: The service has a system to collect information for service management purposes and to meet contractual obligations. Information is collected on a consistent and regular basis.

Service standard 25: The design of documents includes a code to allow for audit trails and identification of source.

5.3.8 Clinical audit

Clinical audit can be defined as the systematic critical analysis of the quality of healthcare, including the procedures used for diagnosis and treatment, the use of resources and the resulting outcome and quality of life for the individual (DH,1989).

The purpose of clinical audit is to improve the quality of care. Clinical audit identifies opportunities for improvement in individual care and the mechanisms for realising them. This is done through reviewing the provision of healthcare to identify deficiencies or weaknesses.

The audit cycle includes the following steps:

● observing current practice
● setting standards of care
● comparing practice to standards and implementing change.

This is a continuous process. It has been suggested that audit is similar to research, the main difference is that whilst research aims to influence clinical practice in its totality, audit aims to influence activity on a local level.

Clinical audit can facilitate the change in culture towards evidence-based practice through clinical guidelines. Standards of care in service delivery can be developed using evidence as their base and may become part of the process of adapting guidelines to local use. Clinical audit can also be used to measure the outcomes of care including individual satisfaction.

Many NHS trusts have their own clinical audit departments that are coordinating activities locally. The main purpose of clinical audit remains the improvement of individual care and health outcomes and the effective translation of research into evidence-based practice.

5.3.9 Continuing Professional Development (CPD)

CPD has been defined as a range of learning activities through which professionals maintain and develop throughout their career to ensure that they retain their capacity to practise safely effectively and legally within their evolving scope of practice (HPC, 2004).

HPC and CPD

In July 2005, the Health Professions Council (HPC) put in place rules and standards that require therapists to undertake CPD as part of their re-registration.

The standards specify that a registrant must:

● maintain a continuous, up-to-date and accurate record of their CPD activities

● demonstrate that their CPD activities are a mixture of learning activities related to current or future practice

● seek to ensure that their CPD benefits the service user

● present a written profile containing evidence of their CPD on request.

See the HPC's website for more information at: www.hpc.uk.org

CPD is not yet a requirement for support practitioners as it is for SLTs, but the RCSLT encourages support practitioners to undertake CPD and believes that a reflective approach is as appropriate to them as to qualified therapists.

In July 2009, the HPC will begin an audit of SLTs' CPD records. This will require therapists selected for audit to submit information on the preceding two years of CPD activity (2007-2009). This audit cycle will repeat thereafter on a two yearly cycle.

RCSLT and CPD

The RCSLT has set standards on CPD which mirror those of the HPC, in addition to setting a standard on minimum number of hours required (see below).

The RCSLT provides the systems and tools to enable members to comply with the both the RCSLT and HPC requirements on CPD. A CPD toolkit will be available to support members in undertaking CPD and keeping records of their CPD.

See: www.rcslt.org/cpd/toolkit

The RCSLT also provides an online system of record keeping. This allows members to record information for different purposes more efficiently and is linked with the HPC and the KSF developmental review. The online system includes a diary or "log" of activities, a record of reflections and will allow members to generate reports on their CPD.

The CPD framework takes an outcomes-based approach to CPD in line with developments in the wider CPD context. Members are required to write reflective commentaries on the impact of their learning on practice in addition to keeping records of the activities.

Personal learning portfolios
Service standard 26: All staff maintain personal learning portfolios and reflect on learning gained through practice, both individually and in teams.
Included in the folio is a personal development plan (PDP).

Personal development plans (PDP)
Every practitioner (including support practitioners) should have a PDP. The PDP should identify areas of development and how these developments could be met. The PDP should be reviewed and updated on an annual basis in parallel with the appraisal process.
Service standard 27: All staff have access to a personal development review at least once every twelve months.
Managers should ensure that clinicians have the appropriate competence to undertake the roles and responsibilities of the post they are appointed to. Practitioners are responsible for ensuring they work within their level of competence; they contribute to identifying their development needs and actively seek learning opportunities. The responsibility for engaging in ongoing appropriate CPD should be shared by practitioners and managers.

Providing opportunities for CPD
Service standard 28: The service has an up-to-date staff training and development policy.
This will usually include requirements for practitioners to undertake a range of training that may include health and safety (fire, infection control, moving and handling, dealing with violence, etc), safeguarding children, and the protection of vulnerable adults. Information about educational/training opportunities should be made available to staff and there should be a system for applying for training. The needs of those working part time and on short-term contracts, as well as those of practitioners returning to the profession, should be taken into account in local policies.
Records should be maintained for all training undertaken, and benefits evaluated and opportunities and funds for training should be equitably managed.

Minimum time commitment to CPD
The minimum required personal commitment for full-time practitioners to their continuing CPD activities covering specific areas

of clinical interest, and in line with the business objectives of the organisation, is the equivalent of 30 hours per year (pro-rata for part-time staff). This is in addition to mandatory training.

All staff should have access to CPD opportunities complemented by access to appropriate supervision mechanisms.

Range of CPD learning activity

The range of activity that can be undertaken is extensive and includes: work-based learning; professional activity; formal training and education and self-directed learning.

Work-based learning
- learning by doing
- case studies
- reflective practice
- clinical audit
- coaching from others
- discussion with colleagues
- peer review
- gaining and learning from experience
- involvement in wider work of the employers, eg representative on a committee
- shadowing
- secondments
- job rotation
- journal club
- in-service training
- supervision of staff or students
- visit to others' departments and reporting back
- role expansion
- critical incident analysis
- completion of self assessment questionnaires
- project work/management
- action learning set.

Professional activity
- involvement in a professional body
- involvement in a Specific Interest Group (SIG)
- lecturing/teaching

- mentoring
- examiner
- tutor
- branch meetings
- organising journal clubs and other specialist groups
- maintaining and/or developing specialist skills
- expert witness
- member of other professional bodies/groups
- presentation at conferences
- organiser of accredited courses
- research supervision
- national assessor.

Formal training and education
- courses
- further education
- undertaking research
- attendance at conferences
- submission of articles/papers
- seminars
- distance learning
- courses accredited by the professional body
- planning or running a course.

Self-directed learning
- reading journals or articles
- review of books/articles
- updating knowledge via the Internet or the media
- progress files

Other CPD
- public service
- voluntary work
- courses.

KSF and CPD
NHS employers are now asking therapists to show evidence of their CPD for KSF appraisal purposes. Much of the activity, and the records that go with them for KSF, will be the same as those required for the HPC and the RCSLT.

5.3.10 NHS Knowledge and Skills Framework (KSF)

The KSF is a broad generic framework that describes the application of knowledge and skills within the workplace in order to deliver quality NHS services. The KSF is about the application of knowledge and skills and not about the specific knowledge and skills that individuals need to possess.

It provides a single, consistent, comprehensive and explicit framework on which to base review and development for all staff.

The key purposes of the KSF are:

● To facilitate the development of services so that they better meet the needs of users and the public through investing in the development of all members of staff.

● To support the effective learning and development of individuals and teams.

● To support the development of individuals in the post they are employed in so they can be effective at work. Managers and staff should be clear about what is required within a post and managers should enable staff to develop within their post.

● To promote equality for and diversity of all staff. Every member of staff should be using the same framework, having the same opportunities for learning and development open to them and having the same structured approach to learning, development and review.

● To form the basis of the development review process. This is an ongoing cycle of review, planning, development and evaluation for all staff in the NHS which links organisational and individual development needs.

● To inform pay progression within pay bands. In order to progress within pay bands an individual will be required to demonstrate the application of knowledge and skills to meet the demands of the post as described in their KSF outline. This evidence will be presented during the individual performance review process.

For further information on the KSF, visit:
www.dh.gov.uk/publicationsandstatistics/publications

5.4 Resources and Resource Management

Service standard 29: The service has sufficient and appropriate resources to support the principal functions of the service.
This includes:

● Pay and non-pay budgets (for example, in relation to training and

development and purchasing of equipment).
● Accommodation that complies with RCSLT guidance (see section 5.4.1).
● Staffing establishment is adequate to meet the contracted needs of the service. This includes an appropriate skill mix.
● Equipment.

Service standard 30: The financial resources of the service are planned, managed and controlled.
In support of this, there is:
● a clear statement of budgetary responsibility for each section head and line manager
● a clear system of budget allocation and monitoring.

5.4.1 Accommodation
Speech and language therapy is provided in a range of settings in line with the following principle:
Wherever possible and appropriate to an individual's needs/choices, and as indicated by the evidence, services will be provided in settings that will most readily facilitate individual assessment and intervention.
This may involve working within dedicated accommodation or within a wide range of other settings.

Dedicated accommodation for speech and language therapy (available within a range of contexts)
Although for many individuals, an everyday environment where communication occurs naturally is the best context for assessment and intervention, the controlled environment of dedicated speech and language therapy accommodation provides the most appropriate context:
● for objective assessment procedures, eg nasometry
● where objective assessment equipment is not portable
● for aspects of assessment and intervention with a young child
● where videoing is integral to the intervention, eg developing parent/child interaction
● where privacy is paramount, eg discussing personal and sensitive information
● for small group intervention activities
● when intervention is focused on aspects of skill building prior to daily life application

- for audio recording and audio training activities
- for running parent groups or support groups for carers
- valve changing (this needs to take place within a hospital setting with access to medical staff in case of emergency).

For more information see the Department of Health guidelines *Essence of Care: Patient-focused benchmarking for healthcare practitioners,* 2003, available at: www.dh.gov.uk

Therapy areas

General functional and design requirements:
- Accommodation should comply with health and safety requirements.
- Therapy rooms should have a good standard of daylight and artificial light.
- Therapy rooms should have good ventilation.
- Therapy rooms should have adequate space to allow for a variety of activities.
- The temperature in therapy rooms should be well regulated.
- Carpets in therapy rooms should be clean, stain-resistant and securely fixed. Where carpet is used, this should be suitable for children and speech and language therapy staff to engage in therapy activities on the floor.
- For certain individual groups, high quality washable flooring is more appropriate than carpet.
- Rooms should be situated away from the disruptive influence of noisy external activities.

For more information see the NHS estates specification, available at: www.dh.gov.uk

Accommodation for therapy with individuals
One room, or space within a multi-professional work area, as appropriate, should be available for each whole-time equivalent SLT. Allowances may also need to be made for students and assistants. The room should be large enough to accommodate the SLT, individual (possibly in a wheelchair), carer and observer and the minimum size should be 15 square metres.

The room must be quiet with sufficiently low background noise to make it suitable for recording and sound-sensitive equipment. It may be necessary for it to be sound-attenuated.

There should be:

● A table and sufficient number of chairs, of a size and design suitable for the particular individual group. Sharp corners and edges of furniture should be protected.

● A wash basin and, in the case of working with individuals with head and neck cancer, the room should have a second, stainless steel basin for the cleaning of equipment.

● Where there is no wash basin, an alcohol-based cleanser or disposable wipes should be available.

● A lockable storage space for equipment, or the room itself should be lockable and secure.

● As appropriate, a full-length mirror attached to the wall, with a curtain to cover the mirror when not in use

● A sufficient number of accessible power points. In children's clinics, these should have protected sockets.

● A telephone point.

● A good light source to allow the individual and clinician to readily see each other's faces and, as appropriate, to support changing or maintenance of valves.

● As appropriate, security systems should be in place for urgent summoning of assistance and risk management.

An observation room with viewing and audio-visual recording facilities is helpful in support of:

● student training

● Multidisciplinary Team (MDT) training

● parent/child observation, assessment and intervention

● videoing.

Accommodation for group therapy

As appropriate, there should be regular and reliable access to a room suitable for group work. 39 square metres is deemed to be the minimum size for such a room.

The room should be sufficiently large to accommodate up to eight individuals plus an SLT and two assistants. Specific needs should be taken into consideration, eg space for wheelchairs, play area, etc. Tables and chairs suitable for the needs of individuals should be available and accessible. An observation room is helpful as well, as described above.

Access to therapy accommodation

The Disability Discrimination Act (2005) places a duty on public bodies to carry out their functions with due regard to promoting equality for people with disabilities

Further information is available at: www.drc.org.uk

Ideally, outpatient clinics should:

● have good access to speech and language therapy departments by public or hospital transport

● have an external entrance with an easy approach for vehicles

● have adequate parking facilities for individuals and staff

● be located in an appropriate part of the hospital/clinic/school according to individual groups, etc. with reasonable access for individuals attending other departments

● have convenient external and internal access for individuals with wheelchairs/pushchairs/walking aids

● be signposted clearly and appropriately

● be well signposted using the written word and an agreed set of symbols

● have easy access to toilets, including a facility for people with disabilities and baby changing facilities.

Where appropriate to the context, (eg within a hospital or community clinic setting) staffed reception facilities and a waiting area will need to be provided.

Reception facilities and waiting area for speech and language therapy provision

Suitable reception facilities should be available. There should be a suitable waiting area near the therapy rooms, large enough and with sufficient comfortable chairs to accommodate the number of people likely to be waiting at any one time. The waiting area should be more than just a corridor.

The therapy room and waiting area should be sufficiently separated so that noise from the waiting area does not disturb intervention and privacy is maintained in the therapy room. Appropriate toys and materials should be available for children.

Whatever settings speech and language therapy staff are required to work into, each member of staff requires a designated office base and access to a range of resources which will support therapy.

Speech and language therapy staff office base

An office area where current case records can be stored and general administrative work can be carried out will be required. In a small department, the office area and therapy room may be combined.

There should be:

- a desk space or workstation for each therapist using the accommodation
- a sufficient lockable filing space to accommodate current and review case records, administrative information, forms, etc
- a notice board in the department
- privacy to make phone calls when confidentiality is an issue
- ready access to IT facilities including the Internet, the NHSonline.net research databases, email and a fax machine
- ready access to administrative resources, eg a range of stationery.

Arrangements should be made to store non-current case notes securely for the required statutory period (up to 25 years duration for children and eight years for adults).

Staff room

Therapists should have easy access to a room with facilities for making drinks and preparing snacks and where they can take regular breaks with colleagues.

Secretarial/recruitment

Reliable and regular qualified secretarial support should be available to receive enquiries from individuals: to type, copy and send out reports and letters within an agreed local time standard. Staff need to be aware of the range of communication difficulties they are likely to encounter and know how to respond appropriately.

There needs to be a reliable method of taking messages and contacting speech and language therapy staff quickly. This may be by a receptionist, secretary, assistant, answer-phone or voice mail. The speech and language therapy department may need to look at recruiting bilingual staff who speak a community language, if appropriate.

Administrative tasks should, where possible and appropriate, be carried out by administration/secretarial personnel.

Accommodation when working across a range of contexts

Services will be provided in settings that will most readily facilitate individual assessment and intervention. Sometimes this will mean working with the individual within their home or other daily living contexts (e.g. school, leisure facilities, shops, stroke clubs, nursing homes, MDT clinics, day-centres).

Facilities for working need to be consistent with the nature of the intervention and requirements will vary accordingly.

At times, a facility for withdrawal may be required to ensure the optimal attention, concentration and engagement of the individual. The facility will need to provide some of the aspects that dedicated accommodation offers, including:

- quietness
- privacy
- natural light
- safety
- space according to need
- hand washing facilities to facilitate infection control
- storage space for equipment
- appropriately sized table and chairs.

Where these cannot be provided, it should be recognised that there could be a trade off in terms of therapeutic effectiveness and assessment results may be compromised.

5.4.2 Equipment

In support of administrative functions and the development of individual resources, speech and language therapy staff should have access to equipment such as:

- a laminator, shredder and photocopier
- a fax machine, answer-phone, and a method of contact when away from base, for example a pager or mobile phone
- computer equipment with database system, Internet and email access and symbol software
- a digital camera
- a range of stationery items, including appropriately headed notepaper.

In support of assessment and intervention:

Hi-tech equipment

Speech and language therapy staff must have access to an

appropriate range of hi-tech equipment for their client group.
To enable accurate recording and analysis of communication skills,
this is likely to include:
- a tape recorder
- digital video equipment
- a microphone
- a tripod
- a range of communication aids to enable assessment and therapy
trials with individuals.

Services should ensure that a budget is available to maintain and
update hi-tech equipment.

Computer equipment with Internet and email access

Speech and language therapy staff should have access to computer
equipment with Internet and email access at their main site of work
in order to source clinical information and evidence; to seek support
and to network with colleagues.

It is recommended that speech and language therapy staff also have
access to a laptop computer with a range of individual–group specific
assessment and therapeutic software.

In the context of clinicians attending outreach clinics, portable
printers may also be necessary in order to provide advice sheets and
assessment information to individuals and their families.

Assessment materials

Although it is recognised that informal assessment may most
appropriately take place in everyday environments where
communication occurs naturally, SLTs will often supplement these
observations by introducing stimulus materials to assess certain
aspects of function.

Assessment materials will include a range of formal and informal
assessments to gather quantitative and qualitative information, as
appropriate to the individual group.

Materials should be age-appropriate and non-discriminatory in
terms of culture, gender, linguistic or religious background of the
individual.

Assessments should reflect the regional variations of the languages
used by the individual.

Local adaptation to informal assessment material should be made when appropriate, without compromising the assessment criteria. The latest editions of any standardised test materials, perceptual and instrumental assessments should be available.

Equipment for an oral examination should include:
● tongue depressors
● a pen torch
● a portable mirror
● protective gloves
● sterile wipes.

Ready access to appropriate clinical specialist services is required (eg videofluoroscopy, nasendoscopy, hearing assessment, FEES).

Therapy materials

Often the most appropriate therapy material will be provided through access to everyday situations where communication opportunities arise naturally, (eg having access to transport for individuals, a telephone, local shops, leisure and social centres and negotiated access to other therapy resources, [eg therapy kitchen, hydrotherapy pool, physiotherapy gym]).

In addition, a range of published and individually prepared therapeutic materials will be required as appropriate to the individual group in order to work on specific aspects of function.

Core materials appropriate to each individual group should be available to speech and language therapy staff to take to outreach settings.

These items should be age appropriate and non-discriminatory in terms of the individual's culture, gender, linguistic or religious background.

Toys and picture materials should reflect the cultural background of the individual.

Service standard 31: Equipment used in therapy is non-hazardous to the individual and conforms to health and safety standards. This includes regular cleaning of equipment in accordance with infection control guidance.

For certain individual groups, specialist equipment is required in order to carry out appropriate functions. As these requirements are likely to change over time, SLTs should advise managers on the equipment and resource needs specific to the individual group.

In support of providing teaching and learning opportunities for

individuals/carers and colleagues, the service should ensure staff have:
● access to appropriate research journals
● access to local and national guidelines and protocols
● access to the Internet
● access to an up-to-date library of relevant text books
● data projector and overhead projector
● flip chart stand and paper
● range of stationery, (eg overhead transparencies, discs, pens and post-its)
● anatomical models as appropriate
● a range of literature for individuals and carers.

Service standard 32: A range of relevant and up-to-date literature is available to support the individual and/or carer in understanding the nature and extent of any given swallowing or communication disorder.

Individual self-help resources:
● Patient UK: www.patient.co.uk
● A-Z Health Guide from WebMD: Support Groups: www.my.webmd.com/hw/cancer/shc12.asp

Service standard 33: The service has a written statement of philosophy, core purpose and operational policy.

Service information for individuals, carers and colleagues should include information on:
● values
● main aims (scope and principal functions)
● who is served
● referral procedure
● process followed on receipt of referral
● service contact details.

Where relevant, this statement should be consistent with the overall objectives of the wider organisation (eg LEA, school, trust, primary care trust).

See also section 1.1 Scope of Practice, in Chapter 1, Professional Framework.

Service standard 34: All staff (including those in remote areas) are aware of available resources and are able to access them as appropriate.

5.4.3 Workload management

Services have a responsibility to ensure that:
● the public and referred individuals are protected from poor quality services
● staff are not subject to stress through excessive workloads.

One way of fulfilling these responsibilities is through ensuring a balance between service demands and staffing establishment.

Service standard 35: The service has a mechanism for ongoing monitoring of staff workloads.

The mechanism for monitoring might include:
● service review, including staffing levels
● sickness/absence review
● activity monitoring
● discussion with individuals as part of an individual performance review process (IPR).

A service may wish to specify maximum contact targets for individual members of staff.

What is workload?

Workload can be thought of in relation to three key dimensions:
● levels of demand or need
● ways of meeting demands and needs
● the staffing establishment (numbers and skill mix) required to meet the demands/needs in particular ways.

Workload is usually expressed as the ratio of work to an individual member of staff or to a team of staff.

However, defining workload is complicated because estimates of need and ideas about the most effective ways of meeting those needs are changing all the time, as a reflection of evolving professional practice.

As far as possible, **workload** should reflect:
● nationally agreed principles
● evidence-based models of working
● local needs
● professional needs
● priorities set in agreement with commissioners and stakeholders.

Estimating the level of demand/need

A consideration of the *current* demands based on an analysis of:
● local demographics and population needs

- the numbers on the caseload
- the numbers of referrals per month
- analysis of activity undertaken
- an estimate of the time taken for different levels and types of intervention
- feedback from individuals
- individual needs, outcomes and benefits
- whether the service meets the priorities of commissioners and stakeholders
- whether professional standards, (eg waiting times) are being met
- risks being faced by individuals or groups of individuals as a result of services as currently configured
- the full range of demands on staff time
- direct individual contact
- travel time
- report writing
- administrative tasks
- preparation of therapy resources
- attending meetings
- service development projects
- development of policies and procedures
- clinical governance
- CPD activities
- supervising and developing less experienced staff
- education of students
- training other professionals
- tier two services, for example, prevention/health promotion.

Consider future demands based on an analysis of:
- national and local strategies and initiatives
- modernisation projects
- demographic trends
- individual and public consultation.

Identifying current ways of meeting the demand/need

The RCSLT recommends that all people referred to a speech and language therapy service should receive models of care that are evidence-based, rather than models of care informed by resource restrictions.

See the *RCSLT Clinical Guidelines (2005)*, available at:
www.rcslt.org/resources and Chapters 6,7 and 8 on Service
Provision for more information.

In terms of profiling current ways of meeting demands, services
may:
● identify the models of service provision that are in use (eg,
consultative/advisory or direct/review or "whole school" approach/
individual children)
● identify how the demand for services is managed
● specify waiting times
● develop prioritisation systems (eg which individuals have high/low
priority within resources available)
● identify where services are provided, (eg acute, community,
school-based, community contexts)
● identify the ways in which speech and language therapy services
work in partnership with other support agencies in terms of roles and
responsibilities
● identify how the skill mix is used in all parts of the service to
support meeting individual needs.

Benchmarking
Speech and language therapy services across the UK do not have
common and agreed systems of measuring and collating activity.
Services do not therefore hold the same data, which means that
benchmarking and comparison of services is problematic.
Models of working vary considerably according to:
● the number of potential individuals
● the range of service locations available
● the type and level of health, education, social service provision
and local demographics.

Estimating required staffing levels
Over the years various methodologies have been used to inform
staffing levels of speech and language therapy services. These have
included notional and actual caseload and workload analyses.
Population figures have long been viewed as an inadequate basis for
calculating staffing establishment. The demography of the local area,
together with information on epidemiology is of paramount
significance.

Staffing requirements, both in terms of numbers and skill mix, will vary according to:
● the number of potential individuals
● the models of service provision employed
● the range of service locations available
● the type and level of other health, education, social service and voluntary sector provision.
Staffing levels will:
● be negotiated locally
● be based on an estimate of demand
● reflect the need to provide safe, accessible, effective and equitable services
● reflect the full range of speech and language therapy roles and responsibilities.

Staffing calculation formula

The formula for estimating the number of sessions available for an individual's contact per year, per whole-time member of staff, is:
5 day working week = 10 sessions
10 sessions @ 52 weeks = 520 sessions
minus 40 days annual leave/public holidays = 440
minus notional 5 days for sick leave = 430
minus 5 days for CPD = 420
Given these assumptions, 420 sessions per year are available per whole-time staff member. This takes account of annual leave, other leave and CPD.
Assuming 50 per cent contact time and 50 per cent non-contact time and estimating that each member of staff will have three direct contacts per contact-session, each extra full-time member of staff will be able to provide 210 sessions and 630 one-to-one direct individual contacts per year.

Workforce planning and staffing levels

In 2005, the RCSLT commissioned a project to support workforce planning and the commissioning of speech and language therapy across the UK. The outcome will be a set of RCSLT national recommendations on workforce planning in 2006. Further information can be obtained from the RCSLT website at: www.rcslt.org

See also Chapter 9, Service Monitoring, Improvement, Evaluation and Development.

Service prioritisation

The RCSLT recognises the right of every individual to have equal access to the services provided by SLTs.

The RCSLT also recognises that most services operate within a framework of insufficient resources in relation to demand and supports the need to focus resources where they will be most effective.

This will, at times, mean that some individuals do not receive a therapeutic care service.

The RCSLT does not believe that the alternative strategy, ie allocating a scarce resource across a greater number of individuals, thereby diluting the service and resulting in clinical inefficiency, poor outcomes and low staff morale, is appropriate.

Local population needs-assessment

When services are operating in a context of insufficient resources to meet demand, it is recommended that an annual needs-assessment of the service-wide population is carried out and linked to an analysis of effectiveness, to ensure that resources continue to be allocated to the most appropriate areas of service.

A re-evaluation of the services currently provided in terms of skill mix is also recommended.

See Chapter 9 on Service audit, improvement, evaluation and development.

The RCSLT considers it inappropriate to make relative judgements regarding the effects of experiencing a potential, or actual communication disorder or swallowing disorder, with or between any particular group of individuals. The policy of prioritising one individual group above another is therefore not supported.

Within any group of individuals, there will exist a continuum of need and an optimum time to deliver therapy. The prioritisation of an identified group of individuals for assessment by, for example, age, disorder or location, does not allow for an efficient assessment and profiling of overall need to be made.

Waiting for triage/screening assessment

The RCSLT, in accordance with the Patient's Charter, recommends that triage/screening assessment of referred individuals be undertaken. Triage assessment allows individuals to have ready access to speech and language therapy services without a lengthy wait and to gain timely access to other facilities as appropriate. It also allows each service to profile the unmet need within any waiting list for therapeutic care. This information can then be used to put forward a case for service development.

Duty of care will only apply once a referred individual is accepted for in-depth assessment and therapeutic care.
See Chapter 1, Professional Framework.

Speech and language therapy services must be aware of other facilities within their locality that can support, enhance and assist with the management of those with communication and swallowing disorders. Knowledge of these local facilities should be borne in mind when drawing up local policies related to triage assessment.

Waiting for diagnostic assessment and therapeutic care
Service standard 36: The urgency or priority of referrals is determined in a systematic and equitable manner. Prioritisation systems are evidence-based as far as possible and clearly documented.

Prioritisation
The RCSLT recommends that a prioritisation policy should be formulated which defines a range of criteria, upon which the decision to fulfil a duty of care will be made on a case-by-case basis.
The range of criteria will normally include the following:
Risk
● immediate health risks if the individual is not seen
● in a mental health context, the risk of suicide and self harm
● risk of secondary sequelae if the individual is not seen.

Timing
● Optimal time for intervention to achieve maximum potential, eg There is evidence that people with long-term neurological conditions have improved health outcomes and better quality of life when they are able to access prompt specialist expertise to obtain a diagnosis and begin intervention (NSF Long-term Conditions, DH, 2005).
● Medical urgency, eg rapidly deteriorating condition.

- Time post trauma (if appropriate).
- Time post surgery, eg post cochlear implant.
- Time of transition, eg about to start secondary school.

Wellbeing
- Anxiety/distress/concern expressed by individual, carer or parent.

Impact
- Effect of difficulties upon an individual's communicative or swallowing function in the current environment and context.
- Effect of difficulties on involvement in everyday activities/quality of life.
- Effect of difficulties on other areas of the individual's functioning (e.g. learning or socialisation).

Predicted outcome in the current context
- Individual/carer's ability to engage with therapy.
- Availability of speech and language therapy resources to provide optimum intensity of intervention as evidenced in research.
- Availability of skilled support to help an individual maintain gains made.
- The individual's potential for change.
- Commitment and motivation of the individual or, in the case of children, of their carers.
- Response to any previous speech and language therapy intervention.

The key factor in relation to prioritising an individual for therapeutic care is the judgement about the level of clinical risk.
However, no one single factor should be taken as an indicator of priority rating, or alternatively as a reason not to prioritise an individual for therapy.

Summary
In these ways, service prioritisation policies will take account of the whole population requiring access to speech and language therapy and will not discriminate against any one group or individual.
The RCSLT recommends that services develop proactive policies and reviews of service in conjunction with their employing authority and commissioners.

5.4.4 Managing staff vacancies

Whenever a vacancy occurs a risk assessment should be undertaken to address the impact of the vacancy on the capacity of the speech and language therapy service. All appropriate stakeholders should be informed on the outcome of the risk assessment. They should also be involved in producing the risk assessment action plan to address the impact of the vacancy. The action plan should be communicated to all concerned.

5.5 Use of Information

5.5.1 Freedom of Information Act 2000, Freedom of Information (Scotland) Act 2000

Role of the SLT

Any SLT receiving a request for information under the aegis of Freedom of Information Act (2000) should immediately inform their manager. The request should be forwarded to the nominated information governance officer/data protection controller for the employing organisation, who will assess the request and ensure compliance with the Freedom of Information Acts.
For further details, see the information relating to Acts of Law. Full details regarding implementation of the Freedom of Information Act is available at: www.foi.gov.uk

5.5.2 Data Protection Act 1998

The Data Protection Act (1998) provides individuals and employees with right of access to personal data about themselves, that is held either in computerised or manual form. Most, if not all, NHS information concerning individuals, whether held electronically or on paper, will fall within the scope of this Act.
The Act imposes statutory restrictions on the use of personal information, including health information. All NHS employees are responsible for ensuring that they comply with the Data Protection Act.
Independent therapists should include data protection information in their practice literature and be registered data controllers.

The data protection principles

The following principles are embedded within the laws relating to data protection:

● Personal data shall be processed fairly and lawfully.

● Personal data shall be obtained only for one or more specified and lawful purposes, and shall not be further processed in any manner incompatible with that purpose or those purposes.

● Personal data shall be adequate, relevant and not excessive in relation to the purpose or purposes for which they are processed.

● Personal data shall be accurate and, where necessary, kept up-to-date.

● Personal data processed for any purpose shall not be kept for longer than is necessary for that purpose.

● Personal data shall be processed in accordance with the rights of individuals under this Act.

● Appropriate technical and organisational measures shall be taken against unauthorised or unlawful processing of personal data and against accidental loss or destruction of, or damage to, personal data.

● Personal data shall not be transferred to a country or territory outside the European Economic Area unless that country or territory ensures an adequate level of protection for the rights and freedoms of individuals in relation to the processing of personal data.

Responding to access requests

All requests for access to health records should be referred to the speech and language therapy manager, who will process the request according to the organisation's policy and procedures.

A request for access must be made in writing, and no reason need be given. Subject to any applicable exemption, the applicant must be given a copy of the information and, where the data is not readily intelligible, an explanation (eg of abbreviations or medical terminology). A charge may be made for the application and copying charges, but not for any explanation required.

There is a requirement to be satisfied that the applicant is either the individual, or, if the applicant is applying on behalf of an individual, that the person has been authorised to do so.

The service manager should determine whether any exemptions to access rights apply following receipt of a request for access and liaise closely with their organisation's information governance officer to ensure that requests for access to records are managed in line with the requirements of the Act.

Employee data

The rights of access and data protection principles outlined above apply equally to employees. All records in computerised or manual form are subject to the same requirements for confidentiality, accuracy, fairness, relevance and adequacy. All employees have an entitlement to:

● be informed whether personal data is processed (which includes being held or stored)
● a description of the data held, the purposes for which it is processed and to whom the data may be disclosed
● a copy of the information constituting the data
● information as to the source of the data.

Information sharing

A working group at the Department of Health is developing national guidance to assist NHS bodies and local authorities on the principles and practical issues involved in sharing patient records for service delivery and of using such aggregated data for planning, commissioning, managing and monitoring. In the interim there may be locally developed policies and protocols in place for sharing information. In the absence of these, speech and language therapy managers should seek advice form their information governance officer or from their organisation's legal advisor.

For further information on the Data Protection Act (1998), see the information relating to Acts of Law or see the Information Commissioner's website at: www.informationcommissioner.gov.uk

5.5.3 Record Keeping

What is a record?

A "record" is a document, which contains information (in any medium) that has been created or gathered as a result of any aspect of the work of NHS employees. This includes paper records, audio and videotapes, as well as photographs.

Clinical records, including electronic ones such as the electronic patient record (EPR), are routinely created and logged for each individual when they first visit a clinician. With the development of EPR there will be a need to identify every item which is patient-related with the relevant NHS number to provide the necessary links through all electronic records.

The best-practice principles of recording information are:
- legibility
- timeliness
- accuracy
- completeness
- provision of an audit trail

Record keeping

Good record keeping ensures that:
- work can be undertaken with maximum efficiency without having to waste time searching for information
- there is an audit-trail, that enables any record entry to be traced to a named individual of a given date/time with the secure knowledge that all alterations can be similarly traced
- those accessing the record can see what has been done, or not done and why
- any decisions can be justified or reconsidered at a later date.

This is vitally important in cases such as:
- providing patient care
- clinical liability
- parliamentary accountability
- purchasing and contract or service agreement management
- financial accountability
- disputes or legal action.

Service standard 37: Written records are kept of each individual's care.

Service standard 38: The service has clear standards of record keeping in line with Data Protection Act (1998) principles and RCSLT guidance that are reviewed and audited on a regular (at least annual) basis.

Each clinical record should contain:
- the name and identifying number of the individual on both sides of each sheet

● important, relevant and complete information, including: referral source and reason; correspondence; case history information; clear aims; an entry for each contact (direct and indirect); reports, and evaluations.

Entries within the records should be:
● written in black ink
● legible
● accurate
● comprehensive
● contemporaneous
● dated
● signed

In addition, there should be no deliberately left blank pages or gaps. If they do exist, they should be scored through, dated and signed. There should be a method of identification for signatures, and there should be a key available for any abbreviations used in the case notes.

If necessary, information should be shared rather than copied in order to reduce risks to confidentiality.

The role of the practitioner:
When creating a patient record, or making entries into an existing patient record, it is the responsibility of the SLT or support practitioner to:
● conform to RCSLT and local guidance
● routinely discuss the information they are recording with the person to whom the record relates, or in the case of children, with their parent/s, at the time of making the entry, wherever possible.
If the SLT makes an entry in the record which he/she has not shared with the individual to whom it relates, the reason should be clearly recorded.

Keeping records of an individual's care within the context of multidisciplinary or multi-agency working

There is no single multi-agency model for the way in which an individual's health record should be documented.

A review of existing standards related to record keeping was undertaken by the NHS Health Records and Communication

Practice Standards (HR&CPS) Group. This survey involved scoping the guidance from three regulatory bodies (Nursing and Midwifery Council, the General Medical Council and the HPC), together with guidance from a range of professional bodies.

The standards in common fall into four categories:
- confidentiality and disclosure
- communication of information
- process principles
- personal and professional knowledge and skills.

For more information see the NHS Health Record and Communication Practice Standards for Team-based Care (2004), available at: www.connectingforhealth.nhs.uk/crdb/docs/scrrdocument.doc

These standards do not address **the content** of a shared record of care. This is currently the focus of the various groups who are developing and implementing the electronic patient record strategies. There is no single model for which details of care should be contained within a shared record and within a uni-professional record.

The following notions may be helpful in guiding team decision-making about the content and level of detail to be included in shared records within different working contexts:
- certain information is core to the individual and core to the work of all the team
- shared documented information should have relevance to team decision-making
- certain levels of detail are meaningful only to a given profession and therefore belong within a uni-professional record of care.

Diaries

Diaries are used to record the daily activity of health professionals in the course of their duties.

Diaries issued by the employing organisation are the property of that organisation and they and their contents should be stored securely to ensure the confidentiality of the information in them. Information recorded about individuals in a diary forms part of the record of that individual. A diary also meets the definition of a "record" in its own right. All diaries with individual related information should be kept for eight years.

Diaries may be audited by the employing organisation and should reflect the work undertaken in the course of the working day. In addition, information relating to the practitioner must also be recorded, including:
- annual leave
- sick leave
- overtime
- meetings attended/cancelled
- conferences/courses attended
- study leave
- supervision of students/assistants
- administration
- research activities
- court appearances
- rotas.

This list is not exhaustive.

The principles for good record keeping that apply to individual records also apply to diaries.

Electronic patient records (EPR)

All four UK countries have a strategy for establishing EPRs within the NHS over the next few years.

Healthcare records, appointment details, prescription information, and up-to-date research into illnesses and intervention will be readily available to all individuals and health professionals. EPR systems will support individual choice and allow first hospital outpatient appointments to be made at a time, date and place to suit the individual. Although each country will make its own decision about the adoption of standards and datasets in relation to EPRs, core patient data such as name, address, NHS number, date of birth, plus basic details on hospital visits and known reactions to drugs, is likely to be held on a national database, with a signpost to the full local records.

The guiding principle for the development of quality health information and information systems is that individual patient information should be as accurate, up-to-date, easy to find and as free from duplication and fragmentation as possible.

For further details see the following websites:

www.connectingforhealth.nhs.uk

www.ehealth.scot.nhs.uk

5.5.4 Records management

Records management is most effective when it is regarded as a professional activity requiring specific expertise.

Records are a valuable resource because of the information they contain. The information is only useable if it is correctly and legibly recorded in the first place, is regularly updated and is easily accessible when needed.

Information is essential to the delivery of high quality evidence-based healthcare on a day-to-day basis and an effective records management system ensures that such information is properly managed and is available:

- to support individual care and continuity of care
- to support day-to-day business, that underpins delivery of care
- to support evidence-based clinical practice
- to support sound administrative and managerial decision-making, as part of the knowledge base for NHS services
- to meet legal requirements, including requests from individuals for access to their records
- to assist medical and other audits
- to support improvements in clinical effectiveness, through research
- to support archival functions by taking account of the historical importance of material and the needs of future research, whenever and wherever there is a justified need for information and in whatever media it is required.

Legal obligation and good practice

All NHS records are public records under the terms of the Public Records Act, 1958. Chief executives and senior managers of all NHS bodies are personally accountable for records management within their organisation and have a duty to make arrangements for the safe keeping of those records under the overall supervision of the keeper of public records. The Department of Health is the liaison point between them and the Public Record Office (PRO) whose responsibility includes permanent preservation.

Other legal obligations exist in respect of particular classes of records especially those containing personal information.

Confidentiality and data protection

All NHS bodies and those carrying out functions on behalf of the NHS have a common law duty of confidentiality. Everyone working for, or with, the NHS who records, handles, stores or otherwise comes across individual information, has a personal common law duty of confidentiality to individuals and to his or her employer. The duty of confidentiality continues even after death of the individual or after an employee or contractor has left the NHS. In general, any personal information given or received in confidence for one purpose may not be used for a different purpose or passed to anyone else without the consent of the provider of the information.

This duty of confidentiality is long established in common law. However, it is not an absolute duty and can be subject to an overriding public interest.

Medical, historical and epidemiological research is based on individual information, usually the information is anonymised so those individuals cannot be identified. In such cases, the use of information does not conflict with the duty of confidentiality.

Where identifiable information is used, in the absence of consent (express or implied), it is necessary to consider whether any public interest in the research outweighs the duty of confidentiality, having regard to all the circumstances.

Ethical approval must be gained for any research using individual records.

The Caldicott Committee recommends that NHS organisations should be held accountable through clinical governance procedures for continuously improving confidentiality and security procedures governing access to, and storage of, clinical information.

Health information should be treated as confidential in accordance with relevant legislation and RCSLT guidance.

Service standard 39: The service has a clear and up-to-date policy on the confidentiality, use, security and disclosure of health information.

The system for recording and storing individual information will provide effective protection against loss, damage and misuse. Each service should also:

● have guidance for staff
● ensure that staff are aware of their duty of confidentiality and its implications
● provide opportunities for individuals to be seen in private
● ensure that individuals are made aware of and consent to uses of personal information

- have inter-agency protocols for the sharing of information
- have IT records that are password protected
- be registered for data protection
- ensure that clinical records are stored in lockable cabinets.

Individual access to personal records
Standard 40: The service has a clear and up-to-date local policy detailing the process through which individuals (or their advocates) have access to their records in line with the Data Protection Act (1998).
Individuals have a right to access their own records. Practitioners must respect individual's rights to access their own information. However, exceptions may apply where the practitioner judges that to restrict or withhold information would cause serious harm to the individual or others.

Principles of efficient storage
Clinical records should be retained and disposed of in accordance with RCSLT guidance.
Records must always be kept securely and when a room containing records is left unattended, it should be locked whenever possible. A sensible balance should be achieved between the needs for security and accessibility.
The principles of good record management practice apply equally to records created manually and electronically.

Disposing of unwanted records
Service standard 41: The service has a clear and up-to-date policy relating to the length of retention and the ultimate disposal of clinical records, which complies with legislation and RCSLT guidance.
Service standard 42: The service has a clear and up-to-date policy relating to storage and disposal of audio and visual recordings.
Records should be suitably disposed of as soon as possible, subject to national and local retention periods.
The length of the retention period depends upon the type of record and its importance to the business of the NHS organisation. The destruction of records is an irreversible act, whilst the cost of keeping them can be high and ongoing.

Most NHS records, even administrative ones, contain sensitive or confidential information. It is therefore vital that confidentiality is safeguarded at every stage and that the method used to destroy such records is fully effective and secures their complete illegibility. The retention and disposal of records should be in accordance with the requirements of Health Service Circular (HSC) *For the Record* (1999). This recommends minimum periods for the retention of records, both clinical and non-clinical.

Key retention periods are as follows:
● Records relating to children and young people should be kept until the individual is 25 years-old or 26, if the young person was 17 years-old at conclusion of intervention; or eight years after an individual's death, if the death occurred before they were 18 years-old.

● Records relating to mentally disordered persons (within the meaning of the Mental Health Act [1983]) should be kept for 20 years after no further intervention is considered necessary; or eight years after the individual's death, if individual died while still receiving intervention.

● Records relating to other patient groups not covered above should generally be kept for eight years after conclusion of intervention.

● All diaries with patient-related information should be kept for eight years.

Independent practitioners are not subject to the same constraints. The Association of Speech and Language Therapists in Independent Practice (ASLTIP) advises members to seek legal opinion on how long to keep records. The practice decisions should be shared with individuals within the practice literature.

Where possible a review of records in storage should occur on an annual basis. A planned review of records will ensure that records to be retained are both valid and current, available storage facilities are effectively maintained and any unwanted records culled on a planned basis.

Where paper-based documents are to be converted to and stored in electronic form and their originals destroyed, the destruction must be for proper motives, such as clearing storage space.

In the event of a challenge in litigation, this action will protect the evidential value of electronic records and avoid misunderstandings of the reasons for the conversion, including any potential suggestion that paper-based records may have been destroyed deliberately to obscure evidence.

Paper records should be disposed of in a manner that preserves confidentiality by shredding, pulping or incineration.

5.6 Management of Risk

5.6.1 Risk management

What is risk?
Risk is defined as the chance of something happening that will have an impact on objectives. It is measured in terms of consequences and likelihood.

risk = consequences x likelihood

Risk management
Risk Management is an organised and proactive approach of risk identification, analysis, controls and evaluation. It aims to reduce the risks to all persons in an organisation, and ensure limited potential harm to an organisation's business opportunities, physical environment, financial assets or reputation. In doing so it will also provide high quality, safe services to individuals and staff and an effective service by eliminating or reducing unnecessary costs.

The no blame culture
"The single greatest impediment to error prevention is that we punish people for making mistakes" (Leape, 2004).
We need an open and fair, no blame culture in order to report, analyse, and learn from incidents and near misses.

Statutory and mandatory duties of NHS trusts
NHS trusts have a statutory responsibility to evaluate the risks to the safety and health of workers they employ and anyone else who may be affected by trustwork activities, such as individuals, visitors and volunteers. NHS trusts must identify measures for compliance and record the findings of these assessments (Management of Health and Safety at Work Regulations, 1992).

All NHS trusts became individually liable for their actions with the removal of Crown Immunity in 1991. This relates to directly employed provider services.

Health Service Guidance (97) 17 requires all NHS trusts to include a comprehensive controls assurance statement in their annual report. This statement is to assure the public that NHS trusts are being properly managed and that systems are in place to minimise all risks.

All NHS trusts will have developed a local assurance framework, which will include a risk management process.

The risk management process

The management of risk is a continuous process, with responsibilities for all employees/staff. The components of the process are recognising, assessing/measuring, reviewing and managing the identified risk and the learning. In NHS trusts this is undertaken at all levels, trust wide, directorate, departments, teams and sites, etc. All risks identified and assessed are reported through defined structures, such as health and safety committees, and clinical governance committees.

Risk management assessment

NHS trusts have developed generic risk assessment tools used for assessing risks within trusts and which can be applied to clinical or organisational risks.

The principles of risk assessment are to:
- identify the risk
- identify those at risk
- evaluate the risk
- identify a risk remedial action plan.

The risk assessment process can be applied to:
- incident reporting
- health and safety
- personal safety
- infection control
- complaints
- managing vacancies
- business planning
- service developments

● decision-making with individuals, see the section 1.9 Decision-making in Chapter 1, Professional Framework.

The responsibility of the speech and language therapy manager

The speech and language therapy service manager is responsible for ensuring that appropriate and effective risk management is in place within their designated areas and scope of responsibility. He/she needs to ensure that all staff are made aware of the risks within their work environment and of their personal responsibilities and that they receive appropriate information, instruction and training to enable them to work safely. These responsibilities extend to anyone affected by the organisation's operations, including sub-contractors, members of the public and visitors, etc.

Service standard 43: The service has a clear and up-to-date risk-management policy and guidelines.

When preparing specific departmental policies and guidelines the speech and language therapy manager needs to ensure all necessary risk assessments are carried out within their area, and they need to liaise with appropriate advisers as necessary, eg health and safety officer, infection control nurse, Caldicott guardian, medical devices liaison officer, estates personnel, human resources personnel, etc. The speech and language therapy service manager is also responsible for implementing and monitoring any identified and appropriate risk management control measures with their designated areas and scope of responsibility. In situations where significant risks have been identified and where local control measures are considered to be potentially inadequate, managers are responsible for bringing these risks to the attention of the trust committee responsible for risk management.

Independent practitioners should undertake risk assessment and management in relation to themselves and their individuals, seeking advice from colleagues as appropriate.

The responsibility of individual staff

All staff have responsibility in risk management and should report incidents/accidents and near misses, in line with policies within their organisations.

Staff should ensure safe clinical practice in diagnosis and intervention and be aware of duty of care under health and safety legislation, as well as duty of care as defined by the RCSLT. Staff should be familiar with their organisation's risk management strategy and organisational or departmental clinical and health and safety policies and procedures and comply with these.

Staff should neither intentionally nor recklessly interfere with, or misuse, any equipment provided for the protection of safety and health and undertake training on specific equipment prior to use.

Staff should be aware of emergency procedures/guidelines, eg resuscitation, evacuation and fire policies and procedures for their area of work/location.

Incident reporting

The term "incident" refers to any clinical or non-clinical accidents, unexpected events or near misses.

The objective in reporting incidents is to:

● improve and promote a healthy workplace
● improve and promote high quality clinical services
● avoid future similar occurrences.

The reporting of near misses provides valuable information to share within a proactive risk management system.

Lines of responsibility and duties are defined within organisations' policies and procedures on reporting and management of incidents. Speech and language therapy managers responsibilities include:

● Rectifying a hazardous situation as appropriate to their level of skill and responsibility.

● When appropriate, removing equipment from their service.

● Ensuring that the subject of the incident receives appropriate medical attention, reassurance, advice/or information.

● Determining whether investigation is required.

● If appropriate or/required, undertaking investigations.

● Taking all practical steps to ensure to address the conditions responsible for the incident to prevent a recurrence.

● Support and encourage staff in reflective practice and learning.

Investigation

Speech and language therapy managers need to use a structured process for identifying the basic factors, reasons and causes for conditions that result in mishaps. Once identified the conditions can be corrected and future mishaps prevented.

Objectivity and uniformity are increased by following a structured root cause process through which the analyst identifies root causes matched to a specific set of questions. This method of investigation is known as root cause analysis. Further information on this technique can be found on the National Patient Safety Agency (NPSA) and the Department for Health's websites.

5.6.2 Complaints

Complaints and compliments are a way of obtaining feedback from service users and are a source of useful information about the quality of service provided. Complaints offer a positive way to improve services and avoid similar situations.

Service standard 44: The service has a clear and up-to-date local policy and procedures for handling complaints.

The policy will include details of:
● how to respond to verbal and written complaints
● timescale for response
● requirements for record keeping
● how records of complaints are kept and monitored
● evidence of review and action planning related to complaints
● how individuals are informed of the policy and how to complain
● how front-line staff are trained in dealing with complaints.

Independent practitioners should inform individuals within their practice literature of the process for handling complaints, including the role and contact details for ASLTIP.

Principles underpinning effective complaints management

Complaints should be resolved as quickly as possible, particularly through an informal response by front-line staff, or subsequent investigation and conciliation through staff who are empowered to deal with complaints as they arise, in an open and non-defensive way.

Many people in receipt of health services find it difficult to express their concerns, criticisms and complaints and worry that this may affect the intervention and care of themselves or those who they care for. It is therefore essential that procedures ensure people are enabled to communicate their complaints, by being assured they are being listened to with respect and concern, and that the response is swift, impartial and fair.

The role of the speech and language therapy manager in complaints management

In the interest of maintaining a high quality service, the speech and language therapy manager has a duty to investigate, or facilitate the investigation of any complaint or concerns expressed by individuals, families or other users of their service.

The role of the speech and language therapy manager is to hold overall responsibility for operation of complaints procedures within their specific service areas. This involves ensuring that all staff are fully conversant with, and follow the complaints procedure, that satisfactory arrangements are in place for handling complaints, particularly by front-line staff, and supervising the investigation of complaints within their service.

The role of the Health Service Ombudsman in complaints management

In the NHS, with effect from 1 April 1996, the Health Service Ombudsman has the role to investigate complaints, which involve actions taken wholly or partly as a result of the exercise of clinical judgement, as well as complaints about services provided or not provided, about maladministration, and the way complaints have been handled.

The role of ASLTIP in relation to complaints about independent practitioners

Complaints about services received at the hands of an independent practitioner may be made to the Association of Speech and Language Therapists in Independent Practice (ASLTIP).

Training in relation to complaints management

Training is the key to ensuring that complaints procedures are effective and operates smoothly. Speech and language therapy staff at all levels should be made aware of complaints procedures and the roles they play in it.

5.6.3 Clinical Negligence Scheme for Trusts (CNST)

The Clinical Negligence Scheme for Trusts (CNST) was established in 1994 by the NHS Executive to provide a means for trusts to fund the cost of clinical negligence litigation.

The NHS Litigation Authority (NHSLA) administers the scheme, which provides indemnity to NHS trusts and primary care trusts in respect of clinical negligence claims arising out of adverse incidents occurring after 1 April 1995. Trusts pay a contribution to the scheme based on a range of criteria.

It is a requirement of membership of the scheme that all trusts are assessed against the CNST risk management standards within two years of their last assessment and within 12 months for Level zero trusts, new or recently merged trusts.

There are seven standards identified by CNST, against which a trust's performance is measured. Further information is available on the NHSLA website at: www.nhsla.com

5.6.4 Health and safety at work

The Health and Safety at Work Act (1974) requires employers and employees to fulfil a number of requirements, including being aware of their responsibilities for health and safety at work.

Each employing agency will have a health and safety policy statement outlining the levels of responsibility within its own management structures.

Service standard 45: The service has a clear and up-to-date policy related to health and safety of staff and individuals.

There should be a system in place to identify, analyse, prioritise and manage risks to health and safety.

Areas covered by policy should include:

- fire safety and prevention
- first aid facilities
- incident reporting and recording
- access for all staff to confidential occupational health services
- control of infection
- control of substances hazardous to health (COSHH)
- arrangements for maintenance of equipment
- manual handling
- electrical and technical equipment
- violence towards staff
- slips, trips and falls
- stress at work
- lone working

- severe weather policy
- community visits.

There should be a named safety representative and a regular auditing of risk management procedures to ensure effective risk management.

Health and safety issues are a line management responsibility alongside, and of equal importance to, responsibilities for the provision of services and the management of resources.

Key health and safety responsibilities of the speech and language therapy manager may include:

- Encouraging a culture of safety awareness amongst speech and language therapy staff, ensuring they are aware of and adhere to health and safety policies.
- Ensuring there is speech and language therapy representation on relevant health and safety committees.
- Securing appropriate health and safety training for speech and language therapy staff, and maintaining a record of training undertaken.
- Developing risk management policies to cover all areas of activity for the service, and monitoring and reviewing the effectiveness of these policies through an annual programme of risk assessment.
- Reviewing accidents/incidents occurring within the service and ensuring appropriate actions are taken to minimise the risk of recurrence.
- Consideration of all reports and advice from enforcing authorities (eg the Health and Safety Executive, the Medical Devices Agency), and taking appropriate action.
- Working with the health and safety advisor and where appropriate staff side representative, (eg to arrange training).

For more information see the RCSLT *Information Pack for New SLT Managers,* 2005.

SLTs working in NHS trusts, local authorities and the voluntary sector will need to make reference to these organisations' health and safety policy, local policies, eg lone worker policy, fire policy, policies on managing violence, aggression or abusive behaviour, etc.

Practitioners should be aware of and act in accordance with RCSLT guidance and local health and safety policy.

Training

Speech and language therapy managers should ensure that an appropriate health and safety training strategy is in place for staff. This will ensure that competencies are maintained for staff to undertake risk assessment and manage potential risks in all areas of their work. Some of this training will be covered through organisations statutory training programmes, eg manual handling, cardio pulmonary resuscitation, etc.

5.6.5 Personal safety

Zero tolerance to violence

Staff have the right to work in an environment where they feel safe and secure and where the risk of violence in whatever form is minimised. The NHS Security Management Service (SMS) has a remit to protect NHS staff and patients from physical and non-physical assault and has developed a strategy which builds on the *Zero Tolerance Campaign, 1999* and supports services in meeting the standards set out in the *Improving Working Lives* (IWL) programme. Detailed guidance and good practice examples related to risk assessment and prevention strategies can be found in *Safer Working in the Community,* 1998, available at: www.dh.gov.uk/publications and www.cfsms.nhs.uk and in *A Safer Place to Work – protecting NHS staff from violence and aggression*, 2003, available at www.nao.org.uk/publications

Legal responsibilities

Health service employers and managers are committed to caring for the health and safety of all their staff. As with other employers, they have duties with respect to the management of work-related violent incidents, framed both by national and European health and safety legislation and by their common law duty of care. A summary of the requirements on employers, under health and safety legislation, is contained in *Safer Working in the Community* (1998).

Managing the risk

Healthcare staff sometimes face a dilemma with regard to the risk from violence. They have a duty of care to the individuals on their caseload, often within a continuing relationship, and that care can only be withdrawn in exceptional circumstances. Additionally, some may feel that coping with a certain amount of aggression is "part of the job".

However, professional codes of conduct do not require healthcare professionals to put themselves or their colleagues at risk for the sake of individuals.

Part of the purpose of risk management by employers is to develop safeguards, or alternative ways of delivering care, such that healthcare staff do not feel that they have to jeopardise their own safety in order to provide care for individuals.

Organisations' responsibilities

Trusts and similar organisations exist as part of a community and it is important that the services they provide are sympathetic to the needs of that community. According to best practice, it is crucial that consideration is given to the environment and social groupings within which an organisation operates. This is critical to the practicality, effectiveness and success of risk management systems.

Guidelines for personal safety

These guidelines are intended to remind SLTs that care must be taken in respect of personal safety at work. Some aspects of the SLT's work can make the practitioner more vulnerable than others, due to the nature or location of the work.

Managers are responsible for producing guidelines in accordance with local policies on personal safety for staff at work on-site as well as off-site. Managers should ensure that all staff are aware of such policies and also appreciate their vulnerability, particularly in relation to community visits and out-of-hours work.

Safety in designated work settings

When interviewing an individual and/or carer alone, staff should make known their whereabouts to their manager or nominated person.

If a staff member is unavoidably working alone in a designated work location, it is her/his responsibility to ensure personal safety and security. This may include locking the entrance door and having a "Please ring the bell" or "Please knock" sign or by working in a room with a telephone.

Staff are urged to record planned contacts in an open diary in a separate office. Records in the diary should state the time and duration of the appointment, the names of the individuals to be seen and the specific room to be used if not the practitioner's own personal office. All staff should be alert to security issues and use alarm/security systems as appropriate.

Safety in community settings

Planning contacts

Staff must not knowingly place themselves in a hazardous situation. Staff should plan visits according to area or risk. When this is not possible and visits need to be made in "at risk" areas, staff are urged to use their discretion and take the following precautions:

● go with a colleague, if possible

● walk in well-lit populated areas, avoiding short cuts through subways, parks or waste ground

● carry a mobile telephone (if available) or a personal alarm and maintain these in working order

● when driving, keep all car doors locked. Do not leave handbags on the passenger seat. Lock personal items, briefcases and folders, etc in the boot and/or place out of sight. Avoid parking in dark secluded areas

● do not wear excessive jewellery or carry unnecessary amounts of money or valuables such as credit cards or cheque books

● staff who are not car owners are advised to use a transport service when making home visits, and to ensure that the return journey is arranged prior to the visit. The driver should be instructed to knock at the front door rather than wait on the road outside

● do not accept lifts from strangers.

Known individuals

If there is evidence prior to contact that the individual or carer is extremely disturbed and/or the available information indicates that there may be concerns about the person's hostility or aggression, a risk assessment should be undertaken and measures put in place to minimise risk to staff.

This should include seeing the individual with another member of staff present.

In some situations the risks identified may indicate that the individual should be seen in a setting other than their home.

It is recommended that a record of the completed contact is submitted.

During visits

Staff have the right to decide not to enter a home if the situation is not as anticipated and they feel that their personal safety may be at risk. They may need to explain to the individual how the situation needs to be different and that they will make alternative arrangements to see the individual. They should then inform their line manager of their action.

In a situation where actual threatening behaviour or sexual harassment is occurring, the member of staff should always err on the side of caution in her/his response and leave immediately.

Staff should remain vigilant to potential threat, eg signs of agitation and use of abusive language, and remain calm and firm.

See the section below on the management of potentially violent behaviour.

Staff should plan an exit strategy and choose to sit in the chair nearest the door from the start of the visit.

Domestic pets may also be a hazard. Consider requesting that they are removed from the room when visiting.

Should staff be delayed for any reason, they should notify their base or line manager/colleague. If further time is required with the individual than was originally planned staff should either:

● ring their base, colleague or visit sheet holder and confirm this

● terminate the interview at the pre-arranged time, and arrange a further appointment with the individual.

If a serious incident occurs staff should call the police/ambulance. Staff are advised to inform the manager or a nominated person at the end of the visit and to report any incidents in accordance with their employer's accident/incident reporting procedure.

Guidelines for the management of violent or potentially violent behaviour

During the course of a working day, staff may be faced with a potentially violent situation. Staff whose work regularly requires them to come into contact with potentially violent individuals should undergo appropriate training.

Three different types of tactic are helpful:

Avoidance

If someone appears to be becoming angry and aggressive, use any means to avoid confrontation. For example, if an individual has become very angry because he/she does not want to do something and may become violent, staff should back down or leave the room, if this seems the most appropriate course of action. This allows the member of staff time to consult with others and try to understand why the individual has reacted in a violent or aggressive manner.

Distraction

Distraction can also be helpful, but it is important not to be patronising when adopting this strategy. For example, if an individual is reacting very aggressively to being told he/she cannot have something, it may be useful to offer to make him/her a cup of tea or coffee before attempting to discuss the problem further.

Defusing

Defusing strategies can help in averting a confrontation. For example, disclosing personal experiences of anger can be helpful if an individual is becoming angry or aggressive.

Whatever approach is appropriate:

● It is important to behave calmly, to use a firm, non-threatening and unhesitating manner, communicating self-control and confidence.

● Be conscious of your own body language and tone of voice. How you say something can be more important than what you say.

● Listening, talking and explaining must be the first approach and, if used properly, can often avert an incident.

● Help the individual to be aware that you are trying to solve the immediate problem and be truthful about this.

● Approach the individual slowly, speaking to them calmly. Do not surprise them, for example, by approaching from behind. Be sensitive to the individual's personal space and do not encroach on it. Beware of "cornering" the individual and blocking their exit as you approach.

Useful websites:

Department of Health www.dh.gov.uk

Home Office www.homeoffice.gov.uk

Criminal Justice System www.cjsonline.gov.uk

Crown Prosecution Service www.cps.gov.uk

The Suzy Lamplugh Trust www.suzylamplugh.org

5.6.6 Infection control

Healthcare associated infection has recently become the focus of more intensified control measures in the NHS.

Infection is a common but sometimes avoidable complication of any healthcare intervention. It has major implications, not only in terms of cost to an organisation, but also in cost to an individual in lost wages, pain, discomfort, side effects of intervention, etc. The ultimate price that the individual might pay is in loss of life.

Bacteria are everywhere and millions live on and in our bodies. These bacteria usually live in harmony with us and perform many useful functions, such as protection from infection and assisting in digestion. These are known as normal flora.

During times when our natural defences are lowered through illness, age or perhaps surgery or invasive devices, these organisms may access, and cause infections in areas of the body where they would not usually be found. This is **endogenous** infection.

Not all infections are caused by the individual's own resident bacteria (normal flora). Transient bacteria are organisms that are easily picked up from other people or the environment. They are very loosely attached to the skin and can easily be spread from individual to individual.

Bacteria and viruses cannot transport themselves and the most common way has been found to be on the hands of the care worker, visitor or family, or on equipment that has been inadequately decontaminated. This is **exogenous** infection.

These organisms, although easily picked up on the hands, can just as easily be washed off.

Bacteria need certain life support systems to survive and multiply, ie food, warmth and moisture. Removal of one of these life support systems will result in either the inability of the organism to multiply, (giving the body a chance to overcome the invasion), or the death of the organism. Good handwashing and environmental cleaning removes all or some of the life support mechanisms and therefore reduces the risk of cross infection substantially.

SLTs need to be aware of standard infection control precautions to protect themselves and minimise the risk of cross infection.

SLTs should perform a risk assessment on the task that they are about to undertake, ie does this procedure pose a risk to their individual or to themselves. Following this, the member of staff can put into place the appropriate standard infection control precautions which, if carried out correctly, will also serve to protect the next individual to be treated.

Standard infection control precautions include:
- handwashing
- the use of personal protective clothing
- safe handling and disposal of waste
- safe handling and disposal of sharps and management of sharps/exposure injuries
- dealing with blood and blood stained body fluid spills
- safe handling of linen
- decontamination of equipment, including cleaning of toys and therapy material
- personal health and hygiene.

Notifiable diseases
SLTs need to be informed of those diseases that require notification under the Public Health (Control of Disease) Act (1984).
A 'notifiable disease' is legally defined as one of the five diseases referred to in Section 10 of the Act. In addition, food poisoning is made notifiable in Section 11 of the Act.
There are a further 24 diseases which have to be notified by the doctor who has diagnosed them. The term 'notifiable disease' is commonly used for all 30 diseases.
Should an SLT come in contact with an individual suffering or suspected to be suffering from a notifiable disease, the SLT must ensure that this is appropriately reported and seek the guidance of a general practitioner or occupational health department.
Diseases that have acquired a high profile, such as Hepatitis B and HIV and AIDS, also require vigilance both to protect the individual and the SLT.
It is the responsibility of managers to ensure that local policies and procedures regarding control of infection are adhered to and that staff are aware of these policies.

Guidance on infection control in specific diseases
Employing organisations will have guidelines and policies in place to enable SLTs to practice safely, and minimise risk to themselves and

individuals. These guidelines and policies are continually updated, in line with new developments in infection control, and extended to include threat from newly emerging diseases/infections. Typically, guidelines and policies are provided for:

- HIV
- CJD
- MRSA
- Prion disease
- AIDS
- Other common infectious diseases, eg rubella, chicken pox, mumps

SLTs should undertake relevant training in infection control on a regular basis, and ensure that they update their knowledge in line with policies and procedures.

Further information can be obtained from the Department of Health's website, go to the health and social care topics section at: www.dh.gov.uk/PolicyAndGuidance

5.7 Public and Patient Involvement (PPI)

There is a strong and widely held view that involving individuals in decisions about healthcare at both personal and strategic levels is fundamentally important to the improvement of health and social care services, as well as being a basic right (NHS, 2002).

The *NHS Plan* (2000) states that "patients are the most important people in the NHS. The aim of the plan is to redesign services around the needs of patients, and to involve patients and carers at every level of healthcare. This will enhance accountability to patients and the public, and secure national improvements in patients' experience."

Within the NHS a number of new bodies have been established and initiatives developed to support patient and public involvement at a national and local level. These include:

- the National Commission for Patient and Public Involvement in Health (CPPIH)
- the Local Independent and Advocacy Services (ICAS)
- Patients' forums
- the Patient advice and liaison services within NHS Trusts (PALS)
- the Expert Patient Programme
- INVOLVE (engagement in research).

Service standard 46: The service involves service users in the evaluation and development of services.

The aim of involvement of public, patients and carers in the planning and provision of services is to achieve the following benefits:

● better quality services that are more responsive to the needs of individuals, leading to better outcomes of care and improvements in health and wellbeing

● policy and planning decisions that are more focused on the individual

● improved communication between organisations and the communities they serve

● greater ownership of local health services, and a stronger understanding of why and how they need to change and develop.

The NHS Modernisation Agency publication *Improvement Leaders' Guide: Involving Patients and Carers* 2002, provides a useful overview of PPI, and also describes some approaches that have been used to involve individuals in improving care. More information is available at: www.modern.nhs.uk/improvementguides/ reading

The approaches described include:

● critical incident techniques

● focus groups

● individual shadowing

● individual diaries

● discovery interviews

● improving practice questionnaire and critical friends groups.

PPI strategy

NHS trusts have commonly developed their own local strategies, setting out objectives and plans for engagement of parents, users, carers, staff, the local authority and the voluntary sector.

National Institute for Health and Clinical Excellence – individual carer involvement

The National Institute for Health and Clinical Excellence (NICE) has established the NICE Individual Involvement Unit which provides information support and training to individuals and carers (both organisations and individuals) that have an interest in NICE guidance.

The NICE offers opportunities for individual and carer involvement at a number of levels, including national individual/carer organisation, including two lay members on all NICE committees and providing guidance in a format for individuals and public. More information is available at: www.nice.org.uk

SLTs' role in PPI:

● To determine the concerns, interests and priorities of people in relation to their communication and/or eating and drinking and how these have been addressed.

● To enable individuals and families to address issues that affect their communication and eating and drinking.

● To involve individuals in decision-making processes surrounding their own care.

● To promote self-management, especially in relation to long-term conditions. This includes:

● Enabling individuals and families to identify the factors that affect their communication and eating and drinking.

● Enabling individuals and families to identify options for optimising their communication and eating and drinking.

● Enabling individuals and families to put their informed choices into action.

● Reviewing with individuals and families the effectiveness of addressing issues that affect their communication and eating and drinking.

5.8 Press and the Media

Service standard 47: The service has a clear and up-to-date policy for dealing with media enquiries.

SLTs employed by the NHS should be aware that, unless they are authorised to do so, speaking to the press or the media may contravene their contract of employment and could result in disciplinary action by the employing authority.

The RCSLT plays a major role in dealing with the media on behalf of the speech and language therapy profession.

One of the RCSLT's strategic communication aims is to increase awareness of the educational, medical, emotional and social effects of communication and swallowing difficulties, and the role of speech and language therapy with the public, government, other professions and the media.

For more information see the *RCSLT Strategic Plan* available at:
www.rcslt.org/about/strategicplan

The RCSLT has developed a *Communications Strategy* that identifies target audiences and the key messages for each of these audiences. From this, the RCSLT communications team has developed an annual action plan for engaging the media. This is reviewed twice a year and adapted according to requirements.

The RCSLT deals with the media on a regular basis either reactively, providing comment on issues raised or by facilitating contact between specialist SLTs and journalists or proactively, by sending out media releases detailing the RCSLT viewpoint.

The RCSLT communications team is available to help any SLTs who have to deal with the media. This includes help with media responses, including writing press releases, or doing radio or TV interviews.

5.9 Partnership Working

5.9.1 The interface between speech and language therapy agencies

The RCSLT produced the document *Working in Harmony*, following a policy review forum in 2000. This was updated in November 2005 and is available at: www.rcslt.org/resources/professional_standards/documents

The document sets out general principles and guidance to facilitate cooperation between SLTs wherever they are employed to ensure a consistently high standard of informed care for all individuals. It is recognised that SLTs may be employed within the NHS, by LEAs, charities and the voluntary sector, or as independent practitioners. The general principles and guidance set out in *Working in Harmony* are as follows:

Choice for individuals

● Individuals are entitled to seek speech and language therapy from an NHS provider and also to seek it from an independent provider.. However, they are not entitled to seek a service from more than one NHS provider.

If an individual chooses to receive therapy both from the NHS and from an independent service, it is in the individual's best interest for the SLTs to collaborate and, with client or parental permission, make

assessment results available to each other. The aim is for th
therapists to agree on a complementary approach.

● It is recommended good practice to advise any potential client o
the availability of speech and language therapy intervention within
the NHS to avoid situations where a member of the public may be
unaware of the existence of statutory provision.

Beyond this, independent practitioners should avoid involvement in
discussions relating to the levels and merits of local provision.

Similarly NHS speech and language therapists should not
recommend individual independent SLTs, but may suggest reference
sources such as business and telephone directories, or to contact
the ASLTIP.

If an SLT is seeing an individual as part of their role within the NHS,
they should not see the individual privately at the same time.

Collaborative working

The role of ongoing communication between all SLTs is to:
● facilitate the therapeutic process
● resolve potential conflicting professional issues
● provide appropriate knowledge of local and national speech and
language therapy service provision
● allay the individual's anxiety
● develop mutual trust.

Good working practices between SLTs will allow complementary
intervention to be developed. After discussion and joint planning, it
may be appropriate for one SLT to take the lead role in managing an
individual's care.

In order to provide continuity of care, all SLTs should have the
opportunity to contribute to planning meetings or case conferences
concerning an individual.

It is not ethical for an independent practitioner to undertake
assessments, provide therapy or give advice to NHS or LEA
colleagues without knowledge of the individual's current speech and
language therapy management within the NHS.

In these circumstances, it is recommended that the SLT and the
NHS or equivalent speech and language therapy manager meet
together with the individual or their representatives to resolve
potential conflicts and agree future speech and language therapy
provision.

to follow different or perhaps conflicting approaches,
cussed with the individual. The individual should be
which approach they wish to pursue. Individuals should
hat they are free to return to the second practitioner
pletion of the chosen therapy.

Individuals seeking second opinions

Individuals may seek a second opinion at any time.

Where an individual seeks a **confidential** second opinion from an independent practitioner, they should be informed that recommended good practice is to notify the NHS department/s. The possibility of test score invalidation and any negative effects of possible conflicting approaches should be explained.

The SLT may request that the individual signs an insertion to their records agreeing or requesting that the consultation remains confidential to the practice.

Setting up in independent practice

SLTs who leave NHS employment to set up in independent practice may work with individuals seen formerly in the NHS. However, these individuals should be aware that they could continue to access their NHS service. In these circumstances, independent practitioners should ensure that any recent reports or background information included in NHS case notes remain with, and are the property of, the NHS. Copies of recent reports should be provided by the relevant speech and language therapy department at the request of the client or their family.

Any independent work should not bring an individual therapist into conflict with their NHS employer. SLTs should not use NHS time or personnel to advertise or develop their private practice, and any NHS equipment or assessment materials utilised must be agreed with their NHS manager.

Further information is available at: www.helpwithtalking.com

5.9.2 SLTs and support practitioners in partnership

Speech and language therapy assistants and bilingual co-practitioners are highly valued and integral members of the speech and language therapy team, often employed directly to act in a supporting role under the direction of a professionally qualified SLT. SLTs also work in partnership with support practitioners who are employed by other agencies (for example, support practitioners in schools).

When working in partnership with support practitioners to provide care for an individual, SLTs should:
- share information, knowledge and skills to an appropriate level
- ensure adequate support and supervision of support practitioners, delegating to them only such duties as fall within their competence
- facilitate support practitioner development and education as appropriate.

When working in partnership with SLTs, support practitioners should:
- maintain a clear sense of their personal scope of practice and competence
- indicate to the SLT when delegated tasks are beyond their personal scope of practice
- seek further advice or training in order to maintain or extend their competence.

For more information see:
Intercollegiate Position Paper on Supervision, Accountability and Delegation of Activities to Support Workers, 2006
RCSLT Standards for Working with Speech and Language Therapy Support Practitioners, 2003
RCSLT Competency Framework for Support Practitioners, 2002
All available at: www.rcslt.org

5.9.3 SLTs and students in partnership
Pre-registration education is now regulated by the HPC and certified by the RCSLT. The RCSLT works with higher education institutions (HEIs) to ensure that their programmes meet the needs of the profession.

The RCSLT has developed standards for practice-based learning, the *National Standards for Practice-based Learning (SPLs).*
These aim to be an explicit articulation of the standards associated with all aspects of practice-based learning, involving all partners in the process: the HEI, the placement provider, the individual placement educator and the student.

The standards are intended to ensure that the patient/individual is the central focus of the student's learning experience and that practice-based learning should foster a culture of reflective practice. They allow for different educational philosophies, but include a statement of the overarching values, beliefs and attitudes underpinning practice-based learning.

The RCSLT uses the following terms, in respect of the partners in pre-registration education:

HEI refers to the higher education institution where the speech and language therapy pre-registration course is located.

Placement provider refers to the speech and language therapy service, that is providing the practice-based opportunity.

Placement educator refers to the individual SLT who is acting as the educator on the placement. *In a small service, the placement provider and the placement educator could be the same person.*

RCSLT values, beliefs, and attitudes about practice-based learning

● A core value is mutual respect for all partners. Central to this is a priority at all times for the wellbeing of the individual and compliance with the ethical codes around confidentiality and consent.

● Students are perceived, treated and respected as part of a collegiate partnership between HEI, placement providers and the individual placement educator. It is recognised that students bring value to the learning partnership.

● It is appreciated that students will have an individual style and pace of learning and will participate in a range of learning opportunities with their placement educators, in order to develop appropriately across all key areas of competence.

● Students are constructively supported by the HEI, placement providers and individual placement educators in the development of professional autonomy, professional and personal skills.

● Students will move through the curriculum developing more self direction and autonomy as they gain experience The placement educator plays a central role in facilitating the student's learning opportunities. Part of the placement educator's role is to help the student access and apply relevant theoretical knowledge for practice. The placement educator will be appropriately prepared and supported by the HEI for taking on this role, and for effectively

managing the placement educator/student relationship.
Practice-based learning, in the form of placements, forms a central part of pre-registration education. The benefits to all partners in adhering to the SPLs are as follows:

Benefits to HEIs
● Universities will be enabled to identify and monitor the quality of speech and language therapy placements.
● Universities will be enabled to secure funding and resources for:
  ● placement coordinators and administrators
  ● continued tutor support for placement learning
  ● support/study days for placement educators
  ● maintenance of essential links with other speech and language therapy courses and with other health professionals
● The design of pre-registration courses, that currently have practice-based education at their core, will be facilitated. Because the standards relate to competencies and Quality Assurance Agency (QAA) benchmarks, they will be a valuable source of reference to HEI staff writing practice-based education programmes, to ensure that students' practice-based education prepares them for the profession.

Benefits to placement providers and placement educators
● The shared responsibility of each of the participants in the placement learning process is detailed.
● They provide a framework for new placement educators and the reassurance of working within best practice guidelines.
● They will be an important resource used by speech and language therapy departments, within their trusts, in order to elicit support for placement education, within a recruitment and retention context.
● They will maintain quality, whilst striving for quantity, as all departments are looking at varying models of placement education to increase throughput.
● They will ensure that the speech and language therapy department is accounting for any possible safety risks within the service.
● All departments will be measured alongside similar services in respect of achievable goals for placement-based learning.

Benefits to students

Practice-based learning, whilst providing crucial learning opportunities and helping apply theory to practice, can be stressful for students. The SPLs will assist in providing safe, supportive environments in which to observe and practise clinical and professional skills. They seek to ensure that:

● students know how to prepare effectively for practice-based learning
● their university provides clear documentation to support that preparation
● students know what they can expect from their placement educators
● progress towards practice-based and personal objectives is monitored.

The provision of clinical placements is therefore a crucial element in the preparation of competent clinicians and the future of the profession.

The RCSLT's key responsibilities are to set out a framework for the provision of practice-based learning, as reflected in the SPLs, and to acknowledge and promote the importance of services providing student placements for the benefit of the whole profession.

One central area is the sourcing and selection of placements:

● Local policies and procedures will be agreed between the HEI and the placement provider with respect to time scales and methods of communication, including alerting the placement providers in appropriate time as to the likely number of placements that will be sought during each academic year. Also, the timing for completion of documentation will be made available by the HEI.
● Sourcing, selecting and allocating placements are normally the responsibility of the HEI, devolved to the placement coordinator. This involves establishing networks and liasing with placement providers and students.
● HEIs will seek input from local placement providers when designing placements in order to maximise capacity.

Speech and language therapy managers have a responsibility to encourage, facilitate and provide practice-based placements for speech and language therapy students.

Specific responsibilities include:

● managing practice-based placements within the service, including keeping statistics of the placements offered and provided

- promoting the importance of placements
- ensuring the role of SLTs as placement educators is reflected in job descriptions
- developing explicit links with at least one higher education institute and pre-registration course commissioning body
- committing the service to a minimum number of student placements over a period of time
- identifying a member of staff to take responsibility for practice-based placements
- working in partnership with the HEI to ensure that placement educators are supported
- ensuring the regional managers group includes representatives from local HEIs
- making student issues a standing item on the agenda at staff meetings
- providing students with an induction to the service
- promoting speech and language therapy as a career.

Service standard 48: The service has a clear and up-to-date policy on the management of SLT student practice-based learning in the service.

SLTs

The RCSLT expects SLTs to take on the responsibility for assuring the future of the profession and the provision of services by providing practice-based placements.

After two years of post-qualification experience, an SLT should commit to taking students. In situations when ongoing support is available from either their own service or the HEI, SLTs may take students after one year.

Students help to develop a therapist's reflective practice. Such activity continues to be recognised by the RCSLT as contributing to an SLT's CPD and may be recorded as part of the annual CPD requirement.

Independent therapists should be recognised as a source for the provision of placements for students. HEIs and local NHS services should therefore be prepared to offer both development opportunities and ongoing support to independent practitioners in their role as clinical supervisors.

Quality of practice-based learning

It is expected that all partners will comply with the SPLs, so that the students can experience placements that are of an acceptable quality. There is a self audit tool, developed from the SPLs, for all partners, available at www.rcslt.org. Examples of good practice, matched to the sections of the SPLs are also available on the RCSLT website.

5.9.4 Professional representation to the wider organisation

Standard 49: Where the service head is not an SLT, there is a system of professional representation to the service manager on matters relating to clinical issues.

5.9.5 Multi-agency team working

Although there will be times when an SLT operates in a uni-disciplinary way to achieve satisfactory outcomes with the service user, most speech and language therapy will be carried out as part of a multidisciplinary team and increasingly, those disciplines will be employed by different agencies. This is the case whether the service user is a targeted at-risk group or a referred individual.

The importance of team working and the difficulty of isolating the impact of one therapy from a rehabilitation or educational programme is recognised (Wade, 2005).

The members of any given multi-agency team will vary according to the local working context and particular circumstances.

Figure 1 provides an idea of the range of people who may be part of the team in given contexts. Not all those listed will be actively involved at any one time and the constitution of the team will vary over time according to changing individual needs.

Levels of multi-agency working in practice

Models of multi-agency partnership working have been reviewed and several levels of operation identified (Sloper, 2004):

● Strategic level working including joint planning, decision making, commissioning and purchasing.
● Consultation and training including professionals from one agency providing consultation and training to practitioners from another agency.
● Placement schemes whereby posts are created to span the organisational divide between agencies.

Figure 1: Multi-agency team working

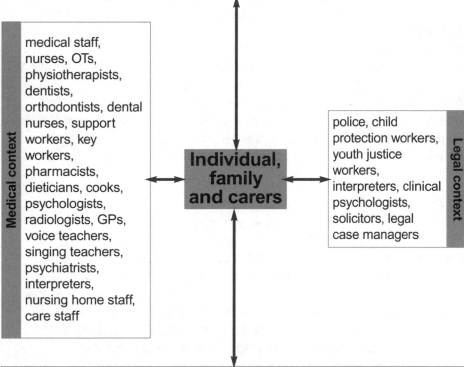

Educational context

teaching staff, SENCos, assistants, dinner supervisors, learning mentors, LEA staff, support teachers, educational psychologists, paediatricians, audiologists, orthoptists, CAMHS workers, clinical psychologists, GPs, health visitors, psychotherapists, interpreters

Medical context

medical staff, nurses, OTs, physiotherapists, dentists, orthodontists, dental nurses, support workers, key workers, pharmacists, dieticians, cooks, psychologists, radiologists, GPs, voice teachers, singing teachers, psychiatrists, interpreters, nursing home staff, care staff

Individual, family and carers

Legal context

police, child protection workers, youth justice workers, interpreters, clinical psychologists, solicitors, legal case managers

social workers, home care organisers, community support staff including nurses, dieticians, health visitors, crèche and child carers, volunteer workers, pre-school and play group staff, audiologists, social workers, child and family psychiatry support workers, voluntary agencies, specialist speech and language therapy services, fostering and housing staff, OTs, physiotherapists, clinical psychologists, portage workers, Sure Start workers, interpreters, bilingual support workers, health advocates, family centre staff, home teachers, educational psychologists, under-5s counsellors, behaviour support workers, child protection staff, child development centre teams, psychotherapists, play therapists, vocational agencies, disability employment agencies, community mental health teams, day centre staff, voluntary employment agencies

Social and community context

Chapter 5

● Centre-based service delivery when one coordinator pulls together services delivered by different agencies.
● Multidisciplinary or multi-agency teams where professionals from different agencies work together as a team on a daily basis.
● Case or care management where an identified lead has the responsibility for ensuring a coordinated service to families.

The aims of working within a multi-agency team (including the referred individual and, where appropriate, parents and/or carers):

● To provide information about the nature of the communication/eating difficulty to team members, gaining additional information from them on these and related difficulties.
● To offer speech and language therapy intervention based on a holistic awareness of the individual's needs and other aspects of care.
● To work collaboratively with the team in planning and implementing individual-centred goals and clinical care.

References

Department of Health. *Essence of Care: Patient-focused benchmarking for health care practitioners*, 2003. www.dh.gov.uk
Department of Health. *HSC 199/053: For the record – managing records in NHS Trusts and health authorities*, 1999. www.dh.gov.uk
Department of Health. *HSG (97)17: Corporate governance in the NHS controls assurance statements*, 1997. www.dh.gov.uk
Department of Health. *Improvement Leaders' Guide: Involving patients and carers – General improvement skills*, 2002. www.wise.nhs.uk
Department of Health. *NHS Health Record and Communicating Practice Standards for Team-based Care*, 2004. www.connectingforhealth.nhs.uk
Department of Health. *The NHS Plan: A plan for investment, a plan for reform*, 2000. www.dh.gov.uk
Department for Health. *NSF Long-term Conditions*, 2005. www.dh.gov.uk
Department of Health. *Our healthier nation: a contract for health*, 1998.
Department of Health. *Prevention and health, everybody's business: A reassessment of public and personal health*, 1976.

Department for Health. *Safer working in the community a guide for NHS managers and staff on reducing the risks from violence and aggression*, 1998. www.dh.gov.uk

Department of Health. *Working for Patients*, 1989. www.dh.gov.uk

Health Professions Council, 2004. www.hpc-uk.org

Intercollegiate Position Paper on *Supervision, Accountability and Delegation of Activities to Support Workers*, 2006.

Leape, L. Making healthcare safe: are we up to it in *Journal of Paediatric Surgery*, 2004, Vol. 39:3.

RCSLT. *Competency Framework for Support Practitioners*, 2002.

RCSLT. *Information Pack for New SLT Managers*, 2005. www.rcslt.org

RCSLT. *Newly-qualified Practitioners Competency Framework to guide Transition to full RCSLT Membership*, 2005. www.rcslt.org

RCSLT. *Returners Pack*, 2005. www.rcslt.org

RCSLT. *Standards for Working with Speech and Language Therapy Support Practitioners*, 2003.

RCSLT. *Starting your career as an SLT: An essential guide*, 2004. www.rcslt.org

RCSLT. *Working in Harmony*, 2005. www.rcslt.org

Sloper, P. *Facilitators and barriers for coordinated multi-agency services in Child: Care in Health and Development*, 2004:30; pp571-580.

Taylor-Goh, S. *RCSLT Clinical Guidelines*. RCSLT, 2005. www.rcslt.org

Wade, D. Randomised clinical trials in clinical rehabilitation in *Journal of Clinical Rehabilitation*, 2005:19; pp133-136.

Acts of Parliament

All available at: www.opsi.gov.uk
Data Protection Act 1998
Disability Discrimination Act 2005
Freedom of Information Act 2000
Freedom of Information (Scotland) Act 2000
Health and Safety at Work Act 1974
Management of Health and Safety at Work Regulations 1992
Mental Health Act 1983
Public Health (Control of Diseases) Act 1984
Public Records Act 1958

Chapter 6

Service Provision: Part 1 Care Pathway

Introduction to Service Provision

The purpose of any given speech and language therapy service is to provide evidence-based services that anticipate and respond to the needs of individuals or at-risk groups who may experience speech, language, communication or swallowing difficulties.

Services work in partnership with these individuals and their families and with other professions and agencies to reduce the impact of these often isolating difficulties on people's wellbeing and their ability to participate in daily life.

See chapter 1, section 1.1 Scope of Practice and chapter 5, section 5.1 Definition of Health.

6.1 Levels of Service Provision

The notion of service levels (or tiers) is being used across health, social and educational domains.

See figure 1: Tiered model of UK health, social and educational services (right).

The tiered framework allows for ready consideration of:
● complexity of need (increasing from Level 1 through to Level 4)
● types of support provided in relation to need (eg for speech and language therapy services, intervention will vary from general advice at Level 1 to highly specialised and individualised advice at Level 4)
● numbers of individuals being targeted at different levels (eg whole populations at Level 1 through to small numbers of individuals at Level 4)
● costs (increasing costs per head from Level 1 through to Level 4).

The model also contains the notions of:

a) **self-managed care** which reflects the concept of health as the responsibility of the individual, as well as of society or government. This has been increasingly emphasised in government strategy documents from as far back as *Prevention and health, everybody's business: A reassessment of public and personal health* (1976).

b) **a journey or pathway** that individuals take, accessing services at different levels according to needs that will naturally vary over time.

6.2 Level 2 Services: Targeting the Needs of At-risk Groups (see Figure 2)

6.2.1 Health promotion

Many speech, language, communication and swallowing difficulties

Figure 1: Tiered model of UK health and social services

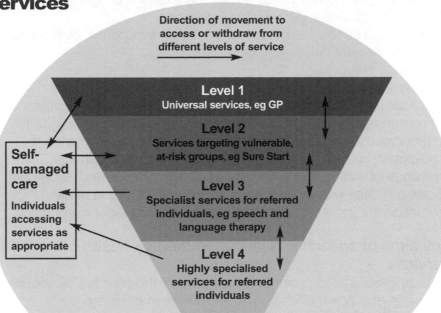

Direction of movement to access or withdraw from different levels of service

Level 1
Universal services, eg GP

Level 2
Services targeting vulnerable, at-risk groups, eg Sure Start

Level 3
Specialist services for referred individuals, eg speech and language therapy

Level 4
Highly specialised services for referred individuals

Self-managed care

Individuals accessing services as appropriate

Figure 2: Level 2 Services

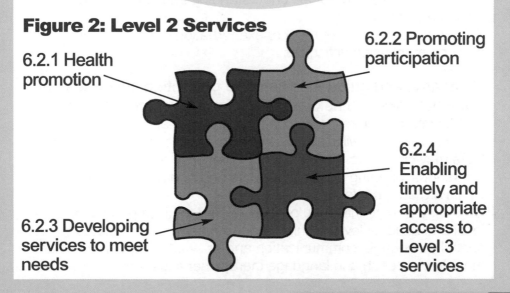

6.2.1 Health promotion

6.2.2 Promoting participation

6.2.3 Developing services to meet needs

6.2.4 Enabling timely and appropriate access to Level 3 services

arise from:

- Medical conditions such as stroke, cancer or a progressive neurological disorder like multiple sclerosis.
- Conditions such as syndromes, eg Down syndrome; cleft palate.
- Developmental delays and disorders.
- Physical impairment.
- Learning disability.

Therefore many speech, language and communication difficulties are not preventable in a primary sense. However, all speech, language, communication and swallowing difficulties can be exacerbated or ameliorated by certain lifestyle choices and factors within the environment, including the responses of others to the individual. These issues are dealt with by a range of strategies, including health promotion and working with others on developing inclusive practice.

Key aims of speech and language therapy health promotion services

- As appropriate, to promote awareness of the process of speech, language and communication development in children.
- To promote awareness of potential risks and risk indicators related to speech, language, communication and/or swallowing difficulties within given populations.
- To make health information accessible and support health self-advocacy through individuals understanding and communicating their own health needs.
- To prevent the development or exacerbation of speech, language and communication difficulties.

Standards and guidance related to promoting awareness of potential risks and risk indicators for a given population

Written information regarding the potential risks and risk indicators for a given population will be made available to potential referring agents. SLTs may choose to present this information in the form of workshops targeting at-risk individuals and/or other referring agents within a given population.

SLTs may work to influence policies related to given populations at a local and national level, highlighting the potential risks related to speech, language, communication and/or swallowing difficulties and the role of speech and language therapy services.

Standards and guidance related to the prevention of speech, language and communication difficulties

Therapists may collaborate with others, including voluntary sector agencies and multidisciplinary teams to develop health promotion materials suitable for the needs of the targeted at-risk group.

Examples of at-risk groups are:
- teachers and lecturers at risk of developing voice disorders
- pre-schoolers in areas of high economic deprivation

SLTs may run awareness raising workshops for at-risk individuals and, in the case of children, their carers.

SLTs may work in a number of different ways within the team that are targeting the needs of at-risk populations.

Methods may include:
- joint-working with other professionals
- training others in the use of appropriate preventative strategies

Standards and guidance related to preventing the exacerbation of speech, language, communication and swallowing difficulties

This guidance will apply to the whole population of individuals with recognised difficulties, as all speech, language, communication and swallowing difficulties can be exacerbated by certain lifestyle choices and factors within the environment, including the responses of others to the individual.

SLTs may work in a variety of ways to influence others in the use of appropriate preventative work and strategies. This may include:
- influencing the development of agency-wide or inter-agency policies and strategies
- providing training workshops for others in the use of appropriate curriculum/work content and environmental or interaction strategies

6.2.2 Promoting participation

Key aims of promoting participation:
- To promote the participation of individuals with speech, language, communication and swallowing difficulties in a full range of life activities.
- To work in partnership with relevant others to support the development of effective communication in given population groups.
- To provide training to those working with people with communication difficulties to maximise inclusion.

● To contribute to raising public awareness of communication/eating and drinking difficulties.

● To promote the participation of the individual with communication/ eating and drinking difficulties in a full range of life activities through working in an advocacy role with services/groups.

● To develop the capacity of services/groups to manage or provide services to specified groups of individuals with communication and/or eating and drinking difficulties. This may involve strategic partnership working with local or national voluntary agencies.

● In the case of the pre-school population, to promote the participation of parents and carers in a full range of life activities with their children.

Guidance related to promoting participation

SLTs may work in a number of different ways within teams or agencies that must include the needs of individuals with recognised difficulties. Examples of working contexts are:

● schools
● further education services
● medical services
● youth justice
● advice services

Methods may include:

● joint-working with other professionals
● training others in the use of appropriate preventative work and strategies
● influencing agency-wide and inter-agency policies and strategies
● advising on communication-support materials appropriate to a given context, eg use of graphic symbols, signing, voice output communication aids
● advising kitchen staff on presentation of food in a range of consistencies

6.2.3 Developing speech and language therapy services to meet needs

Key aims of developing services to meet needs:

● To ensure that speech and language therapy services are

providing a range of secondary and tertiary level services to appropriately meet local speech, language, communication and swallowing needs.

● To inform the process of identifying local health, education and social needs.

● To highlight to commissioners the needs and impact of potential communication and eating/drinking difficulties:

● within care groups
● within care pathways
● within wider population groups

Principles underpinning the development of speech and language therapy services

Services need to be planned taking into account national policies and guidelines, current evidence-based practice, research findings and expert opinion, as well as user consultation within the local context. In planning services, speech and language therapy service managers should take account of the relevant key points in multidisciplinary care pathways where speech and language therapy services are essential or beneficial.

Standards and guidance related to developing services to meet needs

SLTs have a lead role to play in the:

● Commissioning of services for people with communication/swallowing disorders. For example, advising on appropriate resources to meet identified client group need, including appropriate skill mix.

● Formulation and implementation of across-agency policies pertaining to swallowing/communication disorders.

Speech and language therapy managers will be responsible for reviewing the range, appropriateness and effectiveness of speech and language therapy services in relation to local need.

Speech and language therapy managers will be responsible for alerting service commissioners where current service arrangements are not meeting local need.

This will include an assessment of risk to individuals and to the employing organisation.

Service Standard 50: Where there are gaps or shortfalls against standards in the service, there is clear evidence that the service is taking steps to develop and improve the service.
Service standard 51: The service has a strategy in relation to health inequalities and is able to demonstrate actions taken to reduce these inequalities.
See Chapter 9, Service Monitoring, Improvement, Evaluation and Development.

6.2.4 Enabling timely and appropriate access to speech and language therapy Level 3 services: responding to referrals

Key aims of enabling access to Level 3 services:
● To enable appropriate and timely access to speech and language therapy Level 3 services as the clinical need arises.
● To work with other professionals/agencies in the identification of risk/need via the single shared assessment process.
● To provide information about speech and language therapy services.
● To enable easy access to speech and language therapy through ensuring appropriate referral mechanisms are in place.
● To enable equal access to the service for all groups regardless of ethnicity, age, social class, disability, language or location.

Principles underpinning the enabling of access to Level 3 services
Access to speech and language therapy Level 3 services is equitable, non-discriminatory and based on clinical need.

Standards and guidance around referral to speech and language therapy services
This may include transfer from specialist regional units.
Service Standard 52: There are clear and up-to-date written policies on admission to and discharge from Level 3 services.
● Referral procedures will ensure that all individuals have access to the service, irrespective of age, language, gender, race, presenting communication difficulty or location.
● In the case of specialist cleft palate services, access to local

services may be possible even when the parents have chosen a cleft centre other than their local one.

● Written information regarding the scope of tertiary services to a given client group is made available to potential referring agents, including other agencies and targeted groups within the general public.

● This includes information on the referral procedure and the re-referral of individuals who have been previously discharged by the service.

● Standard local response times to referrals will be specified.

● Information should be available in a range of formats to address people's communication needs.

● SLTs may discuss the appropriateness of a referral to speech and language therapy with individuals considering self-referral or with professionals considering referring on an individual for assessment.

● Speech and language therapy services will need to use a range of methods to help individuals engage with services and provide for timely access.

● Responsibility for the acceptance of referrals to Level 3 services remains with a fully registered SLT.

● An open referral system will operate in many parts of a speech and language therapy service. Where this is the case, referrals will be accepted from any source, including self-referral.

Specialist services for particular client groups may apply locally-agreed referral criteria or referral procedures, taking into account the following RCSLT recommendations:

Adults with learning disability: referrals are made through the community learning disability team (CLDT), although SLTs may receive and bring referrals to the team.

Child development centres: referrals are usually made in writing by the individual's GP.

Cleft palate: referrals are accepted from the time of birth notification.

Dysphagia: referrals are made in writing by any member of the multidisciplinary team or by the individual's GP. Professionals involved will usually have received some training in dysphagia identification from the SLTs. **A written medical referral is no longer requisite.**

Head and neck: referrals are made by the medical/nursing team as a part of a tumour staging and management plan.

I CAN nurseries: referrals are made to this tertiary service by an SLT.

Voice disorder: referrals are made by an ENT surgeon or specialist voice therapist following laryngeal examination.

Referral to speech and language therapy requires the consent of the individual or, in the case of children, the consent of a parent/guardian. Exceptions to this may occur where:

● the individual is deemed to lack the capacity to consent
● the individual is an inpatient under section 3 of the Mental Health Act, 1983

Triage: assessing the appropriateness of referrals

Purpose of triage:

● To establish the appropriateness of referral to a particular speech and language therapy service in terms of meeting admission/ acceptance criteria, eg age, medical condition, scope of service provision.

● To allow consideration of factors that may increase or reduce the effectiveness of therapy intervention at that point.

● To identify meaningful management aims.

● To identify the individuals' views on need, urgency, timing and expectation.

● To provide the individual/carer with information on the scope and aims of the service in order to aid their decision making about a choice to proceed with the referral.

● To reduce the anxiety which may arise from a long wait for a first appointment with a therapist by offering a first appointment within standard response times.

● To allow for a timely referral onto another professional, if this is indicated.

● To avoid the development of lengthy waiting lists at the point of entry to speech and language therapy services.

● To provide timely information regarding levels of need of referred individuals that may then be used to inform service organisation and delivery.

● To allow the therapist to judge the relative priority of the individual's need in relation to the needs of others requiring intervention.

● To identify need for referral to a different and more appropriate service.

Service standard 53: The service has links with voluntary organisations, vocational/employment agencies, and local support groups, to complement the work of the service

Principles of triage:
- Triage does not replace the initial assessment stage, but complements it.
- By using triage as a caseload management strategy, therapists can retain an overview of the needs of the caseload as a whole in order to plan for most effective use of limited resources.

Standards and guidance around triage:
- It is recommended that an experienced therapist is best placed to carry out triage. This is because the task requires the complex synthesis of information in a short period (often 30 minutes), taking full account of the individual's/carer's views in making a decision about the appropriateness of referral.
- Referral agents should be informed that a triage system is in use so that they can inform individuals/carers at the time of initial discussion with the individual.
- Referrals received will be examined by an experienced therapist prior to any appointment being arranged to judge whether a triage appointment is appropriate. A decision may be made to proceed with acceptance of the referral and an in-depth assessment based solely on the information given.
- The referral will be acknowledged by the individual/carer.

Timing of triage:
- Triage appointments are arranged as soon as possible after the receipt of referral, within local standard response times.
- Wherever possible, individuals/carers will be asked to make their own appointment on a day, time and setting that is convenient for them.
- The triage appointment will be shorter than an assessment session because it does not include formal testing as a matter of routine.

Form of triage:
- The purpose of the appointment is explained to the individual/carer.
- The therapist will discuss the background to the individual's

difficulty and gain an understanding of the individual's/carer's concerns and wishes in planning for intervention.

● This discussion will include detail of individual's/carer's observations and the pattern of change.

● Within paediatric triage, clinical settings are most valuable when there are facilities for viewing interaction between parents and child using a two-way mirror and sound link. Observation of interaction is key to understanding the child's presentation and the nature of the parent's concerns. Materials selected for parent and child to play with will be culturally and age appropriate.

● As appropriate, triage may be combined successfully with hearing tests in the same location.

On completion of the triage appointment:

● The results of the triage appointment will be reported to the referral agent by letter including details of the next step and timescales.

● If an individual does not attend, the referral agent will be informed and may be requested to encourage the individual/family to contact the service to initiate the appointment.

6.2.5 Guidance on the provision of general advice

● All advice should be evidence or consensus based.

● Advice is based on general strategies to facilitate speech, language and communication development. It should not be targeted at specific individuals nor based on a skills profile generated from assessment.

● If more specific advice is required, the therapist should encourage the individual or responsible adult to consent to referral so they can be registered with the speech and language therapy service. Information or advice given is then recorded in the usual way as part of speech and language therapy intervention.

● If individuals or families express or demonstrate reluctance to be registered with a speech and language therapy service because of perceived stigma or other reasons, the SLT has a responsibility to support their understanding of what registration means. This may include:

● the SLT's ability to give specific targeted advice

● that records are confidential and that information in most instances will only be revealed to others with their express consent
● they will receive a copy of all correspondence
● if they wish, they may have access to read what is recorded in their file (in most instances)

Strengthening accountability for general speech and language therapy advice

The RCSLT recommends that:
● Clinical teams have a standard presentation or a set of key evidence-based statements around which a presentation can be structured. This may include a series of pre-prepared responses to frequently asked questions (FAQs).
● The presentation and/or fact sheets are approved by a local clinical governance committee.
● A policy states the requirement of staff to adhere to the pre-agreed information in all appropriate situations.
● Anonymised notes are recorded, containing a minimum data set of date, time, location, numbers attending, approximate age of individual/s at whom the advice is aimed and the nature of the advice given.
● Anonymised records are peer reviewed every four months for:
● adherence to standardised guidance
● appropriateness of advice given
● Additional information highlighted by regular audit is added to the standardised package.
For further details, see the RCSLT paper on *Accountability for Professional Advice Given to Non-registered Patients,* 2005.

6.3 Level 3 Services: Targeting the Needs of Referred Individuals

6.3.1 Care pathways
● Care pathways set out the anticipated course of care towards positive outcomes for an individual within a designated care group, for example, individuals with progressive neurological disorders or school-aged children with a speech, language or communication disorder.

● Care pathways are important because they help to reduce unnecessary variations in individual care and outcomes. They also support the development of care partnerships and, through increased transparency around service provision, empower individuals and, where appropriate, their carers, to be involved in the choices around care.

Service standard 54: At a local level, there should be clear care pathway for each speech and language therapy care group that reflects and anticipates the needs of referred individuals, many of whom have enduring, complex and multiple health and social needs.

Service standard 55: Where specialist services are not available within the immediate service or local district, there is a pathway and clear procedures for individuals to access these outwith the service.

● Speech and language therapy care pathways will reflect and be integrated into local and national guidelines/pathways developed for specific groups, such as stroke, traumatic brain injury, Parkinson's disease, multiple sclerosis, cancer care, pre-school population.
This will enable speech and language therapy, wherever appropriate, to be part of a multi-agency seamless service that is able to respond to the needs of the individual.

● Where specific national guidelines have not been developed or remain a matter of debate (eg facial palsy), care process maps and practices are derived from general principles of best practice and adapted from existing pathways (see below).

● Although there are circumstances when the SLT is the sole person working with a client, pathways will generally reflect team working and the multi-, trans- and inter-disciplinary processes involved. At the same time there will be maps of care process that are specific to speech and language therapy involvement that feed into the team.

● Variations in the way an individual experiences their route along a care pathway in terms of timing, intensity, aims and content occur as clinical freedom is exercised to meet the needs of the individual.
These variations are shaped by factors such as the choices exercised by the individual; the levels of actual and anticipated risk; rate and type of development; patterns of change in overall medical condition; the impact of this on individuals and their response/s to it; changes in life circumstances and in demands.

● The overall care pathway in speech and language therapy is referral: diagnostic assessment; followed by formulation of, and negotiation of, short- and long-term goals with all parties involved; episodes of speech and language therapy intervention with ongoing monitoring of progress towards goals; reassessment at key junctures; planned and measurable discharge or transition to self-management/other form of care and clearly stated, workable onward and sideways referral criteria.

The key elements of a Level 3 care pathway are set out in figure 3 on page 198.

6.3.2 Acceptance of referrals

Procedures for responding to referrals will follow local policy appropriate to the nature of the specific client group.

Any prioritisation of accepted referrals should be determined in a systematic and equitable manner.

Factors will vary according to context but include:

● assessment of risk

● importance of timing, particularly in relation to risk reduction, health needs and surgery

And as appropriate the:

● need to ensure access to other services

● need to ensure appropriate school placement

● timescales of other agencies

See 5.4.3 Workload management.

Figure 4 on page 199 outlines recommended referral-response times. However, services may wish to set local standards within these limits according to local needs. Services should ensure that these local standards do not fall outside national standards as set, for example, within England in the National Service Frameworks.

Individuals will be informed within two weeks of receipt of the referral, if the date for a first appointment is likely to be outside the standard response time.

Where appropriate, and with the consent of the individual, the SLT may establish with the referring agent if a medical diagnosis and prognosis exists and whether the client/carer is aware of this.

Wherever possible and appropriate, and with the consent of the individual, referrals will be discussed with the team and relevant other professionals known to be involved with the client.

Figure 3: Key elements of a Level 3 care pathway

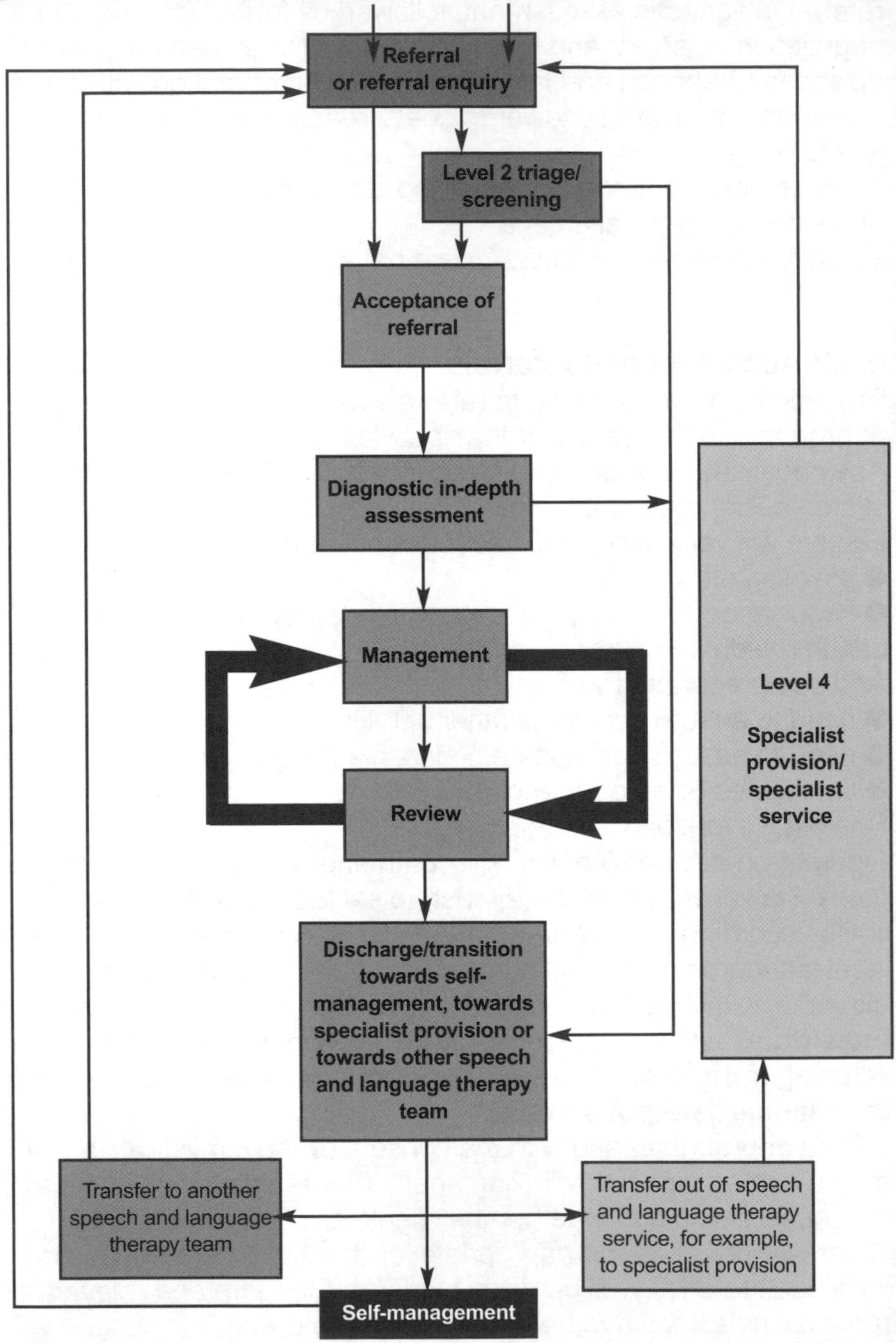

Referral or referral enquiry

Level 2 triage/screening

Acceptance of referral

Diagnostic in-depth assessment

Management

Review

Discharge/transition towards self-management, towards specialist provision or towards other speech and language therapy team

Level 4

Specialist provision/specialist service

Transfer to another speech and language therapy team

Transfer out of speech and language therapy service, for example, to specialist provision

Self-management

Figure 4: Recommended response times from receipt of referral

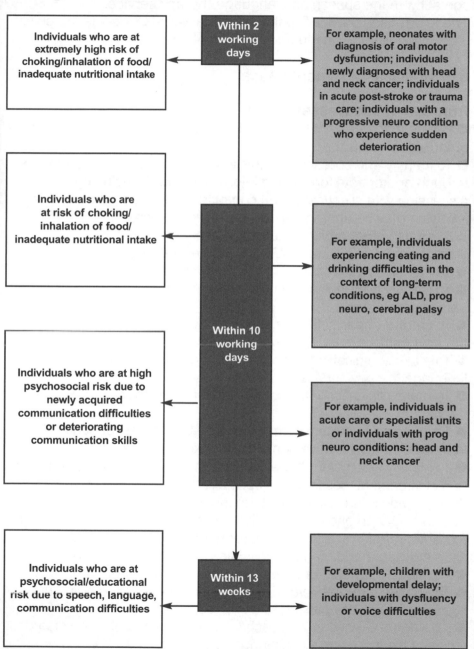

The individual, or in the case of children, their parents, should be informed about what will happen during their first appointment/contact with the speech and language therapy service.
The information provided to the individual will also include the policy regarding failure to attend and its implications.

6.3.3 Initial assessment phase

Purpose of initial assessment:
● Where triage has not been used, to decide on the appropriateness of individual referral.
● To identify and collect the requisite range of relevant information through appropriate formal and informal methods including discussion with client/carer and consultation with colleagues. The following may be appropriate as part of this process:
● referral to other professionals for advice
● involvement of bilingual SLTAs and interpreters
● To identify any immediate risks the individual is facing.
● To identify how the individual's involvement in everyday activities is being compromised.
● To identify capacity for change, both by the individual and within the environment.
● To make a clinical judgement about the need for speech and language therapy service involvement.
● To make clinical prioritisation judgements regarding the client's needs.
● To judge and advise where, when and what form speech and language therapy involvement should take.
● To identify whether further evaluation of the individual's presentation and environment, possibly by a specialist therapist, may be helpful.
● To provide information about the individual's difficulties and possible speech and language therapy care options to the individual /carer/team/referral agent as appropriate.
● To anticipate and manage possible problems.
● To inform individual of potential problems as appropriate.
● To provide information/advice to promote development and prevent exacerbation of any difficulties as appropriate.
● To diagnose whether a speech/language/communication disorder exists in the individual's first language.

- To assess the exact nature of any swallowing disorder that exists.
- To provide a baseline of skills, together with current and predicted needs against which the effects of intervention can be measured.
- To open discussion with individual/carer about ultimate goals and discharge criteria which will be reconsidered and may then be modified throughout episodes of intervention.
- To agree with individual, or in the case of children, their parents, the profile of needs; how they can be met and the role of speech and language therapy within this.
- Initial assessment may have very specific objectives for certain client groups, eg in the case of specialist cleft palate services:
  - to diagnose the existence of a cleft-related speech/language/communication/swallowing disorder
  - to discuss whether surgical intervention is appropriate
  - to make recommendations regarding the appropriate timing for surgical intervention to the surgeon
  - to advise the local speech and language therapy service on the appropriate type and timing of speech and language therapy intervention
  - to provide information and resources for the local speech and language therapy service
  - to support, advise and affirm parents in the care of their child with cleft-related difficulties

Principles underpinning assessment:
- Assessment is informed by the best available evidence and underpinned by client consent.
- Factors related to aetiology, medical needs, time of onset and personal/family context should be taken into account when considering the likely prognosis for an individual.
- Health benefits will be maximised when assessment and intervention include the full and informed involvement of carers.
- Differential diagnosis of speech and/or language disability is informed by assessment in all the languages a client hears and/or speaks.

Standards and guidance around initial assessment stage
A comprehensive assessment will be undertaken with the consent of the individual and/or carer.

As far as possible and appropriate, the purpose of initial assessment will be explained to the individual before assessment begins. In the case of children, an explanation will be given to the child's parent/guardian.

Timing of assessment

An initial assessment may take place over several sessions. Post-operative assessment will be carried out only when the individual is sufficiently medically stable. In the interim, monitoring of the situation may take place through liaison.

Involvement of others in the assessment

As far as is possible and appropriate, the purpose of initial assessment will be explained to the individual before assessment begins.

In the case of children, an explanation will be given to the child's parent/guardian.

Unless the individual does not require the involvement of others, at least one other person who knows the client well will be involved in the assessment process.

Where English is an additional language, an interpreter or bilingual co-worker should be involved in the process as appropriate.

In the case of children, it may be advisable to see the parents on a separate occasion in order to allow for a full and open discussion of all factors. Wherever possible, it is preferable for both parents to attend.

Assessment will include a consideration of the individual's expectations and, where appropriate, the carer's expectations of therapy.

Initial assessment may involve joint/multi/inter-disciplinary assessment with other professionals, which may be through a joint visit or by meetings/liaison.

Where available and relevant to speech/language/communication, the findings of other professionals will be included within the assessment process.

Form of the assessment

Assessment will include a full case history and consideration of functional skills and communication needs within daily life.

Assessment should include an evaluation of the factors in the individual's environment that support or may be perceived as barriers to the individual's functioning. A trial of intervention may help to establish the potential for change.

Assessment should take account of the range of contexts within which the client normally functions and may function in the future.

To assist in the gathering of information related to assessment, the SLT should have open access to:

● inpatient medical notes when working in that context
● educational notes when working in that context

Assessment may include the use of standardised tests, criterion referenced measures, informal assessments and qualitative methods including observations and discussion as appropriate.

Materials will be chosen for their linguistic, cultural and age-appropriateness. The latest editions of any standardised test materials should be used.

Appropriate speech/language and communication assessment material in the required languages should be used where available. As language assessments do not readily translate from one language to another due to cultural bias and linguistic differences, these should not be used unless fully validated and standardised. Where possible and relevant, the initial assessment should be repeatable to allow for a re-assessment at a later date.

On completion of the assessment

The assessment records will be stored, depending on context, either in the SLT's case notes with a record in the multidisciplinary team, educational or medical notes, or single recording and storage may occur.

A written report/summary stating findings, recommendations and agreed action will be forwarded to the referral agent and other relevant professionals.

In concordance with the DH guidance on sharing information with individuals and, in the case of children, parents/carers will be asked if they wish to receive correspondence relating to their care.

Reports/letters should then be provided in an appropriate and accessible form and in accordance with their wishes.

As deemed appropriate, individuals/carers will be made aware of any key pieces of evidence-based appraised literature and websites pertaining to their diagnosed condition.

As deemed appropriate, individuals/carers will be made aware of any national/local support organisations appropriate to their diagnosed condition.

Individuals/carers will be provided with information about how to contact the speech and language therapy service should queries/concerns arise.

Advice should be sought from a specialist SLT or specialist centre when a highly expert perspective or investigation is required, either because the limits of the therapist's competence have been reached or because of the nature of the individual's needs and difficulties. Examples of this are:

● When it is considered that assistive technology is of potential benefit to enhance the communication, educational, social and vocational opportunities of the individual.

● When a child presents with a velopharyngeal disorder.

● When an objective assessment is required, eg videofluoroscopy or nasendoscopy.

Referral to other professionals or agencies may be deemed appropriate and should be done with the knowledge and agreement of the individual/carer.

Examples of this are:

● When it is felt that an individual would benefit from an intensive and focused period of multidisciplinary rehabilitation.

● When an assessment by another professional would add to the understanding of the individual's difficulties and needs, eg referring a child to an educational psychologist

● Where there is a fundamental disagreement between the SLT and individual or parents/carers in relation to needs, priorities, and ways of addressing needs, individuals should be informed of their right to a second opinion from within the service.

6.3.4 Management phase

Purpose of management

To implement an appropriate, timely and integrated approach to the management of the individual's difficulties involving the individual, the family, other professionals and key people in the individual's environment. Intervention may be in English, in another language, bilingual or carried out through an interpreting service.

A judgement of what is appropriate will be based on individual circumstances, evidence-based guidance where available and professional consensus opinion on what is appropriate for particular conditions and settings.

SLTs should be aware of any national service pathways that apply to their care group and how this might impact on an individual's care plan.

Principles underpinning management of referred individuals:

● Intervention is informed by the best available evidence and underpinned by the consent of the individual and/or carer.

● Speech and language therapy works to encourage individual autonomy and to discourage dependency on the therapist thereby enabling individuals to take an active role in managing their condition wherever possible.

● Speech and language therapy works to reduce the health, educational and psychosocial risks faced by the individual.

● Speech and language therapy works to promote individual access to and participation in everyday life activities.

● Person-centred intervention is based on an holistic understanding of the individual and all aspects of their life.

● Intervention should be based on individual need and should take account of available evidence and consensus guidance on effective practice. Intervention should promote individual safety and that of carers and staff.

● An intervention plan is likely to include work to change or maintain the individual's functional ability as well as work to address the impact of their condition when participating in community life. Speech and language therapy intervention aims to be efficient as well as effective.

● Continuity of care is an important aspect of effective practice. Intervention will take full account of the individual's preferred language, culture, lifestyle and environment, including the role that carers can play.

● Whenever appropriate, intervention should be provided as part of a multi-agency team. Where there is a choice, intervention should be provided in the most conducive setting for optimising effectiveness.

● The most effective approach for working with individuals involves integrated and coordinated working across community and acute settings (see the Department of Health's *NSF for children, young people and maternity services*, 2004)

● The service complies with RCSLT guidance on working relationships between independent and public sectors. See the document *Working in Harmony,* available at: www.rcslt.org

● Intervention should be matched to the needs, strengths and capacities of each individual and modified as these change over time.

● Communication and eating/drinking are fundamental rights, meaning that SLTs should ensure that such disorders do not preclude opportunities for self-determination, fulfilment and participation in community life.

● Intervention aims to make communication and eating/drinking as positive an experience as possible.

● Speech and language therapy values and incorporates all means of communication within intervention planning.

Standards and guidance around management phase

Planning options
A management plan should be established in conjunction with the individual and/or key people in the client's life whenever possible and appropriate.

Physical and/or sensory impairment should not restrict consideration of AAC systems given the advances in technology, however in some cases such disability may be a significant barrier.

An individual, their family and the team should be provided with all relevant and necessary information pertaining to the rationale behind the intervention programmes in order to make informed decisions regarding their care.

Written consent should be obtained when intervention involves:
● heightened levels of risk (for example, invasive procedures)
● participating in teaching or research projects
● photographic or audio-visual recordings of the individual
● where a client is unable to give consent, this should be sought from legally authorised parties

All written and spoken information should be clear and accessible to the recipients.

To include carers whose preferred language is not English, the services of an appropriately bilingual therapist or SLT co-worker may be required. Where this is not possible, interpreting and translation services should be used. This will require time in the session for briefing and de-briefing the interpreter.

Where the care is provided as part of a multi-professional approach, management plans may also be multidisciplinary.

Where many professionals are involved with an individual, one named person will take the role of coordinating the assessment and management amongst a large and sometimes geographically fragmented group. In this situation, speech and language therapy should be provided in conjunction with the key support person.

If appropriate and agreed with the individual, the speech and language therapy management plan will be shared with members of the multi-professional team.

The management plan will take account of the individual's environment and priorities and, in the case of children, the priorities of the carer **and will be made available to the client within two weeks of the completion of the assessment process.**

Setting aims as part of the management process

Aims should derive from a consideration of the individual's needs and wishes as well as the therapist's opinion based on comprehensive assessment and reference to the evidence base. Therapists will advise on what is likely to be achievable in the short and long-term taking all the relevant factors into account. This may involve:

● resolving a particular aspect of communicative/swallowing function
● achieving optimal improvement of function (as estimated by taking all factors into account)
● maintaining optimal function, for example, through the use of compensatory strategies
● enabling increased independence through making changes within the individual's environment
● avoiding the development of secondary difficulties

In support of this the therapist may, with the individual, plan to work on one or more of the following aims, to:

● enable the individual/carer to access relevant systems/services/learning environment

- optimise participation in educational, social, work and recreational activities as appropriate
- inform others about the nature of the impairment and the process of intervention
- advise and assist the individual/others in the use of facilitative strategies
- help maximise the individual's communication/eating and drinking skill development
- recommend an appropriate augmentative communication system as appropriate and enable its use
- train others in the use of supportive strategies or teaching tasks
- provide information for individual/carer on the possibility of further difficulties
- advise on ways of preventing the development of further difficulties
- advise on risk reduction
- support the individual/carer in coping optimally with the present condition
- help the individual/carer come to terms with difficulties
- implement an agreed programme of therapy/intervention, whether directly or indirectly through training and advising other agents to conduct a specific programme (which an SLT will monitor and adjust as necessary)
- continue to discuss ultimate goal and discharge criteria

Where appropriate, for example, in the context of a deteriorating condition, the following aims may apply:
- to work with and through others in support of the individual in order to maintain stability and prevent deterioration for as long as possible
- to advise on risk reduction
- to provide the individual with strategies to maintain stability
- to support the individual and carers in coping with a sudden or a slowly deteriorating condition
- to provide physical, psychological and social support as part of the team

Setting goals as part of the management process
The individual management plan should involve establishing clearly defined goals of intervention.
The plan will include goals that are:
- centred on the needs and wishes of the individual
- relevant
- agreed with the individual wherever possible

- specific
- achievable
- measurable
- time limited
- recorded in the notes
- reviewed at an agreed time

Where the individual's condition is changing, goals will take account of the rate of change.

Factors within the individual's environment which influence communication and/or swallowing may be the focus of intervention.

Outcomes of intervention

The SLT will decide how outcomes for the individual will be ascertained and should make sure baseline measures are detailed.

Timing of intervention

A time frame for the plan should be specified.

Ways of working with the individual

Models of delivery include:
- individual input: direct or indirect, (ie working with and through others)
- group therapy
- review appointments for advice, support and monitoring. This may be in the context of specialist clinics or support groups
- joint sessions with other professionals/workers
- carer education and training
- consultation/liaison services
- carer support groups
- workshops and training sessions for people who may then act as agents of change

Intervention involves giving advice, making recommendations, leading therapy activities, as well as providing support and education for the individual, their family, carers and the multidisciplinary team. Carers may be the legitimate focus of intervention.

Review and discharge procedures should be discussed as part of the management plan

The agreed plan of action should be made clear within the case notes, dated and signed.

Continuity of management

As appropriate, and with the consent of the individual, the SLT will ensure that any other agency involved with the individual is kept informed of speech and language therapy involvement.

Wherever possible, care should continue until it has been established that optimal recovery or function has been achieved.

Care is often episodic in nature. Where there are several episodes in a care pathway, particular attention should be paid to ensure that the individual and parents feel clear about the process.

6.3.5 Review phase

Purpose of review

● To allow time for independent management of difficulties as appropriate.
● To allow for key support role to be taken by others.
● To allow for consolidation of skill development.
● To allow natural course of development to occur.
● To allow for other, medical or social, priorities to be addressed by others.
● To wait for optimum time for intervention.

Standards and guidance related to review phase

Although continuous monitoring is an integral part of intervention, a formal review may take place at any point in the therapeutic process and be used to:

● gauge the outcomes of intervention
● gauge the appropriateness and effectiveness of intervention
● monitor the pattern of progress
● consider the need for further investigations or, in some cases, instrumental assessments
● terminate intervention
● determine the need for further intervention in response to changes in the client's ability/circumstances/personal goals
● determine the next step
● agree a different focus for therapy
● agree a different pattern of intervention
● decide on timing of review/reassessment periods for maintenance of gains

- re-evaluate assistive devices as appropriate
- provide further support and information to individuals and carers as appropriate
- provide a second opinion

When an individual is undergoing a period of self-managing their condition, the individual or an identified key worker/carer, may be given the responsibility to ask for a review appointment.

Review of intervention may include repeat assessments to evaluate progress. A review time frame should be agreed when initiating this process.

In the case of specialist cleft services, formal reassessments are required for audit records at five, 10 and 15 years of age.

At key times during the period of intervention, the SLT will ensure that any other agency involved with the individual is kept informed about management and progress made, with consent from the individual/carer.

6.3.6 Discharge/transition/transfer phase

Purpose of transition phase towards discharge/transfer:

- To agree a point of closure with individual/carer. NB This may be a team decision and should be part of a unified, person-centred, care planning approach.
- To support the individual through the process of ending therapy.
- To carry out local discharge procedure, including providing information about referral back into the service.
- To communicate results of episodes of care to relevant others.
- To inform individual/carer of routes for re-referral should it be necessary and of further support agencies and services.
- In the context of transfer from a specialist speech and language therapy provision to a local speech and language therapy service, to provide information regarding individual and care received and specialist advice as required.
- To help individuals feel empowered to self-manage any needs that no longer require ongoing intervention.
- To evaluate the degree to which the aims and goals have been met and explore reasons for variance.

Standards and guidance related to discharge phase/transition towards self-management/transfer to a specialist provision

● Discharge will be at the discretion of the SLT after full consultation and agreement with the patient/client and carer.

● Discharge may be initiated by the SLT or at the request of the individual or, where appropriate, the carer.

● SLT initiated discharge may be for a number of reasons. These may include:

● aims of intervention have been achieved

● communication and/or swallowing issues are no longer a priority

● the individual has reached a point where they are able to self-manage their condition

● the individual will be transferring to specialist care

● individual non-compliance

● intervention not indicated at the present time

● the individual has failed to attend appointments and will therefore be discharged in accordance with local policy and, in the case of children, with due respect to child protection implications

● Where discharge is initiated by the SLT, the reasons for this will be explained fully to the individual and the carer.

● Where discharge is initiated by the individual/carer, the SLT must explain any risks resulting from this course of action, together with information about the re-referral route to speech and language therapy.

● When the individual receives input from a multi-professional team, discharge procedures will take into consideration those agreed by the team.

● As appropriate, and with the agreement of the individual/carer, the SLT will consult with other professionals involved with the individual prior to discharge.

● The decision and reason to discharge will be recorded in the notes.

● Where appropriate, carers and staff should be familiar with strategies for continuing the emphasis on maximising communication in the client's environment after discharge.

● A report will be completed at the point of discharge/transition and included in the case notes. This may include:

● details of initial communication status, including any communication disorder diagnosis

● medical and social details

- medication
- summary intervention including aims, goals and objectives
- principles of supporting communication
- items needing to be reviewed including AAC, hearing aids
- progress since assessment, including any influencing factors, such as medication or temperament
- reason for discharge
- guidance on re-referral
- any arrangements for crisis support
- recommendations for other services taking over intervention/providing support
- a clause indicating that the individual may be contacted in the future for service evaluation purposes
- A discharge report should be sent to the individual or, in the case of children, to the carers within three weeks of the point of discharge/transition.
- With the knowledge of the individual or, in the case of children, with the knowledge of the carers, copies of the discharge report should be sent to relevant others including the individual's GP.
- It may be appropriate for this to be a uni-professional SLT report or to be a report from the team.
- The individual should be made aware of relevant national societies, voluntary organisations and local groups for support of ongoing needs.
- For some client groups, individuals and carers need to understand that re-referral may be necessary during major life transitions.
- Duty of care to the individual is terminated through completion of the discharge procedure or, in the case of an individual being transferred to another service, the duty of care will rest with the new service.

References

Department of Health. *NSF for children, young people and maternity services*, 2004. www.dh.gov.uk
Department of Health. *Prevention and health, everybody's business: A reassessment of public and personal health*, 1976. www.dh.gov.uk
RCSLT. *Accountability for Professional Advice Given to Non-registered Patients*, 2005.

RCSLT. *Working in Harmony*, 2005. www.rcslt.org
RCSLT. *Returners Pack*, 2005. www.rcslt.org

Acts of Parliament
Data Protection Act, 1998
Mental Health Act, 1983

Chapter 7

Service Provision: Part 2 Working Contexts, Tasks, Techniques and Strategies

7.1 Guidance related to Working Contexts

The following working contexts have been identified as key for SLTs:
- **Integrated teams**.
- **Community:** Level 2 services, eg Sure Start; Level 3 services, eg homes, work, leisure and day opportunities.
- **Primary and secondary healthcare environments**, eg community clinics; GP practices; acute hospitals; outpatient departments.
- **Specialist healthcare settings**, eg secure units; rehabilitation centres; hospices; forensic services, mental health services; autism spectrum disorder units/services; child development centres.
- **Education**, eg pre-school facilities; schools; colleges of further education; adult education.
- **Independent practice**.

7.1.1 Integrated teams

In line with government strategy, many SLTs now work in multi-agency teams, which may include health, education and local authority staff.

Integrated teams may be multidisciplinary or inter-disciplinary and may be line-managed by non-health staff. This may have a significant impact on models of caseload management and prioritisation.

It is recognised that integrated and coordinated working across community and acute settings is the most effective approach to supporting individuals with health needs (DH, 2004; 2005). This is supported by integrated team working, where liaison, joint working/visits, sharing information, joint planning and understanding of others' roles ensure an holistic approach is adopted.

Input should occur in the most natural and comfortable setting for the individual. This may be the home environment or educational/day opportunities, leisure and work environments accessed by the individual on a regular basis. Alternatively, hospital or specialist centres may be the most appropriate context for support.

SLTs should familiarise themselves with environmental policies and procedures when working across a range of community and acute settings. In particular they should familiarise themselves with strategies of risk management and health and safety procedures.

The context for SLT working continues to change in line with government policy. Therapists need to keep up to date with these changes and understand the likely impact on working practice.

7.1.2 Community

Level 2 community services (for targeted at-risk groups)

Speech, language, communication and swallowing difficulties can be exacerbated or ameliorated by certain lifestyle choices and factors within the environment, including the responses of others to the individual. These issues are dealt with by a range of strategies, including health promotion and working with others on developing supportive and inclusive practice.

For example, pre-schoolers in areas of high economic deprivation are at risk of speech, language and communication difficulties that will impact on their social development and learning in school. Speech and language therapy services form part of the government 'Sure Start' programme and are provided primarily through working in local activities set up to meet the health and social needs of families in a given geographical area.

For further information see Chapter 6, Level 2 services.

Level 3 community services (for referred individuals)

Level 3 community services are those offered to individuals in their own homes, whether this is the family home, a residential/group home, supported living accommodation or a nursing home, and other community settings for example, work, leisure activities, shops, etc.

Services may be provided by one team but link in with other agencies, in order to provide an overall management approach. These services include:

● Specialist community neuro teams providing rehabilitation and support in the home and local environment (provided by specialist community neuro-rehabilitation teams).

● Outreach from specialist centres.

● Generic community teams providing rehabilitation and support to people with many different conditions in the home or local environment (DH, 2001b; 2005).

Through offering services to people in their own environments community input can be directed at specific problems in context and as identified by the individual and carer. Thus addressing the restrictions they experience in daily living, maintaining their optimum independence and enabling social participation. This is supported by the recommendations in the NSF both for long-term conditions and specifically for stroke individuals (DH, 2005, 2001).

Input is often individual led and incorporates approaches to facilitate maintenance of independence and function, quality of life and participation in life roles.

Joint visiting/working may be appropriate to ensure individuals receive holistic care and multidisciplinary input, for example, a physiotherapist and SLT assessing positioning and swallowing management. This may also cross service boundaries, for example, social services and voluntary organisations.

The GP and all disciplines involved with the individuals, for example, social worker, district nurse, allied health professionals (AHPs) should be kept informed of the plan for intervention.

SLTs must be aware of and comply with organisational guidance related to:

- risk assessment
- risk management including personal safety strategies
- cultural considerations and respect for the individual's home environment
- dealing with challenging behaviour
- medical emergencies, eg if an individual suffers an epileptic fit
- visiting at appropriate and convenient times
- child and adult protection

For further information see 5.6 Management of Risk, with particular reference to 5.6.5 Personal safety.

Supported living/group homes

A service provided to individuals living in homes of their own or in group homes with the support of care staff. A range of therapeutic services may be provided to the individuals.

SLTs should recognise that this location of service delivery is first and foremost the individual's home.

Training of and liaison with all levels of staff is a priority.

Day opportunities

Day opportunities refer to any daytime occupations that are engaged in by an individual. For the SLT it will involve input into a wide range of community settings which are accessed by the individual either independently or with support, (eg leisure centres, work places, day services).

The focus of the SLT input is to enable staff to work effectively with people with communication and/or eating and drinking needs. Speech and language therapy will be affected by the purpose and organisational culture of the service provider but is likely to be consultation and training based, time limited and negotiated around mutually agreed outcomes for either the communication environment or for individuals.

Intermediate care

Intermediate care links with the services described above but provides the opportunity for speech and language therapists to work across acute and community settings.

Introduced in the *NHS Plan,* 2000b, intermediate care services are designed to provide a new range of services to build a bridge between hospital and home. The policy was developed to promote the independence of older people through a range of services to be delivered in partnership between primary and secondary healthcare, local government services, social care and the independent sector (DH, 2001a).

Intermediate care services should (DH, 2001b):

● Target people who would otherwise face unnecessarily prolonged hospital stays or inappropriate admission to acute patient care, long-term residential care or continuing NHS inpatient care.

● Be provided on the basis of a comprehensive assessment resulting in a structured individual care plan that involves active therapy, treatment or opportunity for recovery.

● Have a planned outcome of maximising independence and typically enabling the individual to resume living at home.

● Be time limited, normally no longer than six weeks and frequently as little as one to two weeks or less.

● Involve cross professional working with a single assessment framework, single professional records and shared protocols.

Service models include:

- Rapid response – to prevent avoidable acute admissions.
- Hospital at home – intensive support in the individual's own home.
- Residential rehabilitation – short stay, short-term rehabilitation in residential setting care home/community hospital.
- Supported discharge – short-term period of nursing/therapy package in the individual's own home.
- Day rehabilitation – short-term programme in day hospital/day centre.

More information is available on the following websites:
- Department of Health www.dh.gov.uk
- The King's Fund www.kingsfund.org.uk
- The Change Agent Team www.changeagentteam.org.uk

7.1.3 Primary and secondary healthcare environments

Many SLTs work within or interface with aspects of primary and secondary healthcare.

Example 1: Acute hospitals

Speech and language therapy services may be provided in a hospital setting to both inpatients and outpatients. Outreach services may also be provided in association with primary healthcare and education teams.

The SLT based in a hospital has the responsibility of representing the needs of individuals with communication/swallowing problems to the multidisciplinary team. This will involve liaising effectively with all the professionals involved, both on-site and off-site during the acute episode of care, including facilitating and coordinating transition of care to the next stage of intervention.

Example 2: Community clinics

A service delivered from a community clinic/health centre to the local population, where the speech and language needs of the individual can be met most efficiently and effectively by services provided in local settings.

As attendance at a community clinic/health centre is a routine part of the well-person's lifestyle, it is essential that the SLT working in such a location actively seeks out the other professionals who are relevant to the individual at the time of the speech and language therapy referral.

The establishment and maintenance of these relationships are paramount to the holistic multidisciplinary approach to the individual's needs. By definition, the individual attending clinic is part of the community 'at large' and therefore there is no finite list of professionals with whom the SLT will liaise.

It is incumbent upon the SLT, as part of the assessment procedure, to identify other professionals with whom formal/informal contact must be made. Contact may be made in writing, by phone or by face-to-face contact and is facilitated by attendance at primary healthcare team meetings, liaison committees, etc.

Example 3: Hospices

A residential and/or day care unit where individuals may go for periods of care/support and/or respite care. Individuals may choose to be in a hospice during the palliative care stage of their illness. SLTs will manage communication and swallowing problems regardless of aetiology and whether the problems are transient, persistent or progressive.

SLTs will focus on rehabilitative and supportive care for the individual and their family, aiming to achieve optimum quality of life. This will be done in the context of close collaboration with other members of the team. Decisions regarding management and quality of life will all be taken in partnership with others, bearing in mind the rapidly changing circumstances and the fact that these individuals may be facing end-of-life issues.

Example 4: Services to critical care

Critical care refers to the level of care given to a group of individuals who are deemed to be critically ill.

The division into high dependency and intensive care services based on beds, is now replaced by a classification (Intensive Care Society, 2002) that focuses on the level of care that individual's need, regardless of location (DH, 2000a).

Level 0

Individuals whose needs can be met through normal ward care in an acute hospital.

Level 1

Individuals at risk of their condition deteriorating, or those recently relocated from higher levels of care whose needs can be met on an acute ward with additional advice and support from the critical care team.

Level 2
Individuals requiring detailed observation or intervention including support for a single failing organ system or postoperative care, and those 'stepping down' from higher levels of care.

Level 3
Individuals requiring advanced respiratory support alone or basic respiratory support together with support of at least two organ systems. This level includes all complex individuals requiring support for multi-organ failure.

Many individuals who are critically ill have requirements for the support for their neurological, respiratory and digestive systems, all of which can impact on their ability to communicate and swallow independently. Presence of technologies to prolong life/enable clinical management of the individuals with critical illness such as mechanical ventilation, tracheostomy tubes, naso-gastric tubes and naso-pharyngeal airways as these may also impact on communication and oro-pharyngeal swallowing abilities.

For more information on the role of speech and language therapy, see section 8.10 on Critical Care.

Example 5: Services to palliative care
Palliative care is an approach that improves the quality of life of individuals and their families facing the problems associated with life-threatening illness, through prevention and relief of suffering by means of early identification and impeccable assessment and treatment of pain and other problems, physical, psychosocial and spiritual (WHO, 2006).

For more information on the role of speech and language therapy, see section 8.17 on Palliative Care.

7.1.4. Specialist health services
Specialist health services are dedicated healthcare services to a particular individual group with defined specialist health needs and approaches to treatment.

SLTs need to be effective at working as part of the specialist healthcare team, whilst maintaining a broad perspective. The SLT may be working as a lone SLT practitioner. Regular SLT liaison and support networks should be sought to prevent professional isolation.

Example 1: Child development centre
A specialist multidisciplinary assessment and diagnostic centre for children and their carers.
This assessment results in the evolution of an individual centred plan of care to meet the child's identified needs. The centre may provide an assessment or assessment and intervention service.
Due to the multidisciplinary nature of child development centres, the SLT will work in close collaboration with all team members by attending team meetings and case conferences.
The SLT may act as a key worker for particular children with whom she/he is centrally involved.

Example 2: Rehabilitation centre
A centre that exists to provide intensive therapeutic rehabilitation to a designated individual group. The rehabilitation centre may be a local provision or a regional specialist centre.
Services are offered to enable individuals to reach their potential and therefore maximise their long-term functioning. The therapeutic services are provided within an inter-disciplinary framework.
In most instances, the individuals are medically stable and may be at any stage in their recovery.

Example 3: Specialist outpatient centre
Specialist outpatient referral centres provide services to individuals where a further opinion has been requested by the individual, carer, SLT or other professionals.
The SLT at a specialist centre will need to consider what additional value speech and language therapy within the centre offers compared to that provided in local or other settings.
Only if an individual is considered to be able to make greater progress within a specialist centre and funding has been agreed, should therapy be offered within that location. If intervention is to be offered in a local setting, the local service must ensure that recommendations made can be effectively implemented and the specialist centre informed of the position.

When the individual is discharged from the specialist centre it is likely that intervention may be continued at a local location. The SLT at the specialist centre will need to liaise with the local SLT to ensure continuing care and to ensure that the individual/carer is informed about and prepared for any changes in the models of care.
However, it may be that shared care, with ongoing support from a specialist tertiary centre, may be the most effective way of providing support for the individual.

7.1.5 Education

Education includes all contexts that provide educational opportunities and courses, including children's centres and extended schools. Whilst taking account of individual need, educational contexts are primarily curriculum focused. Therapists need to provide integrated and inclusive services that promote access to learning opportunities and the development of functional social relationships.

Example 1: Pre-school facilities

A day provision that is exclusively for pre-school children. Facilities may include social service/health service day nurseries, educational day nurseries, neighbourhood centres, opportunity playgroups and state and independent day nurseries.
Pre-school facilities may vary greatly according to working philosophy, ratio of staff to children, turn-over of staff, qualifications and training of staff.
The linguistic diversity of the provision will also vary, as will the length of stay and type of placement for each child. As a result, the SLT will need to familiarise her/himself with the particular context.
The SLT will need to liaise with the key worker for the child and the head of the service to negotiate an appropriate model of working. Ongoing liaison with all members of the team for the child will be important in maintaining integrated support services.

Example 2: Mainstream schools

A service delivered within a mainstream school to children who need support for and development of their communication skills.
Speech and language therapy in a mainstream school is a specialist service and not simply a speech and language therapy 'clinic' located in a school.

Services should be provided in such a way as to enable education staff to incorporate the aims of speech and language therapy in the planning of an individual educational programme within the context of the broad curriculum.

Intervention will include facilitating access to the National Curriculum/the 5-14 Curriculum and supporting staff to make environmental changes to support inclusion. This is most effective through collaborative working strategies including joint assessment, planning and working, as well as through training workshops, provided as part of the school in-service training (INSET) programme.

Example 3: Special schools and resourced provision

A speech and language therapy service provided to a special educational establishment or resourced provision for children with statements of special educational needs/additional support needs. The children's primary educational needs may be the result of a specific speech and language disorder or may be the result of general learning and/or physical difficulties.

The service is usually based within the school and operates at different levels:

● Level 1: Working with the whole school body to identify and implement school improvement objectives related to meeting the needs of children's speech, language, communication and/or swallowing needs.

This will usually involve being a member of task-groups; participating in, or leading, in-service training sessions.

● Level 2: Supporting individual members of staff or staff groups to make environmental changes to optimise the inclusion of all children within class activities. This will usually involve joint-planning, co-working and training sessions and will take account of the highly developed expertise of staff working in these settings.

● Level 3: Collaborating with staff and parents to review the progress of individual children; to advise and to provide intervention as appropriate. This will usually involve joint goal setting, agreeing strategies and planning for how speech and language therapy targets can be integrated into the child's daily life activities in school and at home. Certain children may need regular and continuing help from an SLT, either individually or in a group. In other cases, it may be appropriate for staff at the child's school to deliver a regular and discrete programme of intervention under the guidance of an SLT. Intervention includes supporting the development of children's functional communication; facilitating children's access to the school curriculum and supporting staff in their use of inclusive strategies. Effective practice will be facilitated by the SLT being seen as part of the school team and, where possible, attending staff and parent meetings.

For further information see chapter 8 on Working with Specific Client Groups.

7.1.6 Independent practice

A growing number of SLTs are self-employed or work as part of an independent group practice. The RCSLT advocates that all therapists who practise independently are members of the Association of Speech and Language Therapists in Independent Practice (ASLTIP).

Members of ASLTIP are certified members of the RCSLT and are registered with the HPC. Membership of ASLTIP represents a commitment to agreed standards of professional conduct and performance within independent practice.

Regular SLT liaison and support networks should be sought to prevent professional isolation.

See section 5.3.3.on Supervision and Supporting Staff and 5.3.9 on CPD.

An independent practitioner should have at least two years' recent post-qualification clinical experience before practising independently. Therapists running large independent practices may employ newly qualified therapists.

For further guidance on recommended procedures see 5.3.4 on Competence and the NQP.

If an SLT has had a break from professional practice of over two years and wishes to practise independently, she/he should satisfy the requirements of the HPC and the RCSLT. SLTs who have not practised professionally for more than two years should apply to become a returner member of the RCSLT. This status is held for a year prior to transfer to the full membership list.

The RCSLT's *Returners Pack* is available at: www.rcslt.org

See also the 5.3.4 section on Competence and returners to practice.

Ethics of independent practice

Practitioners should observe the courtesy of contacting all established independent practitioners within an area when intending to establish a new independent practice.

An SLT, on leaving a group practice, should not canvass individuals who were referred to that practice to move with them.

For further guidance on setting up in independent practice, refer to the ASLTIP website: www.helpwithtalking.com

Independent practice management

Practitioners should take steps to protect themselves from suspicion of unethical conduct by careful consideration of their activities. SLTs who have any current NHS involvement with a particular individual may not undertake the private management of that case.

Independent practitioners should also pay serious consideration to the following:

- clinical record keeping
- practitioners should register under the Data Protection Act (1998)
- emergency procedures
- premises and equipment
- legal and business protection, contracts
- advertising and marketing

See 5.5.3 on Record keeping and 5.6 on Management of Risk.

The practice should define its scope and objectives, and make this clear in any literature describing the practice. Account should be taken of the responsibility of practitioners to offer assessment and management only in areas where adequate clinical experience has been gained.

The practice should publish terms and conditions of therapy and scale of charges. Details should include information on any additional charges for the provision of reports and mileage charges for home visits. This information should be made available to prospective and actual individuals before the initial consultation, so there is full awareness of expectations for fee settlement and what constitutes a therapy session, in terms of duration and content.

After initial assessment, individuals should be given, where possible, a cost and time estimate for therapy.

Practitioners should ensure that accurate accounts and receipts are kept of all individual and practice transactions, and that those records necessary for annual financial audit are in place.

The practice or practitioner should consider implementing a quality assurance programme. This provides a systematic way of evaluating the quality of services provided and offers an opportunity to address identified weaknesses. Practices are advised to undertake regular internal audits to include examination of administrative and clinical procedures.

This may involve the practitioner requesting a liaison agreement with a senior NHS therapist to discuss service and professional issues. ASLTIP strongly advises that members actively seek this type of arrangement to promote cooperation between service providers. These recommendations should not interfere with the independent practitioner's right to provide services that may differ in style and organisation from those provided by NHS employed counterparts. For further information on service audit, see Chapter 9 Service Monitoring, Improvement, Evaluation and Development.

Interface with members of the team, including other SLTs

SLTs in independent practice should be aware of the need to liaise fully with other professionals who may also be working with the individual.

See 5.9 Partnership Working and 5.9.1 Interface between speech and language therapy agencies and the RCSLT *Working in Harmony* document, available at: www.rcslt.org

Communication with the individual's medical practitioner should be maintained at appropriate stages of the intervention. The therapist should send a communication stating that an initial consultation has taken place and outline the planned course of action arising from this. A note of discharge should follow when applicable.

Independent practitioners should advise the appropriate speech and language therapy service of the names of any individuals being seen, although due consideration must be taken of individual circumstances. In certain instances, for example where an individual seeks a confidential second opinion, the practitioner should make discretionary decisions in order to act in their individual's best interests. Serious and due consideration of the possibility of test score invalidation and any deleterious effects of possible dual involvement should be borne in mind in such circumstances.

In summary, recommended good practice is notification to health service departments. In discretionary circumstances the procedure may be circumvented. In these instances the therapist may consider requiring the individual to sign an insertion to their records agreeing or requesting that the consultation remains confidential to the practice.

It is recommended good practice to advise individuals of the availability of speech and language therapy within the health service, to avoid situations where a member of the public may be unaware of the existence of statutory provision. Beyond this, independent practitioners should avoid involvement in discussions relating to the levels and merits of local provision.

Where it is considered in the individual's best interests to receive professional help from two practitioners, one must undertake the lead role in the coordination of case management. This responsibility should be delegated after discussion, and steps should be taken to clarify with the individual the nature of the arrangement that has been reached.

Written permission to circulate reports should be obtained from the individual. Practitioners may decide to recommend the sharing of information in a covering letter, but leave the responsibility to do so with the individual.

7.2 Guidance related to Specific Speech and Language Therapy Tasks, Techniques and Strategies

7.2.1 Augmentative and alternative communication

Communication may be defined as the transmission and reception of meaning between one individual and another, or between an individual and a group – where 'meaning' is taken to include social and affective intentions and reactions, as well as propositional content. The mode or medium of the exchange (speech, non-verbal signals, symbols, signs, writing, electronic code, etc) does not alter this definition of the central essence of communication.

Augmentative and alternative communication (AAC) refers to methods of communicating which supplement or replace speech and handwriting. The term refers to a function, not to any specific communication systems or methods. In practice, augmentations and alternatives to speech often overlap and go together, but it should be recognised that they are not interchangeable terms.

AAC is a means by which an individual can supplement or replace spoken communication. Communication may range from any movement or behaviour which is observed and interpreted by another person as meaningful, to the use of a code agreed upon between people where items have specific meanings, ie a language.

AAC encompasses various types of communication, both aided and unaided systems. Unaided communication refers to the use of systems involving the user's body, such as body movements, facial expressions, gestures, signing, eye-pointing and vocalisations. Aided systems refers to the use of additional resources and/or equipment, such as objects, photographs, symbols and voice-output communication aids (VOCAs).

AAC includes four strands:

i) Communication medium – how the meaning of the message is being transmitted. This might be via aided or unaided systems.

ii) A means of access to the communication medium, through hand/eye pointing, a keyboard, joystick, switches for direct selection/switch accessing.

iii) A system of representing meanings, ideas and concepts, eg signs (British Sign Language, Signalong, Makaton Vocabulary, etc) and/or symbols (Picture Communication Symbols, Widgit Rebus, Makaton Vocabulary, Blissymbols, traditional orthography, etc).

iv) Strategies for interacting, eg initiating conversations, maintaining a conversation by turn-taking and using questions, repair strategies when communication breaks down.

Use of AAC in relation to client groups

The use of AAC is not exclusive to one client group, but is a strategy that can be used by individuals with significant communication difficulties, irrespective of the aetiology.

It is not possible to provide figures for the numbers of individuals who require AAC as they do not come from any one identifiable individual group.

However, the most common congenital conditions likely to require

this type of support are cerebral palsy, autism, learning difficulties and developmental apraxia of speech (Mirenda & Mathy-Laikko, 1989).
To obtain an idea of the incidence and prevalence for conditions that may require individuals to have access to AAC/total communication, see the following sections on specific client groups described in chapter 8:

8.1 Acquired Motor Speech Disorders
8.2 Adult Learning Disability
8.3 Aphasia
8.4 Autism Spectrum Disorder
8.6 Brain Injury
8.7 Cerebral Palsy
8.10 Critical Care
8.11 Deafness
8.12 Dysfluency
8.15 Head and Neck Cancer
8.17 Palliative Care
8.18 Pre-school Children
8.19 Progressive Neurological Disorders
8.20 School-aged Children
8.21 Specific Language Impairment
8.22 Specific Speech Impairment

Some individuals who require AAC/total communication will use AAC and total communication throughout their lives; others will only need to use some of these tools for a limited time as their underlying condition and skills change, improve or develop. There is no research to provide figures.

Prevalence of use of AAC

The following points give a general idea of the number of people requiring access to AAC/total communication at some point in their lives.

There have been several studies carried out in America (Beukelman & Ansel, 1995; Blackstone & Painter, 1985; Matas et al, 1995) including one that identified 0.4% of the population as having AAC needs.

In reviewing the research from America and the UK, it can be concluded that there is an estimated range of 0.3-1.4% of the total population who require the use of AAC systems.

AAC within the school population

A 1990 estimate of 0.2-0.6% of the total school population requiring the use of AAC (Blackstone, 1990) has been considered to be a conservative figure by today's expectations, considering advancing technology. However, this estimation is in line with the figures presented below:

● A survey of the special schools and mainstream schools in 11 London boroughs, estimated that the prevalence of the need for AAC systems was in excess of 10% of all statemented children (0.3% of the total school population) – (Norwich & Grove, 1997).

This is supported by 2003 Department for Education and Skills (DfES) figures, which indicate that at least 0.2 % of children have a long-term communication difficulty.

Risk issues

Individuals requiring AAC may be at risk of the following, if the introduction of AAC is delayed. Reduced opportunities for:
● social interaction
● control of one's environment
● development/restoration of language skills
● initiating communication
● learning
● developing of life skills
● participating in education/employment

This may result in:
● lack of/loss of identity
● depression
● passivity
● reduced learning opportunities
● increased isolation
● increased risk of harm/abuse
● failure to develop skills to full potential, resulting in many lost life opportunities

If the SLT does not work as part of a multi/inter-disciplinary team and/or has minimal knowledge of AAC/total communication, individuals are at risk of the following:
● provision of an inappropriate communication system
● inappropriate use of a communication system

- inappropriate access system
- unsafe and/or ineffective mounting of VOCA

This may:
- restrict language development/restoration
- restrict opportunities for interaction and communication
- prevent effective control of one's environment
- prevent/restrict participation in education
- possibly lead to physical damage due to poor positioning/access

Failure to develop skills commensurate with abilities, can lead to reduced opportunities for:
- social interaction
- effective control of one's environment
- developing language skills
- initiating communication
- learning
- development of life skills
- participation in education/employment

This may result in:
- loss of identity
- depression
- passivity
- increased isolation
- increased risk of harm/abuse
- failure to develop skills to full potential resulting in many lost life opportunities

SLT responsibilities in relation to AAC equipment:
- **Safety checks**: are essential to ensure that the equipment is well maintained and any problems are resolved before the problem becomes more severe.
- **Decontamination**: equipment must be kept clean and decontaminated. There should be guidance for each piece of equipment and appropriate wipes available.

Care pathway
Further details of the AAC care pathway, outlined below and developed by the South Birmingham PCT, can be accessed at:
www.wmrc.nhs.uk/act/AAC_pathdocs.html

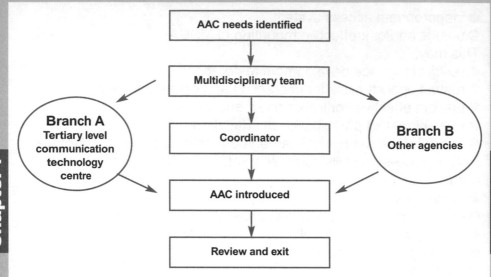

Key sources of additional information and support on AAC:
● ACE Centre Advisory Trust www.ace-centre.org.uk
● The CALL Centre www.callcentre.education.ed.ac.uk
● Communicability www.communicability.smartchange.org

7.2.2 Counselling

What is counselling?

Counselling may be thought of as the process through which an individual is assisted to make a decision from the many choices available in an understanding and confidential atmosphere.
Individuals are encouraged to express their thoughts and feelings in order to understand their feelings and to clarify their situation so that they can come to terms with a difficulty more objectively and with a reduction in anxiety and tension.
Counselling has developed as a branch of psychological clinical practice, offering a range of therapeutic communication skills, and also has its own knowledge base and body of human science research. It is therefore a profession in its own right.

Regulatory bodies for counsellors:
● British Association of Counselling and Psychotherapy
www.bacp.co.uk

- UK Council for Psychotherapy www.psychotherapy.org.uk
- British Confederation of Psychotherapists www.bcp.org.uk

Counselling skills within speech and language therapy

Use of counselling skills (as opposed to being a counsellor) relates to where there is intentional use of specific interpersonal skills that reflect the values of counselling, and when the practitioner's primary role (for example, SLT or support practitioner) is enhanced without being changed.

Thus the individual perceives the practitioner as acting within their primary professional or/caring role, which is not that of being a counsellor.

Counselling is part of the SLT's repertoire of clinical skills. The extent to which a counselling approach is adopted will depend on the needs of the particular individual in the therapeutic process.

It may be appropriate for the SLT to use counselling skills to address emotional issues brought up by individuals, providing the issues are related to the communication disorder.

Standards and guidance in relation to use of counselling skills

All SLTs should have undertaken basic training in counselling, listening and communication skills.

Counselling should be part of a holistic approach to intervention for a communication disorder.

All SLTs should have access to support and clinical supervision. See 5.3.3 Staff supervision and support.

Where counselling skills are used as a main therapeutic approach, it is vital that:
- the focus of therapy is explained and agreed with the individual at the outset of the contract
- the SLT has undertaken a postgraduate counselling skills course
- the SLT has enhanced access to clinical supervision and support

SLTs using counselling skills as a primary therapeutic intervention must ensure that their manager is fully aware of their practice and that this is reflected in their job description.

If advanced postgraduate counselling skills are essential for the job, then the grade as well as the job description should reflect this responsibility.

SLTs considering an advanced counselling training should have an experience of personal therapy themselves and also an opportunity to role play an individual via experiential learning.

SLTs should not pass on information gained during counselling to colleagues without the individual's permission.

If the SLT feels uncomfortable in a counselling role, supervision may either clarify the need to refer the individual on, or eliminate the need. The SLT may have the appropriate skills but lack confidence.

All SLTs should be aware of the limits of their competence in the counsellor role, and should refer on if necessary.

The SLT needs to be sensitive to the fact that suggesting the individual needs to be referred on can give the impression that the individual's problem is too big for either the SLT or the individual to cope with.

SLTs should inform individuals of the number of sessions they can have, and they should prepare individuals for their last session, rather than it be presented suddenly. It may be advisable to recommend that the individual can return for an SLT review after a course of counselling.

SLTs may need to consider whether it is the individual who has difficulty leaving therapy or the SLT's own difficulty about letting go of an individual.

Some agencies for referring individuals on to:
- GP
- child and adolescent mental health service
- psychology or psychiatry department
- some voluntary bodies employ counsellors, but their training may vary

7.2.3 Writing legal statements relating to court inquiries

What is a statement?
A statement is an accurate account of a person or professional's involvement with an individual adult, child or family for a professional reason during the course of undertaking their duties.

Who might request a statement?
- the employing authority

- a solicitor
- a social worker
- a guardian ad litem (an officer appointed by the court to represent the interests of the child)
- others

Principles:
- The statement should be truthful, accurate and factual.
- The facts should, to the best knowledge of the therapist, be verifiable.
- The statement should be made from the records.

Standards and guidance related to providing a statement

Before making a statement, the professional should first establish the employing authority's policy for professionals making a statement. This will usually include contacting a line manager in the first instance.

When writing a statement, the following format should be followed:
- date of statement
- name, professional address and qualifications, position and employing authority
- name, address and relationship of family and member/s about whom the statement is written
- the sequence of events in chronological order, eg sub-headings with dates of each contact and an explanation of what took place or was observed. A record of any clinical measurement/treatment should be included
- in chronological order, any other communication or attempted communication, eg telephone calls, visits, failed appointments, contact with other agencies/disciplines

The above should be in short paragraphs to facilitate reading. Advice should be taken from the legal officer retained by the authority.

7.2.4 Writing medico-legal reports

What is a medico-legal report?
A medico-legal report is a written professional assessment of a given individual's strengths, needs and situation.

It will contain professional judgements supported by evidence and expertise.

Standards and guidance related to medico-legal reports

Preliminary steps:
- Gain clarity about who is asking for the report and why.
- Ensure the instructions received are clear. Seek any necessary clarification.
- Check that there is no conflict of interest. If so, this must be declared.
- If asked to be an expert witness, therapists must not take on a case if they have insufficient expertise in the area in question.
- Request further reports or information as required.
- Ensure that the time scales can be complied with.
- Confirm acceptance of instructions, or otherwise, within five working days.
- Inform the solicitor of contractual terms, (ie fees and payment method and timing). As appropriate, this will need to be discussed with any manager.
- Clarify who is to arrange the assessment appointment with the individual.
- Inform the solicitor once a date is set.

Process related to preparation of report and preparation for court appearance:
- Read instructions/documentations carefully.
- Have all necessary documentation available at the assessment.
- Allow time for seeking out additional information, (eg contacting an RCSLT adviser or finding out about local availability of therapy services).
- Be prepared to attend meetings, sometimes at short notice.

Report format
The report should:
- contain a statement detailing the substance of instructions
- contain a declaration that duties have been understood and complied with
- provide a 'range of opinion'
- be a statement of truth

- be objective
- be professionally set out
- use numbered paragraphs with headings
- refer, on a separate page, to all the documents that have been seen
- contain a separate summary and recommendation
- be signed and dated

Therapists may need to include an estimate of short and long-term therapy requirements.

Process once the report has been prepared:
- Check the report carefully before submission.
- Submit the report, plus any requisite copies, to the solicitor.
- Submit an invoice as appropriate.
- Be prepared to enter the witness box, give evidence and be cross-examined.

7.2.5 Appearing in court as a witness

SLTs who anticipate any involvement with regard to the making of statements, medico-legal reports or appearing in court should seek help from their employing authority's legal department.

Before giving evidence, the witness is required to swear an oath or to affirm that the evidence that she/he will give is the truth. Questions will be asked on the basis of the written statement which the professional will have been asked to make prior to appearing in court. Professionals will not have a copy of their statement while giving evidence.

In some cases, the statement will have been written months earlier. Under these circumstances, a witness may wish to refresh her/his memory by referring to contemporaneous records.

It is necessary to obtain permission from the employing authority to take the records to court. Under normal circumstances, permission is given as the witness summons or the subpoena may stipulate that the practitioner attend court with the relevant records.

A witness should not attempt to give evidence from memory in the absence of a record in an attempt to be helpful.

A witness who has no relevant records available but who has received a witness summons or subpoena should attend court. Refusal to attend could be seen as contempt of court.

If it is necessary to refer to contemporaneous records or notes whilst giving evidence, a witness must ask leave of the judge or magistrate. If there are no objections, the witness may refresh her/his memory.

It is important to note that if the records or notes are referred to in court, they become part of the evidence in the case and may be examined by the other solicitors and the judge/magistrate.

The professional can be cross-examined by the solicitor of the defendant on matters contained in the records that may not have been referred to orally.

When giving evidence, technique is important. A witness is advised to:

● speak slowly and clearly, in a loud voice
● address all answers to the judge
● remember everyone is nervous in court

The SLT may be asked to explain any clinical terms used. The evidence given by the SLT may be weighed against that of an expert witness (independent therapist) or the SLT may be called as an expert witness. In such instances, it is vital to be clear and specific when giving evidence.

7.2.6. Writing professional advice on children with speech, language and communication difficulties

Speech and language therapy advice for education

The context and processes for supporting children with special needs or additional support needs are subject to review and change. Members are advised to review the up-to-date guidance on the relevant educational websites.

The government departments responsible for education in England, Northern Ireland, Scotland and Wales, are as follows:

● England: the Department for Education and Skills
www.dfes.gov.uk
● Wales: the National Assembly for Wales Training and Education Department (NATED) www.learning.wales.gov.uk
● Northern Ireland: the Department of Education (DE)
www.deni.gov.uk
● Scotland: the Scottish Executive Education Department (SEED)
www.scotland.gov.uk/About/Departments/ED
See also 3.2. Acts of Relevance to the profession.

Whatever the specific requirements placed on members through the law and codes of practice, professional advice should be guided by the following principles and report structure.

Duty of care
Members are reminded that they have a duty of care for any child they are writing advice for. Advice should be written with the needs of the child in mind, not the available resources.

Principles underpinning the writing of advice:
● Any models of intervention, facilities and resources recommended should relate to the speech, language and communication needs of the child and not to the speech and language therapy resources available.
● Advice should be full enough and clear enough to give other professionals, and particularly the child's parents, an understanding of the child's needs.
● Terminology used in reports should be unambiguous.
● Where it is necessary to use professional terminology, it should be defined.
● SLTs should advise only within their sphere of expertise and where necessary seek opinion from more experienced therapists.
● Parents should be included as partners in the process of identifying the support needs of the child.
● All aspects of advice provided should be justifiable and supported by evidence wherever appropriate.

The report detailing professional advice should set out:
● Brief details of the level and type of SLT involvement to date.
● An analysis of the child's speech, language and communication impairment including:
  ● a positive statement about the child's strengths
  ● statements about the child's difficulties that are supported by clear evidence in the form of examples or standardised test scores as appropriate an indication of the child's rate of progress
  ● language and communication levels in relation to other non-verbal abilities, where this information is reliably known
  ● where the child has experience of two or more languages, the first language should be noted, whether or not an assessment has been made in that language

● A description of the impact, or predicted impact, of these difficulties on the child's social participation, learning and accessing the curriculum.
● A broad description of the speech, language and communication outcomes being sought for the child.
● A description of the required resources and features of the educational setting which will best help the child achieve the outcomes being sought. This should include detail of:
● facilities, (eg provision of a small quiet room for developing listening skills)
● modifications, (eg information presented primarily through visual means, including the use of symbols and signing)
● resources, (eg provision of a hi-tech communication aid; symbol software available in school)
● staff knowledge and skills, (eg knowledge and experience of teaching children with autism)
● A description of the speech and language therapy provision required to help the child achieve the desired outcomes:
● SLT advice should specify the appropriate model of therapy provision, (see section below on models of intervention)
● Where a regular and discrete speech and language therapy programme of intervention is required for the development of specified skills, therapists should state how frequently and by whom the programme should be carried out and monitored
● Where a receiving educational establishment is not immediately able to provide the appropriate environment to help the child achieve the desired outcomes, additional speech and language therapy provision may be required to work with school staff in the development of an appropriately supportive and inclusive environment
● Where an individualised programme of intervention will not be effective without the requisite resources and features of the educational setting, this should be stated

Models of intervention:

● Supported inclusion of the child.
Supporting individual members of staff or staff groups to make teaching-style changes or environmental changes to optimise the inclusion of the child within class activities. This will usually involve joint-planning, co-working and training sessions.
● Child skill development through inclusive means

Supporting individual members of staff or staff groups to carry out programmes of work with the whole class or small groups in order to develop targeted language or communication skills
● Child skill development through the integration of individualised targets
Collaborating with parents and members of staff in order to integrate individualised speech, language or communication targets into the child's daily life activities in school and at home
● Child skill development through individualised programmes of work
A regular and discrete programme of individualised intervention aimed at developing specified speech, language and/or communication skills. This may need to be provided directly by an SLT or SLTA, or it may be appropriate for staff at the child's school to provide the programme under the guidance of an SLT.
For those children requiring regular and continuing speech and language therapy input, this will usually be provided in the context of an inclusive approach which seeks to support the child by embedding targets and modifying aspects of the social and learning environment.
In order to be effective and to have maximum impact on the child and their family, speech and language therapy interventions are part of a wider package of support and may change over time (RCSLT, 2006).

Involvement of parents in the process
Parents are an essential part of the multidisciplinary team, as the 'experts' on their own child. They should receive appropriate support and guidance to enable them to play a full and appropriate part in supporting their child, as part of the team.
Parents should be given details of any voluntary agencies appropriate to their child's needs, which can assist them with understanding special educational needs procedures, information and support.

Resourcing recommended levels of provision
As stated above under **Principles**, any models of intervention, facilities and resources recommended should relate to the speech, language and communication needs of the child and not to the educational and/or the speech and language therapy resources available.

Any mismatch between need and available resources should be recorded and monitored as part of a regular service audit. This information should be brought to the attention of the appropriate authorities, eg local education authorities or commissioners for children's services, as part of an improvement and development process.

Communication and liaison

Effective action on behalf of children with special educational needs/additional support needs will depend upon close cooperation between various agencies with local authorities taking the lead (DH, 2005).

The importance of good communication with and between all members of the child's team cannot be overstated. Liaison with colleagues will:

- allow the therapist to share concerns about a child who may have special educational needs
- ensure weight is given to the therapist's view about the child
- enhance the effectiveness of provision
- form the basis of a collaborative and integrated support plan for the child

7.2.7 Writing reports on referred individuals

A report is a written account designed to convey information and ideas for a specific purpose.

A report must be timely eg if the SLT is making an onward referral, a report should accompany the referral.

Each report must have:

- an introduction, identifying the purpose of the report
- a middle section, which covers relevant information and actions taken or planned
- a final section, which includes a summary, conclusions and recommendations

The report may be:

- an initial report following an assessment
- a closure report at the point of discharge or transfer
- an interim report as and when necessary following acceptance of a referral

Hallmarks of a good report include:

- clarity (sentence structures are short; headings are provided; jargon is avoided)
- completeness (all relevant information is provided; the report is fit for purpose; all recipients are listed)
- accuracy (statements are truthful, accurate and factual; sources of information are given)
- consistency (the terminology and information is consistent and cohesive)
- logical progression (from past to present to future; content is well-structured)
- conciseness (details are brief but incisive and intelligible)

Once the report has been prepared in line with the principles listed above:

- the information must be checked
- the grammar and spelling must be checked
- the report date must be checked
- the report, or the SLT section of the multidisciplinary report, must be signed

Duty of care

SLTs have a duty of care for the individual they are writing a report on and may be called to account for what they have written. SLTs are reminded that reports that are incomplete or inaccurate can mislead and have unexpected and undesirable consequences for an individual. See also Section 7.2.4 Writing medico-legal reports and Section 7.2.6 Writing professional advice on children.

References

Beukelman, D & Ansel, B. Research priorities in augmentative and alternative communication in *Augmentative and Alternative Communication*, 1995:11; pp131-134.

Blackstone, S. Populations and practices in AAC in *Augmentative Communication News*, 1990:3(4); pp1-3.

Blackstone, SW & Painter, MJ. Speech problems in multihandicapped children in JK Darby (Ed.), *Speech and language evaluation in neurology: Childhood disorders*. Grune & Stratton, 1985; pp 219-242.

Department of Health. *Comprehensive Critical Care*, 2000a. www.dh.org.uk

Department of Health. *Health Service Circular*, 2001. www.dh.gov.uk

Department for Health. *The NHS Plan: a plan for investment, a plan for reform*, 2000b. www.dh.gov.uk

Department for Health. *NSF for children, young people and maternity services*, 2004. www.dh.gov.uk

Department of Health. *NSF for long-term conditions*, 2005. www.dh.gov.uk

Department of Health. Standard 3 in *NSF for older people*, 2001a. www.dh.gov.uk

Department of Health. Standard 5, Stroke in *NSF for older people*, 2001b. www.dh.gov.uk

Gascoigne, M. *Supporting children with speech language and communication needs within integrated children's services* – position paper. RCSLT, 2006. www.rcslt.org

Glennan, S. and De Coste, D. *A Handbook of AAC*. Singular Publishing, 1998.

Intensive Care Society Standards, 2002.

Matas, J, Mathy-Laikko, P, Beukelman, D & Legresley, K. Identifying the non-speaking population: A demographic study in *Augmentative and Alternative Communication*, 1995:1; pp17-31.

Mirenda, P & Mathy-Laikko, P. Augmentative and alternative communication applications for persons with severe congenital communication disorders: An introduction in *Augmentative and Alternative Communication*, 1989:5; pp3-13.

Norwich, B and Grove, N. *The Use of AAC systems in London Schools*. Institute of Education, 1997.

RCSLT. *Returners Pack*, 2005. www.rcslt.org

World Health Organisation (WHO), 2006. www.who.int/cancer/palliative

Acts of Parliament

Data Protection Act, 1998

Every Child Matters Childcare Bill, 2005

Chapter 8

Service Provision: Part 3 Working with Specific Client Groups

This information on services to specific client groups is designed to support speech and language therapy services undertaking reviews of service organisation and provision.

Each subsection follows the same basic format although the form and emphasis varies somewhat:

- definition
- national guidance and sources of further support and information
- aetiology
- prevalence and incidence
- vulnerabilities of individuals: risk issues
- speech and language therapy value
- references

Therapists seeking detailed clinical guidance in relation to specific client groups are advised to seek this level of detail within the *RCSLT Clinical Guidelines* (2005), position papers and the *Reference Framework: Underpinning Competence to Practise* (2003), available on the RCSLT website at: www.rcslt.org

8.1 Acquired Motor Speech Disorders

This information is designed to support speech and language services undertaking reviews of service organisation and provision. SLTs seeking detailed clinical guidance are referred to the *RCSLT Clinical Guidelines* (2005), position papers and *Reference Reference Framework: Underpinning Competence to Practise* (2003), available on the RCSLT website: www.rcslt.org

Definition

'Acquired motor speech disorders' is a general label that covers

Chapter 8

several distinct disruptions to speech arising from illness or injury to the central or peripheral nervous system.

Speech changes resulting from problems of muscle function or the nerve-muscle synaptic junction are also subsumed within the group of disorders. Two broad classes of disorder fall under the label:

● **Dysarthria**, denoting a difficulty, due to neuromuscular changes, in producing or sustaining the range, force, speed and coordination of the movements needed to achieve appropriate breathing, phonation, resonance and articulation for speech.

● **Apraxia** of speech, representing a disruption to the selection, programming and online control of the movements for speech.

There exist subtypes of neuromuscular disruption to speech, at least at the impairment level, related to site of lesion, eg cerebellum, brain stem, basal ganglia, upper motor neurone.

Speech changes associated with focal or generalised dystonias also fall under the dysarthria label. There are also subtypes of disruption to speech motor programming and online control.

Dysarthria and apraxia of speech may occur separately or concurrently.

Cross-referencing with further chapter sections below is recommended:

8.3. Aphasia
8.5. Bilingualism
8.6. Brain Injury
8.12. Dysfluency
8.13. Dyslexia
8.14. Dysphagia
8.16. Mental Health
8.19. Progressive Neurological Disorders
8.24. Voice
7.2.1 AAC

National guidance and sources of further support and information:

The following national guidance should underpin all service delivery and developments:

● Scottish Intercollegiate Network Guideline on *Management of individuals with stroke: Rehabilitation, Prevention, Management of Complications and Discharge Planning.* SIGN 64, 2002. www.sign.ac.uk

● Scottish Intercollegiate Network Guideline on Dysphagia. SIGN 78, 2004. www.sign.ac.uk
● *Guidelines on Stroke* (2nd edition), Royal College of Physicians, 2004
● National Service Framework for Long-term Conditions (NSF), Department of Health (DH), 2005.
● *Older People's Services NSF*, DH.
● *RCSLT Clinical Guidelines* section on Dysarthria, 2005. www.rcslt.org/resources/

The following websites are a useful source of information on neurological conditions and links to relevant societies that will provide support in the form of information and advice:

The Neurological Alliance:
www.neural.org.uk/pages/about/members.asp

National Academy of Neuropsychology
www.nanonline.org/nandistance/nanneuro/NeuroIII/index.html?neuroIIImain

National Institute of Neurological Disorders and Stroke
www.ninds.nih.gov/disorders/disorder_index.htm

National Institute on Deafness and Other Communication Disorders
www.nidcd.nih.gov/health/voice/index.asp

National Spasmodic Dysphonia Association
www.dysphonia.org/(spasmodic dysphonia)

Glaxo Neurological Centre (hub for neurological disorders groups in Great Britain)
www.glaxocentre.merseyside.org/index.html

Aetiology

Acquired motor speech disorders may arise in association with any neurological changes that affect the planning or realisation of movements required for speech.

The more common aetiologies seen are: stroke; traumatic brain injury; progressive neurological disorders, (eg Parkinson's disease and atypical Parkinson's syndromes, multiple sclerosis, motor neurone disease, hereditary ataxias); nervous system infections; brain tumours; focal dystonias; and isolated cranial nerve and spinal cord lesions.

Incidence and prevalence

Few reliable figures exist for the incidence and prevalence of acquired motor speech disorders from any aetiology, though one source cites them as being the most prevalent communication disorder of all.

In stroke or brain injury more than 50% of people have been described as having dysarthria or apraxia of speech, though this figure clearly diminishes during the period of recovery.

In progressive neurological illness speech may be the first presenting sign; at other times speech changes are a late manifestation. In some neurological conditions speech disorders are an inevitable consequence but in others, speech changes are a rare sequel (see section 8.19 Progressive Neurological Disorders).

Incidence and prevalence figures based on the screening of motor speech performance have a further drawback as regards the true number of speakers who may require services because of dysarthria or apraxia of speech: speech impairment changes do not necessarily predict impact on communication. Mild changes or changes imperceptible to the listener may cause maximum disruption to the life of one speaker and be a priority for change; severe impairment may have little impact on another speaker and low priority for intervention; for most aetiologies motor speech disorders exist as part of a complex picture of disability.

Vulnerability: risk issues

SLTs must be fully aware of any risks that are specific to an individual's condition.

Cross refer to sections on Traumatic Brain Injury (8.6), Adult Learning Disability (8.2), Progressive Neurological Disorders (8.19), Head and Neck Cancer (8.15), and Dysphagia (8.14), in relation to an individual's health, psychosocial and emotional vulnerabilities.

Speech and language therapy value

Enabling an individual to achieve a mode of communication fitting to their age, gender, social circumstances and desires, within the limitations dictated by their neurological condition.

Principles

Aiming for optimum intelligibility may involve work at impairment level on eg range, force, sustainability of movements, but intervention and aims at this level are subordinate to effecting change in activity limitation and participation restriction.

Return to pre-morbid mode of communication, even in medical conditions which can improve, may not be possible. In progressive conditions speech and language therapy will not halt the inevitable overall decline. Accordingly, a general principle is to aim for compensated intelligibility by maximizing the communication potential possible within the speaker's current resources through strategic manipulation of speech and non-speech variables.

Speech is only one medium of communication. It may be relevant to supplement or supplant speech with other methods of communication. Refer to section on augmentative and alternative communication (see section 7.2.1).

As communication always involves a listener as well as a speaker, it is clear that speech and language therapy input supports listeners as well as speakers.

Care pathway

As acquired motor speech disorders are almost invariably part of a more complex picture of change, speech and language therapy care pathways will reflect and be integrated into local and national guidelines/pathways developed for specific groups, such as stroke, traumatic brain injury, Parkinson's disease, multiple sclerosis, cancer care. Where specific guidelines have not been developed or remain a matter of debate, (eg facial palsy), pathways and practices are derived from general principles (see section 6.5.1.) and adapted from existing pathways (see figure 1, pages 254-255).

It is unlikely that the SLT is the sole person working with an individual, as care pathways involve multi-, trans- and inter-disciplinary processes. At the same time there will be care pathways specific to speech and language therapy involvement that feed into the multidisciplinary team (MDT).

Accordingly, SLTs must be cognisant both of the national and international guidelines on best practice for their area of work, as well as local service agreements.

Development of care pathways for speech and language therapy involvement is shaped by the evolving underlying medical picture and the evolving real and perceived impact of changes on communication for the individual as she/he and their carers learn of, react to and adjust to, altered circumstances.

The elements of timing, intensity, aims and content of speech and language therapy pathways of care for different groups are shaped by: patterns of change in the overall medical condition; the impact of this on individuals and their response/s to it; evidence for best practice concerning timing, intensity, aims and content of intervention.

The overall pathway in speech and language therapy is diagnostic assessment; followed by formulation of and negotiation of short and long-term goals with all parties involved; episodes of speech and language therapy intervention with ongoing monitoring of progress towards goals; reassessment at key junctures; planned and measurable discharge; and clearly stated, workable onward and sideways referral criteria.

The flow chart in figure 1 (pages 254-255) illustrates a sample model pathway of care.

8.2 Adult Learning Disability (ALD)

This information is designed to support speech and language therapy services undertaking reviews of service organisation and provision. Therapists seeking detailed clinical guidance are referred to the *RCSLT Clinical Guidelines* (2005), position papers and *Reference Framework: Underpinning Competence to Practise* (2003), available on the RCSLT website: www.rcslt.org

Definition and aetiology

The **World Health Organisation** (WHO) define learning disability as "*a condition of arrested or incomplete development of the mind, which is especially characterised by impairment of skills manifested during the developmental period, skills which contribute to the overall level of intelligence, ie cognitive, language, motor and social abilities*", (1992).

More recently (2001), DH definitions have been based upon functional descriptors and the level of support required by the individual.

Learning disability includes the presence of:
● A significantly reduced ability to understand new or complex information, to learn new skills (impaired intelligence), with
● A reduced ability to cope independently (impaired social functioning); which started before adulthood, with a lasting effect on development.

Figure 1: Level 3 Services for Acquired Motor Speech Disorders

Referral received

↓

INITIAL ASSESSMENT:
(Standardised and informal methods)
• establish appropriateness of referral
• determine views of individual/carer

↓

DIAGNOSTIC ASSESSMENT

Establish baseline measures on all key variables using valid, reliable, repeatable formal and informal assessments

All or some of the following are appropriate according to needs • speech motor examination • perceptual assessments • instrumental assessments

They will cover: • respiratory function • phonation • resonance • articulation • prosody • intelligibility

Assessment also encompasses repeatable measures of:
• communication skills profile • self and other perceptions of dysarthria/apraxia • psychosocial impact on speaker and family • conversational partners

Audio/video records are recommended as well as score sheet summaries from other assessments.

Appropriate assessments of language and other cognitive variables

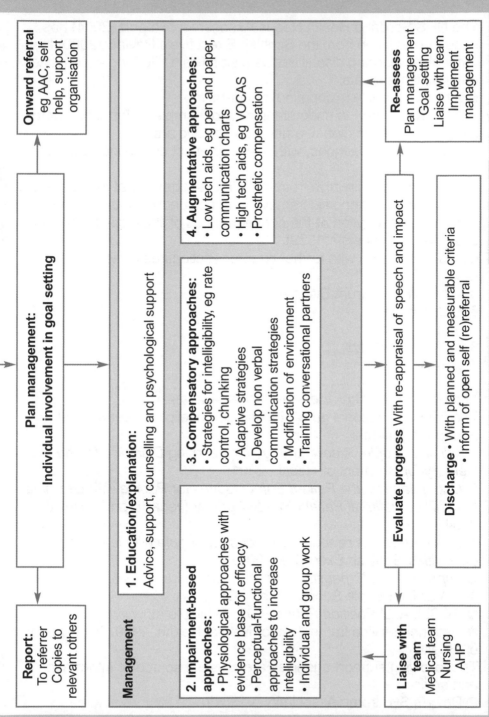

Report: To referrer Copies to relevant others

Onward referral eg AAC, self help, support organisation

Plan management: Individual involvement in goal setting

Management

1. Education/explanation: Advice, support, counselling and psychological support

2. Impairment-based approaches:
- Physiological approaches with evidence base for efficacy
- Perceptual-functional approaches to increase intelligibility
- Individual and group work

3. Compensatory approaches:
- Strategies for intelligibility, eg rate control, chunking
- Adaptive strategies
- Develop non verbal communication strategies
- Modification of environment
- Training conversational partners

4. Augmentative approaches:
- Low tech aids, eg pen and paper, communication charts
- High tech aids, eg VOCAS
- Prosthetic compensation

Liaise with team Medical team Nursing AHP

Evaluate progress With re-appraisal of speech and impact

Discharge • With planned and measurable criteria
• Inform of open self (re)referral

Re-assess Plan management Goal setting Liaise with team Implement management

The NHS Scotland Health Needs Assessment Report (2004) has used the definition from the Scottish Executive's Review (2000) that recognises learning disabilities as a significant, life-long experience that has three facets:

● a reduced ability to cope independently
● a reduced ability to understand new or complex information or to learn new skills (in global rather than specific areas)
● onset before adulthood, with a lasting effect on the individual's development.

The most recent directive from the WHO suggests that that there is a need to use a "diagnostic framework in conjunction with one that provides a description of the consequences of the disability on everyday functioning." (1999).

Cross-referencing with further chapter sections below is recommended:
8.4. Autism Spectrum Disorder
8.7. Cerebral Palsy
8.14. Dysphagia
8.16. Mental Health
7.2.1 AAC

National guidance and support agencies

The following national guidance should underpin all service delivery and developments:

● *Valuing People: A new strategy for Learning Disability for the 21st Century.* Department of Health, 2001.
● *Understanding the Patient Safety Issues for People with Learning Disabilities National Patient Safety Agency.* Department of Health, 2004.
● *Same as you: A review of services for people with learning disabilities.* Scottish Executive, 2000.
● *Improvement, Expansion and Reform: Ensuring that "all" means "all".* Valuing People Support Team, DH 2004.
● RCSLT. ALD *Position Paper,* 2003. Available at: www.rcslt.org
● National Service framework for Mental Health, 1999. Department of Health.

The following support agencies are a useful source of information and advice:
● Down's Syndrome Association www.downs-syndrome.org.uk

- Fragile X www.fragilex.org.uk
- Home Farm Trust www.hft.org.uk
- British Institute of Learning Disabilities (BILD) www.bild.org.uk
- Foundation for people with learning disabilities www.mentalhealth.org.uk/fpld
- Learning Disabilities UK www.learningdisabilitiesUK.org.uk
- SENSE www.sense.org.uk
- Mencap www.mencap.org.uk
- National Autistic society www.nas.org.uk
- MIND www.mind.org.uk

Incidence and prevalence

It is difficult to be precise about the number of people with learning disabilities. Prevalence figures vary depending upon the definitions applied, the age of the population and level of severity of learning disability, (McLaren & Bryson, 1997; Welsh Health Planning Forum, 1992; Farmer et al, 1991. The Department of Health (2001) estimated that in England there were 210,000 children and adults with severe and profound disabilities and 1.2 million with mild and moderate disability

In Scotland, Scottish Executive (2000), there are thought to be 120,000 people with learning disabilities; about 20 people in every 1,000 have mild or moderate learning disabilities and 3-4 people in every 1,000 have severe or profound learning disabilities.

The Foundation for People with Learning Disabilities (2000) notes that:

- Up to 90% of people with learning disabilities have communication difficulties.
- About 60% of people with learning disabilities overall have some skills in symbolic communication, such as speech, signs or picture symbols.
- About 80% of those with severe learning disabilities do not acquire effective speech.

Vulnerability: risk issues

- People with learning disabilities are at risk from being unable to exercise their right to communicate, as they require very specific assessment and support around all modalities of communication (ASHA, 1992; Bradley, 1998).

● People with learning disabilities are at risk from being unable to exercise real choice in their lives, as they may not have the means or the opportunities. They need to be enabled to be more independent and empowered to achieve the greatest possible autonomy (DH, 2001).

● People with learning disabilities and communication needs are at risk from being unable to consent to intervention, life issues, etc (DH, 2001). Harm may result if a person with a learning disability is unable to understand information relating to illnesses, intervention or interventions (NPSA, 2004).

● People with learning disabilities have greater health needs and risks when compared with the general population (NPSA, 2004; DH, 2004);

● People with learning disabilities have an increased uptake of medical and dental hospital services but a reduced uptake of surgical specialities compared to the general population, with a similar overall rate of hospital admissions and a reduced length of stay.

● People with learning disabilities are vulnerable in general hospitals. Lack of training for generic health staff in specific health concerns suggests that there may be missed or wrong diagnoses (NPSA, 2004).

● Much of the health need is unrecognised and unmet. Symptoms are linked to a person's learning disability and not their illness.

● People with learning disabilities are at risk of receiving either no service or an uncoordinated service from either mainstream mental health services or specialist mental health support within specialist learning disability services. This risk is due to the lack of communication between mainstream psychiatry services and learning disability psychiatry services.

● A very high number of people with learning disabilities receive prescribed psychotropic medication, most commonly anti-psychotic medication that has many possible side effects. Communication difficulties make it harder to describe pain or symptoms and to understand medical intervention and implication. People with learning disabilities are at risk from lack of understanding around health information, leading to illness or disease being misdiagnosed or un-diagnosed, and therefore mistreated or untreated (NPSA, 2004). A lack of accessible information creates a barrier to accessing healthcare and appropriate intervention.

● People with learning disabilities have greater health risks than the general population:

● People with learning disabilities are between 8.5 and 200 times more likely to have a vision impairment compared to the general population and around 40% are reported to have a hearing impairment, with people with Down's syndrome at particularly high risk of developing vision and hearing loss.

● The prevalence of dementia is higher amongst older adults with learning disabilities compared to the general population and people with Down's syndrome are particularly at risk of early onset.

● Prevalence rates for schizophrenia in people with learning disabilities are approximately three times greater than for the general population.

● Reported prevalence rates for anxiety and depression amongst people with learning disabilities vary widely, but are generally reported to be at least as prevalent as the general population, and higher amongst people with Down's syndrome.

● There is a high prevalence of epilepsy (NHS, Scotland).

● People with learning disabilities may additionally have specific acquired or developmental speech and language disorders.

● Communication difficulties make it harder to describe pain or symptoms and to understand medical intervention and implication. People with learning disabilities are at risk from lack of understanding around health information, leading to illness or disease being mistreated or undiagnosed, and therefore mistreated or untreated (NPSA, 2004).

● A lack of accessible information creates a barrier to accessing healthcare and appropriate intervention.

● The impact of a communication difficulty in addition to a learning disability increases the incidence of challenging behaviour and/or mental health issues:

● Expressive difficulties are linked to self injurious behaviour (Murphy et al, 1993; Oliver, 1993).

● Language and communication problems are linked with challenging behaviour (Celi, 1986; Chamberlain et al, 1993; Quine, 1986; Richman et al, 1982).

● People with no speech and a good level of understanding have increased behavioural problems (Bott et al, 1997).

● Increased risk of social exclusion – without shared communication there is automatic exclusion and isolation (DH, 2001). Many people with mild learning disabilities who can cope with most of day-to-day living can have poor social networks. Some of these people may withdraw and also experience mental health problems.

● Staff and carers of people with learning disability may lack awareness, information and training around communication. This presents a risk for people with learning disability as their carers do not necessarily have the skills or knowledge base to identify or manage their communication difficulties.

● People with learning disabilities are at risk of not being asked their opinions due to their communication difficulties. There are many day-to-day tasks and events that people with learning disabilities are excluded from, eg choosing day opportunities or choosing who to live with. There is a risk of the client group not being properly represented, ie being excluded from meaningful consultation/ feedback events, being excluded from future research due to consent issues. This is because consultation with this client group is very difficult to achieve effectively.

● There is an increased risk of being both a perpetrator and a victim of crime, people with learning disabilities are more vulnerable to abuse of their human rights, and need support to access the judicial system, both in cases of prosecution and defence.

● People with learning disability are at risk of not understanding information in public places and within the wider community.

● There are issues around stigma and society, and how people with learning disabilities are valued.

Speech and language therapy value

In the context of working collaboratively across agencies, professional groups and the lifespan of the person with a learning disability:

● Promotion of communication skills for independence, choice, inclusion and rights.

● Consideration of communication needs within the social model of disability, respecting and promoting all modalities of communication and linking all speech and language therapy intervention with the life aims of the individual.

● Enabling maximal involvement of the individual.

8.3 Aphasia

This information is designed to support speech and language therapy services undertaking reviews of service organisation and provision. SLTs seeking detailed clinical guidance are referred to the *RCSLT Clinical Guidelines* (2005), position papers and the *Reference Framework: Underpinning Competence to Practise* (2003), available on the RCSLT website at: www.rcslt.org

Definition

Aphasia (sometimes also referred to as dysphasia) is an acquired, multi-modal language disorder resulting from neurological damage. It may affect a person's ability to talk, write and understand spoken and written language, leaving other cognitive abilities intact.

All languages can be similarly affected, including the sign languages used by deaf people. In some individuals, the ability to use non-linguistic communication, such as gesture and drawing, is also impaired.

Aphasia can co-occur with a number of other cognitive disorders that may also affect communication, particularly in the case of traumatic brain injury.

Aphasia is a long-term, life-changing condition, which affects both the individual and others around him/her. Living with aphasia involves individuals and those in their environment in a process of adaptation to change, in terms of communication style, lifestyle, identity and life roles. Although not a feature of aphasia per se, the influence of cultural factors will have an affect on communication style.

Cross-referencing with further chapter sections below is recommended:

8.1. Acquired Motor Speech Disorders
8.2. Adult Learning Disability
8.5. Bilingualism
8.6. Brain Injury
8.10 Critical Care
8.13. Dyslexia
8.14. Dysphagia
8.16. Mental Health
8.17. Palliative Care
8.19. Progressive Neurological Disorders
8.23. Visual Impairment
7.2.1 AAC

National guidelines and sources of further support and information

● *National Clinical Guidelines for Stroke,* 2nd edition. Royal College of Physicians, 2004 www.rcplondon.ac.uk

● *National service framework (NSF) for older people's services.* Department of Health, 2001 www.dh.gov.uk/PolicyandGuidance

● *NSF for long-term conditions.* Department of Health, 2005 www.dh.gov.uk/PolicyandGuidance

● Scottish Intercollegiate Guidelines Network (SIGN):
Guideline 64: *Management of individuals with stroke: Rehabilitation, prevention and management of complications, and discharge planning,* 2005.
Guideline 13: *Management of patients with stroke part I: Assessment, investigation, immediate management and secondary prevention,* 1997 www.sign.ac.uk

● *RCSLT Clinical Guidelines,* 2005 – section on Aphasia. www.rcslt.org

● Mental Health Capacity Act. Department of Health, 2005. www.mca2005.co.uk

● UK Connect www.ukconnect.org

● Stroke Association www.stroke.org.uk

● British Aphasiology Society www.bas.org.uk

● Speakability www.speakability.org.uk

● Aphasiahelp www.aphasiahelp.org

● Communication Matters www.communicationmatters.org.uk

● Different Strokes www.differentstrokes.co.uk

● International Classification of Functioning, Disability and Health-2 http://sustainable-design.ie/arch/ICIDH-2Final.pdf

Aetiology

Aphasia is an acquired problem resulting from a focal lesion in the dominant hemisphere of the brain. In many people this is the left hemisphere but the non-dominant right hemisphere is also known to contribute to language function and damage here can result in aphasia. Conditions such as stroke, brain injury and cerebral tumour can produce aphasia.

Disordered communication can be seen in many neurological conditions such as dementias, acute confusion, nervous system infections, psychosis, traumatic brain injury, but this does not necessarily indicate the presence of aphasia.

Prevalence and incidence

There are no official figures for the incidence and prevalence of aphasia in the UK. Most people who have aphasia have had a stroke. Over 130,000 people have a stroke every year. Stroke affects between 174 and 216 people per 100,000 population in the UK every year and it is estimated that approximately 20-30% of stroke survivors experience aphasia. Six months following a stroke it is estimated that of these survivors, 15% still experience communication problems (Royal College of Physicians, 2004).

Vulnerability: risk issues

Recent research in the UK (Hilari et al, 2003) has shown that the health-related quality of life of people with aphasia after stroke is significantly affected by their emotional distress, their activity level, the severity of their communication disability and their overall health.

Services for people with aphasia should aim to minimise communication disability, address emotional health, and enable participation in an individual's social context and in the community and society more generally (Brumfitt, 1993; Parr et al, 2003, 1997). People with aphasia can have difficulty accessing information, particularly written information, and this can affect their ability to make informed choices. They may be considered incompetent to make decisions or to resume pre-morbid activities owing to their language difficulties.

Services for people with aphasia should aim to facilitate them to participate in decision-making processes including educating the professionals about aphasia and training them on how to facilitate informed consent (Rose et al, 2003; Eames et al, 2003; Kayan, 1995).

Speech and language therapy value

Meeting the needs of individuals with aphasia in maximising their potential for recovery of language, and in developing effective conversation strategies that can be used by both the individual and those they converse with, thereby maintaining their ability to influence their environment, maintain social relationships and quality of life.

8.4 Autism Spectrum Disorder

This information is designed to support speech and language therapy services undertaking reviews of service organisation and provision. Therapists seeking detailed clinical guidance are referred to the *RCSLT Clinical Guidelines* (2005), position papers and *Reference Framework: Underpinning Competence to Practise* (2003), available on the RCSLT website: www.rcslt.org

Definition

Autism Spectrum Disorder (ASD) is a life-long developmental disability affecting communication and social skills. People with ASD may also have accompanying learning disabilities but, whatever the level of intelligence, everyone with the condition shares a difficulty in making sense of the world.

ASD includes the condition Asperger syndrome. People with Asperger syndrome are of average or above average intelligence and generally have fewer obvious problems with language. However, their expressive language is affected by underlying problems related to ASD, including a very literal understanding of language, involving difficulties in understanding metaphor and some inflexibility of thought. This is likely to impact on communication and social relationships (NAS, 2005).

Certain characteristics of ASD will be more prominent at certain ages than at others, so the way that an individual presents will vary during their lifetime.

Many children with ASD may show impairment and delays in development from birth but this may not be recognised by either parents or professionals within the first year. Possibly, one third will show a regressive pattern often around 21 months (varying from 13-23 months), in which word-use is lost, and eye contact and social awareness diminishes. A very few children show normal development to 24 months and beyond, and then regress.

Children with ASD are affected in a variety of ways and to very different degrees. Pragmatic difficulties are always present and are accompanied by a degree of speech, language and general processing difficulty, which may in turn be linked to sensory disturbances. The results of these difficulties may be expressed as anxiety, frustration and challenging behaviour.

The International Diagnostic Standards for Autism Spectrum Disorder are ICD 10 (WHO, 1993) and DSM 4 (American Psychiatry Association, 2000). These relate to the 'Triad of Impairment' (Wing, 1988) involving:

● impairment in communication
● impairment in socialisation (empathy)
● limited repertoire of interest (imagination)
● a developmental disorder with onset prior to 36 months that affects all aspects of life.

Cross-referencing with the chapter sections listed below is recommended:

8.2. Adult Learning Disability
8.5. Bilingualism
8.11. Deafness
8.14. Dysphagia
8.16. Mental Health
8.18. Pre-school Children
8.19. Progressive Neurological disorders
8.20. School-Aged Children
8.21. Specific Language Impairment
8.22 Specific Speech Impairment
8.23. Visual Impairment
7.2.1 AAC

National guidance and sources of further support and information

● *The National Autism Plan for Children* (2003) published by the National Autistic Society (NAS) for the National Initiative for Autism – Screening and Assessment (NIASA), describes a care pathway involving a secondary and sometimes tertiary level of assessment within a multidisciplinary forum.

● *National Needs Assessment for Autistic Spectrum Disorder* (Public Health Institute of Scotland, 2001) contains information regarding a care pathway for adults.

● *Good Practice Guidelines for Services – Adults with Asperger Syndrome* (NAS, 2002).

● The Scottish Intercollegiate Guideline (SIGN) – on assessment, diagnosis & clinical intervention for children and young people with ASD (in print).
● *RCSLT Clinical Guidelines* (2005) – section on ASD. www.rcslt.org
● OAASIS The Office for Advice, Assistance, Support and Information on Special Needs www.oaasis.co.uk
● The ACE Centre Advisory Trust www.ace-centre.org.uk
● Quality Standard for ASD Diagnostic Services www.scotland.gov.uk/Publications/2006/02/28084616/12

Aetiology

The causes of ASD are not known, but research shows that genetic factors are important. In many cases ASD may also be associated with various conditions affecting brain development.

Co-morbidity factors such as epilepsy, hearing impairments, learning disabilities, motor disorders, specific learning disabilities (dyslexia, dyspraxia), attention disorders (attention deficit disorder [ADD], attention deficit hyperactivity disorder [ADHD]) and psychiatric disorders (obsessive compulsive disorder [OCD], anxiety and depression, oppositional defiant disorder [ODD]) need to be identified and addressed.

During the past decade the focus on autism research has increased dramatically aiming to identify factors underlying the disorder and effective methods of intervention.

Prevalence and incidence

The estimated population of people with ASD in the UK is 500,000: an estimated prevalence of 91:10,000 (NAS, 2005).

These figures include those at the higher end of the spectrum who may not need specialist services and support.

In the past the suggested sex ratio was 4:1 males to females (Gilberg, 2002). However, in recent years, more females with ASD have been identified. It is thought that many are missed as children as they tend to be more socially robust (Attwood, 2004).

Vulnerability: risk issues

There is a considerable degree of overlap between children and adults, as far as vulnerability and risk issues are concerned.
In children there is an:

- increased risk of stress and anxiety within the immediate family
- increased risk of difficulties in accessing the school curriculum
- increased risk of difficulties in forming and maintaining friendships.

As children enter puberty and move towards and into adulthood there is an:

- **Increased risk of isolation and loneliness**: difficulties in forming relationships, including sexual ones.
- **Increased risk of social, emotional and sexual abuse** due to poor language, communication and social interaction skills.
- **Increased risk of mental illness (anxiety and depression)**: choice making and access to advocacy and person centred planning may be limited.
- **Increased risk of challenging behaviour and/or self injurious behaviour** due to comprehension and expressive language difficulties.
- **Increased risk of becoming involved in the judicial system** due to their behaviour or responses to other's behaviour being perceived as inappropriate. This can range in severity from slightly odd to offending behaviour. As a teenager or young adult, individuals with ASD are more at risk than their peers.
- **Poor social awareness** may result in difficulties expressing needs and in inappropriate social and sexual habits, eg inappropriate touching of others or masturbation at inappropriate times, stalking.
- **Risk of misdiagnosis leading to inappropriate care and placements**. SLTs have a role in differential diagnosis of primary diagnosis of ASD and in diagnosis of co-morbid conditions such as dyspraxia, dyslexia, deafness, Tourette's syndrome, as there is a risk of diagnosis of ASD overshadowing, ie everything is put down to ASD. Unusual patterns of language use can lead others to form inappropriate opinions, (eg the individual may be diagnosed as having schizophrenia or psychosis).

Speech and language therapy value

- To contribute to the diagnosis of ASD as a key member of the MDT. For children, the core team consists of a paediatrician/psychiatrist, clinical psychologist and an SLT. For adults, the core team consists of a psychiatrist, clinical psychologist and SLT.
- To provide individuals with a means to make free choices, express their feelings, to learn, and to increase their independence.
- To provide an environment which maximizes opportunities for

individuals to develop their receptive and expressive communication skills.

● To provide carers and educators with the means to support individuals.

This includes ensuring that carers and educators are able to use appropriate systems and levels of communication when interacting with individuals, eg use of AAC, communication aids, communication methods such as PECS, comic strip conversations and social stories, narrative therapy and systems to support routine and structure involving an appropriate level of reference (eg objects, photos, pictures, gesture, symbols, etc).

8.5 Bilingualism

This information is designed to support speech and language therapy services undertaking reviews of service organisation and provision. Therapists seeking detailed clinical guidance are referred to the *RCSLT Clinical Guidelines* (2005), position papers and *Reference Framework: Underpinning Competence to Practise* (2003), available on the RCSLT website: www.rcslt.org

Definition
Individuals or groups of people who acquire communicative skills in more than one language. They acquire these skills with varying degrees of proficiency, in oral and/or written forms, in order to interact with speakers of one or more languages at home and in society.
An individual should be regarded as bilingual regardless of the relative proficiency of the languages understood or used.
Any of the conditions listed within this chapter may occur in the context of bilingualism. Cross-referencing with all chapter 8 client group sections is therefore recommended.

National guidance and sources of further information
● *RCSLT SIG Bilingualism Good Practice Guidelines*. RCSLT (to be revised, 2005).
● Race Relations (Amendment) Act, 2000.
● *Sure Start planning pack: Sure Start for all: Guidance on involving minority ethnic children and families.* Department for Education and Employment, 1999.

- *Quality protects: Black and ethnic minority children and their families*. Department of Health, 1998.
- *The NHS Plan: A plan for investment, a plan for reform*, Department of Health, 2000.
- Disability Discrimination Act,1995.
- Human Rights Act, 2000.

Prevalence

Bilingualism is not a disorder and it is not therefore appropriate to be considered as a condition with measurable prevalence.

There are few reliable official statistics on the number of bilingual individuals in Britain and there is virtually no data available on language use in Britain.

The UK Census 2001 indicates that 7.9% of the population is from a minority ethic background and, although caution should be exercised in equating a minority ethnic background with bilingualism, the links between language, ethnicity and culture are widely acknowledged (Battle, 1998; Schott & Henley, 1996).

There are over 300 languages spoken by children in London schools (Literacy Trust, 2000). Winter (1999) reports that 59% of SLTs working with a paediatric caseload in England have at least one bilingual child on their caseload, with 11% of these having 20 or more bilingual children on their caseload.

As bilingualism does not cause communication disorders, there is no reason why bilingual children should have a different rate of speech and language problems from a monolingual population (Crutchley, 1999; Crutchley et al, 1997a, 1997b; Duncan & Gibbs, 1989; Winter 2001).

Speech and language therapy value

- Assessment of the individual's communication skills in all the languages to which they are exposed. This detailed assessment will facilitate the SLT to reach a differential diagnosis and establish if there is a primary communication difficulty that does not arise as a result of acquiring English as an additional language.
- Providing intervention in the individual's mother tongue and support the family in their use of mother tongue when necessary/appropriate, ie when it is the individual's preferred/ dominant language. Language choice should be discussed and

agreed with families. With regard to children, the evidence base demonstrates both the need for mother tongue therapy in cases of speech disorder (Holm & Dodd, 2001; Holm et al, 1999) and the efficacy of therapeutic intervention in the individual's mother tongue in language delay and disorder (Guttierrez-Clellen, 1999).

● Ensuring equal access and equal quality of care for all members of the local population regardless of ethnic or linguistic background. The use of trained bilingual SLTAs/ bilingual co-workers and expertise in working with interpreters will ensure that bilingual individuals have access to all care pathways.

● Ensuring a clear, culturally appropriate explanation is provided in the most appropriate language for individuals with dysphagia and their families in order to minimise the risk of aspiration, chest infections and malnutrition. Guidelines should be provided in the most appropriate medium and language as well as demonstrated and reviewed until fully understood.

Vulnerability: risk issues

Specific language impairment is under-identified within bilingual children in the UK. These children are therefore not accessing speech and language therapy services (Crutchley et al, 1997a, 1997b; Winter, 2001).

Similarly there is evidence emerging that bilingual children with speech disorders are not being identified by referral agents and are therefore under represented on speech and language therapy caseloads (Stow & Dodd, 2005).

Bilingual individuals may be vulnerable to well-meaning, but ill-informed, professionals who advise the abandonment of mother tongue in order to facilitate the development of skills in English. SLTs should not advise individuals and their carers to abandon their mother tongue to facilitate progress in English.

The RCSLT recognises that bilingualism in an adult or child is an advantage and does not cause communication disorders.

With regard to assessment and differential diagnosis, bilingual individuals are vulnerable to misdiagnosis if linguistically and/or culturally inappropriate assessment tools are used to reach a diagnosis. An incomplete picture of their skills will emerge if only one language is assessed.

There is also risk if normative data that has been developed with monolingual populations is applied to bilingual individuals. SLTs should strive to assess an individual in all the languages to which they are exposed. When reaching a differential diagnosis, or writing reports, SLTs should highlight any areas where lack of appropriate assessment tools have prevented a full investigation of an individual's skills.

Lack of therapy material or written information translated into other languages may mean that individuals are not able to access AAC systems and families are not able to fully partake in intervention. As a result, compliance may be reduced.

Understanding the aetiology of a condition may be difficult, if language barriers exist and bilingual co-workers are not present at consultations.

8.6 Brain Injury

This information is designed to support speech and language therapy services undertaking reviews of service organisation and provision. Therapists seeking detailed clinical guidance are referred to the *RCSLT Clinical Guidelines* (2005), position papers and *Reference Framework: Underpinning Competence to Practise* (2003), available on the RCSLT website: www.rcslt.org

Definition and aetiology

The term 'acquired brain injury' (ABI) includes **traumatic brain injuries** such as open or closed head injuries, or **non-traumatic brain injuries**, such as those caused by strokes and other vascular accidents, tumours, infectious diseases, hypoxia, metabolic disorders, (eg liver and kidney diseases or diabetic coma), and toxic products taken into the body through inhalation or ingestion (CARF, 1996).

Certain conditions can be associated with potential for repeated or multiple insults to the brain, eg sickle cell disease, epilepsy, with resultant complex and varied patterns of deficit.

ABI is the most common cause of new disability in childhood. It refers to any injury occurring to the brain after the period immediately around birth (Children's ABI Interest Group, 2003).

Traumatic brain injury (TBI), also referred to as 'head injury', can be described as 'an insult to the brain, not of degenerative or congenital nature, but caused by an external force that may produce a diminished or altered state of consciousness' (National Head Injury Foundation, 1985).

TBI can be a result of either closed or open injury to the head. Closed head injury describes trauma (such as that sustained in a road traffic accident, fall, or non-accidental injury), that does not result in opening of the skull and typically gives rise to diffuse damage. Open head injury or penetrating injury (such as a gun-shot wound), tends to give rise to more focal damage (RCSLT, 1996).

TBI includes the effects of direct complications of trauma, notably hypoxaemia, hypertension, intracranial haemorrhage and raised intracranial pressure (BSRM, 1998).

Table 1: Classification of severity of head injury according to severity (adult population)

Severity	GCS (Glasgow Coma Scale)	Period of altered consciousness	Post-traumatic amnesia (PTA)	Approx incidence/ 100,000 population/ year
Mild	13-15	Less than 15 minutes	Less than 1 hour	250
Moderate	9-12	15 minutes – 6 hours	1-24 hours	18
Severe	3-8	More than 6 hours	24 hours or more	8

Cross-referencing with the chapter sections listed below is recommended:

8.1. Acquired Motor Speech Disorders

8.3. Aphasia

8.12. Dysfluency

8.13. Dyslexia

8.14. Dysphagia

8.16. Mental Health

8.18. Pre-school Children

8.20. School-aged Children

8.24. Voice

7.2.1 AAC

National guidance and sources of further information and support

● *Establishing minimum recommended standards for post-acute brain injury.* Malia, K Duckett, S in *Brain Injury*, 2001, Vol.15, no. 4, pp357-362.

● *Rehabilitation following an acquired brain injury: National clinical guidelines.* British Society of Medicine and Royal College of Physicians, 2003.

● *Vocational assessment and rehabilitation after acquired brain injury. Inter-agency guidelines.* Royal College of Physicians of London, 2004.

● *National Clinical Guidelines for Diagnosis and Management of Stroke in Childhood.* Royal College of Physicians, 2004.

● *NICE Head injury. Triage, assessment, investigation and early management of head injury in infants, children and adults.* Clinical Guidance, 4. June, 2003. www.nice.org.uk

● *The National Service Framework for long-term conditions.* Department of Health, 2005.

● *Supporting People with Longer-Term Conditions. An NHS and social care model to support local innovation and integration.* Department of Health, 2005.

● *Bournewood Consultation.* Department of Health, 2005. www.dh.gov.uk

● The Mental Capacity Act, 2005.

● Child Brain Injury Trust www.cbituk.org

● Headway www.headway.org.uk

8.6.1 Children with Acquired Brain Injury

Definition

Communication disorders in children following brain injury
TBI, both localised and diffuse, is likely to give rise to a complex association of motor, cognitive, perceptual, emotional and communication problems (CBIT, 1996).

There are other factors following a traumatic brain injury that affect speech and language and impact on the child's development and communication skills. These may include medical problems, physical disability as well as difficulties with attention and concentration, memory, speed of information processing, perception, executive functioning (including control, planning and organisation), behavioural and psychosocial issues. (Children's ABI Interest Group, 2003)

As a child with an ABI matures and develops they may continue to learn and communicate and do well in relation to formalised testing, resulting in a misleading picture of recovery, particularly in relation to the school environment. As the child grows, deficits in cognitive-communication and executive skills may lead to difficulties with both new language and learning. As the brain becomes challenged with more complex reading, writing and thinking, the need to both recognise and respond to the increasing complexity of social cues is more difficult. It is therefore important to monitor a child's language development and learning skills through adolescence (DePompei & Blosser, 1998).

Overtime, new difficulties may appear that are directly related to the brain injury. It is harder for people to connect the earlier brain injury with later difficulties with behaviour and learning. For the child who has a brain injury, time reveals instead of heals. (Lash & Associates, 1998).

Prevalence and incidence

Prevalence

Overall, ABI results in at least 3000 previously healthy children acquiring significant disability every year in the UK.

In a large secondary school with 1,500 pupils, one child will acquire a significant disability as a result of TBI every other year, although this may not always be recognised (Children's ABI Interest Group, 2003).

Incidence

Accurate statistics regarding children's head injury are not readily available as most studies focus on population as a whole. (CBIT, 2006).

TBI is the most common cause of death and acquired neurological handicap among children over one year of age in the UK. (Paediatric Epidemiology Group, 2005).

Each year, 160 per 100,000 children are admitted to accident and emergency in the UK with TBI.

During the period 2000-2001, 112,978 hospital admissions in England were made as a result of a head injury. Of these, 30% were children under 15 years old. Estimated figures for Wales show 6,700 people were admitted to hospital, again 30% were children under 15 years old (CBIT, 2006).

Trends

TBI in children is common and one in every ten children will sustain a significant head injury. Head injury accounts for over 150,000 attendances every year of children aged 14 years old, or under, at casualty departments in the UK. More than 40,000 children are admitted to hospital each year with head injuries in the UK.

● Approximately 33% TBIs occur at home, playing or during a sporting activity.

● 15% of TBIs are due to falls.

● 10% of TBIs are caused by road traffic accidents.

● 5% of TBIs occur at school or as a result of assaults (Headway, 2006).

Vulnerability: risk issues

Children return to school (education) at various stages in their recovery from ABI. Some return directly from an acute hospital setting. Others may have participated in a rehabilitation programme and still others may have been at home for extended periods, with or without the benefit of home tuition (Children's ABI Interest Group, 2003).

The age at which the brain injury occurs may be crucial to the results of future recovery. Children are within a developmental continuum and neurological development continues until approximately 20 years old. Damage to specific areas of the brain may not be apparent until skills mediated by those areas would normally develop and this could be years after the initial injury (Children's ABI Interest Group, 2003).

Research has shown that even brain injuries considered as minor can cause significant changes to the injured person's behaviour, personality and ability to learn (Acquire, 2006).

Children and young people are at risk of under-achievement and even failure both at school and in higher education. They can be prevented from gaining an independent lifestyle, successful relationships and future employment (Acquire, 2006).

The lighter size and weight of children makes it possible for many families to care for them at home. Rehabilitation programmes for children are few and far between in the UK, and generally only those who are most severely affected are considered for places (Lash & Associates, 1998).

Younger children are at greater risk for difficulties in the future because early brain development has been interrupted. They also have less life experience and skills to help them to adjust to changes caused by brain injury (Lash & Associates, 1998).

The view that brain damage in children is less impairing than equivalent damage in adults is no longer acceptable (Rose et al, 1997).

The challenges of paediatric rehabilitation seldom if ever fall within the remit of any one professional and necessitate collaboration between various disciplines at experimental and/or clinical levels (Paediatric Rehabilitation, 2001).

For example the greater vulnerability of the developing organism to physical insult and the failures of learning and development have been extensively documented for many years, yet the persistent notion that children do better after brain injury, than adults do, may be responsible for the virtual absence of paediatric rehabilitation and resources in this area (Paediatric Rehabilitation, 2001).

Even a mild brain injury can affect brain functioning. Even when a neurological examination is normal, a mild brain injury can cause changes in learning and behaviour that show up later at home or in school (Lash and Associates, 1998).

Speech and language therapy value

● Provision of rehabilitation services for speech, language, cognitive-communication disorders and dysphagia covering all stages of recovery, from acute care to successful reintegration into an educational setting.

Within acute hospital settings speech and language therapy should form part of an MDT provision.

Within the community, speech and language therapy should be part of a holistic multi-agency provision, including health, social services and education services and address the following aims:

- Development and maximising of overall communication skills in all environments.
- Introduction of sustainable strategies which minimise the impact of cognitive and behavioural changes, subsequent to ABI, which could otherwise impact upon successful reintegration to, and progress in, school.
- Ensuring that schools and the education service providers are aware of the potential long-term consequences of ABI, are alert to possible new difficulties appearing as the child matures, and are aware of how to access re-referral to services if new concerns do arise.
- Promotion of inclusion into school and social contexts.
- Promotion of access to the curriculum.
- Minimising secondary difficulties arising out of cognitive and communication impairments, such as emotional and behavioural difficulties.
- Supporting and educating parents as to the altered nature of the child's cognitive and communication abilities, and enabling them to be proactive in ensuring that the ABI and its consequences are recognised throughout childhood and adolescence.

Speech and language therapy services are also committed to increasing the overall awareness of the broader community regarding the cognitive, communication and swallowing needs of this client group.

8.6.2 Adults with Traumatic Brain Injury

Definition
This section has intentionally focused on TBI and not the full range of brain injuries that come under the term acquired brain injury (ABI), for example brain injury due to stroke. Information about stroke can be found in the Aphasia section above. However much of the remainder of this section will be appropriate to adults following other forms of ABI due to non-progressive or non-traumatic brain injuries, including brain injury due to tumours, haemorrhages, infectious diseases, metabolic disorders and neurotoxic products, as they share many clinical features.

Prevalence and incidence

The acquisition of precise prevalence data is problematic and there is no clear agreement. Few studies exist and results show the overall prevalence as anywhere between 5% and 24% of a given population (McGuire et al, 1998).

The prevalence of severe brain injury is about 100-150 per 100,000 population (Royal Hospital of Neuro-disability, 2001).

Incidence

Head injuries requiring hospitalisation occur in the UK at the rate of about 275 per 100,000 population annually (BSRM & RCP, 2003). Every year 150,000 people in the UK will have a minor head injury, 10,000 will suffer a moderate head injury and 11,600 a severe head injury (Headway, 2006).

For those suffering a moderate to severe brain injury (estimated at 25 per 100,000 population per year):

● 10-20% is likely to have a severe disability or prolonged coma.

● 65-85% will have a good physical (but not necessarily cognitive or psychosocial) recovery (BSRM RCP, 2003).

● Only 15% of people with a severe head injury return to work within 5 years (Headway, 2006).

Aetiology

There is evidence that people who sustain a TBI can be characterised in terms of age (predominantly 17-30); gender (predominantly male) and socio-economic factors, (ie a tendency towards limited education, vocational achievement and a history of risk-taking behaviours) (Rimmel et al, 1990). Alcohol is a major factor in many traumatic brain injuries (eMedicine, 2006).

● Road traffic accidents account for 40-50% and are associated with severe traumatic brain injury.

● Domestic and industrial accidents account for 20-30%.

● Sport and recreation account for 10-15%.

● Assaults account for 10% (Powell, 2004).

Incidence

Cognitive-communication disorders

There are currently no incidence figures available for cognitive-communication disorders (CCD) or cognitive-language disorders (CLD), first described by Hagen (1984), however there is an increasing amount of research and literature on the nature of communication difficulties following diffuse or multiple brain lesions concentrated in the temporal and frontomedial lobes of the brain commonly associated with TBI.

CCD/CLD are difficulties that stem from the relationship between commonly occurring cognitive difficulties following TBI, (eg impaired attention, memory, self-monitoring, judgement, planning) and their effect on language processing, language use and communication behaviour. Like patterns of cognitive impairment post-TBI, these disturbances are highly variable with some characteristic patterns as well as individual variations. These include:

● Altered communication behaviour reflecting reduced application of social rules.

● Changes in the quality and effectiveness of communication including reduction in verbal fluency, word retrieval and the coherence and relevance of information supplied.

● Difficulty with processing complex written and spoken information including understanding of inference.

CCDs may only impact fully when the person is attempting to return to former life roles or activities, reflecting the multiple cognitive demands that accompany many everyday communication activities.

Dysarthria occurs in approximately a third of the traumatic brain injured population according to a US study (Murdoch & Theodoras, 2001). Dysarthria is reported to be the most persistent of communication impairments, resulting in significant impact on the traumatic brain injury victim's ability to regain functional independence (Beukelman & Yorkston, 1991) (refer also to the section on *Acquired Speech Motor Disorder*).

Aphasia is more common when there is more focal brain damage. Data regarding prevalence is dated as it would previously have included some cognitive communication disorders which are now categorized in their own right. Incidence levels quoted vary from 2% (Heilman et al, 1971) to 30% (Sarno & Levita, 1986) (refer also to the section on *Aphasia*).

Apraxia of Speech (AOS) is a disturbance in the programming of movements for speech which can exist without apparent impairments in the speech muscles for non-speech tasks. This often co-exists with dysarthria and aphasia but can emerge as the only speech disturbance where brain damage is more localised.

Due to the more diffuse nature of brain damage after TBI, AOS is more likely to co-occur with other communication disorders. It is nearly always the result of left cerebral hemisphere pathology.

General incidence rates have been difficult to identify due to difficulties with definition and diagnosis criteria, no figures are available for the TBI population alone however, AOS was reported as the primary speech pathology in 9% of the speech therapy caseload (Mayo Clinic, 1987-1990; Duffy, 2005) (refer also to the section on *Acquired Speech Motor Disorders*).

Mutism is a condition in which the person does not speak and makes no attempt at spoken communication despite preservation of an adequate level of consciousness (Lishman, 1998). The individual's presentation needs careful assessment to distinguish it from severe AOS, aphasia, anarthria, aphonia and or severe psychomotor retardation.

Careful medical diagnosis is also required to differentiate mutism resulting from an organic cerebral cause, eg akinetic mutism associated with lesions in the upper brain stem, mutism resulting from lesions in the frontal lobe etc, from mutism resulting from non organic causes, eg affective disorders, psychosis, etc.

Aphonia, following traumatic brain injury, is a frequently reported perceptual feature (Cherney & Halper, 1996; Scholefield, 1987) (refer also to the sections on *Voice and Acquired Speech Motor Disorder* regarding dysarthrophonia).

Dysphagia is a common complication of head injury. The reported incidence of dysphagia in individuals with TBI ranges from 41-61% (Cherney & Halper, 1996; McKay et al, 1999). Dysphagia results not only from disordered physiology of the swallowing mechanism but from compromised cognitive-communicative skills and behavioural disorders (Halper et al, 1999) (refer also to the section 8.14.2 *Adults with Dysphagia: Risk Issues*).

Vulnerability: risk issues
Impact of reduced communication on functional outcome
Some authors have suggested that communication abilities may play the pivotal role in determining the quality of life after TBI (Najenson 1978). Communication disturbances following TBI are becoming increasingly recognised as significant factors in:
● reconstruction of identity (Ylvisaker & Feeney, 2000).

- resuming former life roles, work re-entry, psychosocial adaptation and forming and maintaining satisfying relationships (Marsh & Knight, 1991; Brooks et al, 1980; Isaki & Turkstra, 2000; O'Flatter & Douglas, 1997).
- the person with TBI being identified by members of the general public as mentally ill or learning disabled (Swift & Wilson, 2001).

Impact of reduced communication on carers

Communication disturbances following TBI have been shown to place an increased strain on roles and activities both in and outside care-giving situations (Connolly & O'Dowd, 2001).

A hidden disability

Individuals are at risk of being discharged without adequate follow-up, as more subtle cognitive-communication difficulties may go undetected in the clinical setting (Snow et al, 1995) and the individual themselves may have reduced/lack of awareness of the extent of their symptoms until they return to normal life (Harrington et al, 1993; Moss & Wade, 1996; King et al, 1999).

Neurobehavioural disability

The cerebral frontal lobes are particularly susceptible to deceleration closed head injuries. Individuals with this kind of injury frequently present with disorders of behaviour and cognition that persist long after the post acute phase.

Neurobehavioural disorders can be seen as barriers to rehabilitation as the learning process or application of learnt information is undermined and the individual has difficulty inhibiting behaviour that is offensive or embarrassing to others. The individual experiences emotional distress through being unable to sustain relationships, and presents with a disability that does not fit into conventional or psychological categories of disability (Wood, 2001).

Speech and language therapy value

- Providing early assessment in the acute setting to enable early identification of intervention for communication and swallowing needs and the need for prompt transfer to either inpatient or community based specialist rehabilitation services, (see also the *NSF for long-term conditions* (DH, 2005) – QR 3 & 5).
- Providing well planned and goal orientated rehabilitation in a specialist setting by expert professionals working in a coordinated interdisciplinary team (IDT), (see also the *NSF for long-term conditions* – (DH, 2005) QR 4).

● Providing well planned and flexible discharge to community living which may include communication goals for trial periods in the community, utilising and working with carers in specialist supported living facilities, working in collaboration with providers of community rehabilitation, supporting access to specialist equipment and providing training and advice to care workers so that they can support the individual with their communication or swallowing needs on a day-to-day basis, etc. (see also the *NSF for long-term conditions* (DH, 2005) – QR 4, 5 & 8).

● Providing continued coordinated and goal orientated specialist long-term MDT rehabilitation in the community to improve longer term outcome and self management and reduce hospital readmission or secondary health or psychological complications related to risks associated with communication and/or swallowing difficulties, (see also the *NSF for long-term conditions* (DH, 2005) – QR 5).

● Providing a service that addresses the communication needs of the individual at any time post onset in consideration of the individual's changing life aims and how their communication difficulties impact on their ability to achieve independence and inclusion in their life aim/s. This may be provided using a pattern of 'review-intervention-review' or provision of clearly defined points and procedures for re-entry into speech and language therapy rehabilitation or community services, (see also the *NSF for long-term conditions* (DH, 2005) – QR 4).

● Fostering strong links and work on collaborative goals with other agencies so that the individual with communication difficulties after TBI can be supported in playing a full inclusive role in society, including accessing public services, information, education, careers advice, employment, and health, social and voluntary sector services and/or facilities, (see also the *NSF for long-term conditions* (DH, 2005) – QR 5 & 6).

● Providing intervention that focuses on wider social participation such as leisure and recreational activities including combined working with other agencies in health, education, supported employment, and voluntary sectors, (see also the *NSF for long-term conditions* (DH, 2005) – QR 5 & 6).

● Supporting the individual's family and carers in contributing to and planning their own rehabilitation process, (see also the *NSF for long-term conditions* (DH, 2005) – QR 4, 5 & 10).

● Providing intervention that assists individuals and their carers or support workers develop the requisite knowledge, skills and confidence to enable them to manage their communication difficulties with greater independence This may include regarding accessing speech and language therapy advice, intervention or consultation at a future date as life goals or circumstances change, (see also the *NSF for long- term conditions* (DH, 2005) – QR 4, 5, 10 & 11).

● Raising awareness of the needs of individuals with communication difficulties after TBI within the multi-agencies involved in the post brain injury sequelae so that the individual is able to access appropriate support or training to reach the highest possible levels of communication independence, social inclusion and self determination.

8.7 Cerebral Palsy

This information is designed to support speech and language therapy services undertaking reviews of service organisation and provision. Therapists seeking detailed clinical guidance are referred to the *RCSLT Clinical Guidelines* (2005), position papers and *Reference Framework: Underpinning Competence to Practise* (2003), available on the RCSLT website: www.rcslt.org

Definitions

Cerebral palsy (CP) is persistent disorder of posture and movement, due to a defect or lesion of the immature brain. It is not a specific condition, rather an umbrella term covering a group of non-progressive, though not unchanging, motor impairment conditions, which range from multiple and profound to barely detectable. There are two aspects to the motor impairments:

● The lesions affect the immature central nervous system leading to delayed or arrested motor development.

● There are abnormal patterns of posture and movement due to abnormal reflex activity.

CP includes a variety of conditions. The three main types correspond to injuries to different parts of the brain:

● **Spastic cerebral palsy (spasticity)**

This is caused by impairment in the motor cortex of the brain and is the most common form of CP. It is characterised by constant increased muscle tone and weakness in the parts of the body affected. This increased muscle tone (hypertonia) creates tightness (stiffness) in the muscles, leading to a decreased range of movement in the joints. The effects may increase with anxiety or increased effort, leading to excessive fatigue. This affects 70-80% of people with CP.

● **Dystonic or dyskinetic cerebral palsy (athetoid cerebral palsy)**
This is caused by impairment in the basal ganglia area of the brain. It is characterised by involuntary and uncontrollable muscle tone fluctuations, sometimes involving the whole body. The muscles alternate between being floppy and tense and there will often be difficulty in maintaining posture. The person usually has full range of movement in their joints, but not the stability or coordination to control their movements.

Unwanted movements may be small, rapid, irregularly repetitive, random, and jerky, sometimes referred to as choreic movements. The unwanted movements may also be of a long, slow, writhing nature. Someone with athetoid cerebral palsy will often appear restless and constantly moving, only being still when fully relaxed and sometimes only when asleep.

The movements will often become worse when the person is excited or is attempting to do something.

Speech is nearly always affected to some degree, because of difficulty in controlling the tongue, breathing and vocal chords. Similarly there may be difficulties with eating and, the person may drool (have saliva coming out of their mouth). This affects an estimated 5-10% of people with CP.

● **Ataxic cerebral palsy (ataxia)**
This relatively rare form of CP, which affects less than 10% of people with CP, is caused by impairment to the cerebellum, which is in the base of the brain.

The cerebellum coordinates the actions of groups of muscles and is responsible for, amongst other things, balance. As with athetoid CP, all four limbs and the trunk are usually involved.

This impairment can lead to a general poor sensation of balance, unsteadiness and staggering when walking. Tremors may also be present when the person is attempting a task.

● **Mixed cerebral palsy**
It is not unusual for people with CP to have symptoms of more than one of the previous three forms. The most common mixed form includes spasticity and athetoid movements but other combinations are also possible.

CP can be categorised further, by referring to the parts of the body affected.

The three main categories are as follows:
- **Diplegia**: both legs are affected more than the hands and arms.
- **Hemiplegia** occurs where one side of the body (including arm and leg) is affected.
- **Quadriplegia/tetraplegia**: all four limbs are involved together with, usually, the trunk and neck. It is also known as 'total body involved'.

Occasionally you may come across these categories:
- **Monoplegia**: only one limb is involved.
- **Triplegia**: three limbs are affected – usually both legs and one arm.

It is important to remember that the trunk is involved in all limb and head movements whether voluntary, for balance, or for locomotion. Awareness of this is vital for positioning, both of the person and their impairment.

Individuals with CP have their difficulties compounded by:
- epilepsy (about 10%)
- visual impairments: physical and/or perceptual difficulties
- hearing impairments
- learning difficulties
- a 'specific learning difficulty', ie a problem with a particular activity, such as reading, drawing or arithmetic because a particular part of the brain is affected.

Cross-referencing with the chapter sections listed below is recommended:
8.2 Adult Learning Disability
8.11 Deafness
8.14 Dysphagia
8.18 Pre-school Children
8.20 School-aged Children
8.22 Specific Speech Impairment (dysarthria, dyspraxia, fluency and prosody)
8.23 Visual Impairment
7.2.1 AAC

Sources of further information and support
- The British Association of Teachers of the Deaf (BATOD) www.batod.org.uk
- The Communication Aids for Language and Learning (CALL) Centre www.callcentre.education.ed.ac.uk
- Communication Matters www.communicationmatters.org.uk

Aetiology

Causes of CP can be multiple and complex. Studies suggest that CP is mostly due to factors affecting the brain before birth. Known possible causes include:
● infection in the early part of pregnancy
● difficult or premature birth
● a cerebral (brain) bleed. This is more common following premature or multiple birth
● abnormal brain development
● a genetic link (though this is quite rare).

CP is present prior to birth for about 70% of children who have cerebral palsy, although it may not be detected for months. An additional 20% are diagnosed with CP due to a brain injury during the birthing process. In most cases, the cause of CP is unknown (SCOPE, 2006; UCP, 2001).

Incidence and prevalence

Incidence: approximately one in every 400 births is affected, ie about 1,800 babies are diagnosed with CP in the UK each year (SCOPE, 2006).

Prevalence: CP is a relatively rare condition affecting two or three people in every 1,000 (Griffiths & Clegg, 1988; Parkes et al, 2001; SCOPE, 2006).

Some research as shown that there may be a possible higher incidence of cerebral palsy in some British ethnic communities (Sinha et al, 1997).

Vulnerability: risk issues

Risk	Impact	Management of risk
Lack of recognition of the learning abilities of individuals with CP	Failure to develop the skills and abilities of the person with cerebral palsy to their optimum	Team working
Inadequate seating, positioning and access	Increased physical impairment which may result in short, medium or long term physical damage	Requires a team approach with occupational therapist and physiotherapy
Inadequate identification of additional sensory impairments	Reduced opportunities for communication and learning	Will require input/involvement of experts in these fields as part of the team
Increased risk of eating and drinking difficulties including attention to nutrition	Inadequate nutrition plus increased risk of illness including potential life threatening illnesses, eg pneumonia	Providing timely access to SLT when required
Inadequate skills and knowledge of the specific communication needs of this group (including AAC)	Harm to health, education and wellbeing	Providing timely access to adequately skilled and knowledgeable SLT when required
Lack of AAC supports (when speech is not developing to a point where speech can be understood by most people)	Marked consequences for success in social, educational and vocational aspects of life	Team working

It is essential that the SLT works as part of an inter-/multidisciplinary team to ensure the risks to people with CP are minimised.

Speech and language therapy value

● Promoting the development and use of effective communication and language systems.

● Promoting the social, cognitive and motor skills which contribute to effective communication, eg cause and effect, turn taking, interaction.

● Ensuring that individuals receive adequate nutrition. Individuals should be able to take nourishment in ways that are safe, comfortable and dignified. This may involve referral to a specialist feeding clinic.

● Promoting the development of eating and drinking skills, ensuring safe nutrition.

● Providing information and advice on oro-motor difficulties, including reasons why articulation therapy may be ineffective and counter-productive.

● Providing information and advice/therapy regarding the management of drooling.

● Providing information, support, advice and training regarding therapy procedures for those supporting the individual across the individual's environments.

● Ensuring that individuals with CP continue to have access to speech and language therapy when needed across their lifespan.

● Promoting communicatively responsive environments, hence facilitating communication for the individual with a wider group of people.

8.8 Cleft Palate and Velopharyngeal Disorders

This information is designed to support speech and language therapy services undertaking reviews of service organisation and provision. Therapists seeking detailed clinical guidance are referred to the *RCSLT Clinical Guidelines* (2005), position papers and *Reference Framework: Underpinning Competence to Practise* (2003), available on the RCSLT website: www.rcslt.org

Definition

This group includes individuals born with syndromic and non-

syndromic cleft palate (with/without cleft lip) and those with submucous cleft palate, non-cleft velopharyngeal insufficiency/dysfunction, and oral maxillofacial anomalies but excludes individuals with other craniofacial disorders.
Cross-referencing with the chapter sections listed below is recommended:
8.9. Craniofacial Conditions
8.11. Deafness
8.14. Dysphagia
8.18. Pre-school Children
8.20. School-aged Children
8.22 Specific Speech Impairment
8.23. Visual Impairment
8.24. Voice

National guidance and sources of further support and information

● *Clinical Standards Advisory Group Report* on the care and outcomes in children born with a unilateral cleft, 1998.
● *RCSLT Clinical Guidelines*, section on *Cleft palate*, 2005. www.rcslt.org
● Cleft Lip and Palate Association (CLAPA) www.clapa.com
● Maxappeal Support Group for 22q11 www.maxappeal.org.uk
● Changing Faces www.changingfaces.org.uk
● Contact a Family (CAF) www.cafamily.org.uk

Aetiology

When cleft lip/palate occurs with no other anomaly or associated syndrome it has a multi-factorial aetiology involving both environmental and genetic factors.
Current thinking is that there are probably multiple genes involved which may interact, not only with each other, but also with environmental factors. Environmental factors include certain drugs, alcohol, pesticides, and maternal smoking. Most cases occur as a one-off event in families but a family history is present in about a quarter of cases.
The chances of a sibling of a child with a cleft lip and/or palate also being affected are around 30-40 times the risk of the non-cleft population (Lees, 2000). In the majority of cases the cleft will be the

only defect, but clefts of the lip and palate may also be found in association with other congenital anomalies, or may occur as part of a well-defined syndrome.

More than 400 syndromes include cleft lip and/or palate. The most common syndromes are Stickler and Velocardiofacial syndrome both of which can be associated with Pierre-Robin sequence (Harding and Sell, 2001).

Incidence

Cleft lip and palate is the most common congenital craniofacial abnormality affecting about 1 in 600-700 live births (Gregg et al, 1994; Sandy, 2003).

There is considerable variation in the presentation of clefts of the lip and palate.

Incidence of different cleft types

Cleft lip alone (incidence 25%) may be complete or incomplete, unilateral or bilateral.

When cleft lip occurs in association with cleft palate, unilateral cleft lip and palate (UCLP), or bilateral (BCLP) may result. The incidence of UCLP is 25% and that of BCLP 10%.

Isolated cleft palate has an incidence of 40%. The extent and width is variable. In addition to overt clefts of the palate this client group includes:

i. **Submucous cleft palate**: three characteristic signs are associated with submucous cleft palate: a bifid uvula; a very thin membranous central portion of the soft palate where the levator palatini muscles are wrongly inserted into the back of the hard palate and not joined in the midline; and a palpable notch at the junction of the hard and soft palate.

ii. **Non-cleft velopharyngeal insufficiency/dysfunction** (non-cleft VPI/VPD): can be caused by a muscle dysfunction, ie hypotonia; dysarthria; or discoordination or by a structural impairment, eg increased dimensions of nasopharynx following adenoidectomy; trauma to the soft palate; or disproportionate size of the nasopharynx in relation to sphincter closure pattern.

Classic speech characteristics associated with VPI are described as hypernasality and/or nasal emission with weak/absent pressure consonants (plosives and fricatives) and/or a prevalence of nasal consonants or glottal articulation.

The non-cleft VPI population represents as many as 50% of the cleft specialists SLT caseload (Sell & Ma, 1996).

Issues in classification of cleft palate

Common descriptors of cleft type include complete/incomplete, bilateral/unilateral, hard and soft, primary/secondary cleft palate, and soft palate only.

Use of different terminology can be ambiguous, no firm agreement has been reached for clinical use but for more precise database records, Kernahan's striped Y classification gives a clear diagrammatic display of cleft type.

Vulnerability: risk issues

Feeding difficulties, particularly in infancy and subsequent impact on health and wellbeing.

Atypical speech development with the possibility of persisting speech and/or resonance problems into teens or adult life (Harding & Grunwell, 1996; Russell & Harding, 2001; Sell et al, 1998).

Without specialist therapy input, ineffective therapy can extend over many years and optimal results may not be achieved.

There is mild/moderate fluctuating hearing loss in 90% of children with cleft palate which may contribute to severity of speech difficulties. Repeated grommet insertion and/or hearing aids may be needed. There is some risk of long-term conductive hearing loss.

Atypical dentition/dental malocclusion: most intervention occurs from eight years-old to late teens.

Atypical facial growth affects appearance, causing dental occlusion affecting speech and self-esteem and frequently requires maxillofacial surgery at about nine to 10 years-old and possibly more major surgery is required in late teens.

Dysphonia has a higher incidence in the cleft palate population than the non-cleft population. A history of hearing loss may be a contributory factor; as may hypernasality.

Cleft palate may have a negative impact on psychosocial and emotional development throughout life, but primarily in major social adjustment phases. For example, entrance to pre-school and school with the combination of speech difficulties, a fluctuating hearing loss and, in many cases, visible facial difference, may have significant psychosocial and educational consequences for children born with cleft lip and palate (Nash, 2002).

Non-cleft speech disorders such as phoneme specific nasality/active nasal fricative might be inappropriately referred to ENT and may be misdiagnosed as VPD which could result in unnecessary surgery or inappropriate therapy.

Non-cleft VPI/VPD or undiagnosed submucuous cleft identified in community clinics, may be a feature of undiagnosed syndromes such as Velocardiofacial syndrome or 22q11 deletion syndrome, without referral to the cleft team accurate diagnosis may not be made.

Referral of non-cleft hypernasal resonance and/or nasal emission cases to ENT consultants can result in misdiagnosis and possible unnecessary surgical intervention.

Management of risks at level of service organisation and provision

The national standards of care set by CSAG report (1998) require that all children born with cleft palate should have access to specialist care provided by centres of excellence.

In the event of visible or suspected structural impairment, a specialist therapist's opinion is necessary to assess and advise on specific speech difficulties in relation to structure so that appropriate surgical, prosthetic and/or therapeutic intervention can be planned (modified).

Specialist SLTs liaise closely with cleft team audiologists and ENT services and incorporate principles relating to mild/moderate hearing loss into therapy advice about pre-speech/speech development.

Sufficient and timely specialist-led therapy during key periods of speech development may introduce adaptive strategies to maximise articulatory potential whilst minimising the use of compensatory articulation (Harding & Sell, 2001).

Multidisciplinary discussions and decisions within the cleft palate clinic help to ensure the most appropriate care at all stages of the care pathway (CSAG, 1998).

Suspected cases of non-cleft velopharyngeal dysfunction (VPD) or palate problems in community clinics should be referred to a cleft specialist SLT for an opinion on the need for palatal investigations.

Speech and language therapy value

Facilitation of normal speech, language and communication development in the context of structural abnormality through collaborative specialist interdisciplinary assessment, planning and management within and across specialist multidisciplinary teams for cleft lip and palate and VPI/VPD.
This entails:

● Specialist clinical assessments and advice throughout childhood and adolescence.
● Appropriate therapy offered either in specialist centre or locally under guidance from the specialist practitioner/s based in the surgical centre.
● Appropriate liaison with, members of the cleft team and local health and educational colleagues across the network.
● Collaborative management of speech development in relation to conductive hearing loss.
● Collaborative management of VPI/VPD with cleft surgeons (Sell, 2005).
● Collaborative preparation for maxillary osteotomy with maxillofacial surgeon, orthodontists and psychologists.
● Development of specialist services for specific clinics, eg 22q11 clinics.
● Teaching and CPD for community speech and language therapy teams to extend knowledge and resources in local services.
● Clinical and audit record keeping in accordance with national guidelines.

Care pathway

The care pathway for cleft palate and velopharyngeal dysfunction includes time windows for speech and language therapy contacts related to cleft surgery; national audit data collection and routine monitoring by local and/or central specialist speech and language therapy services.

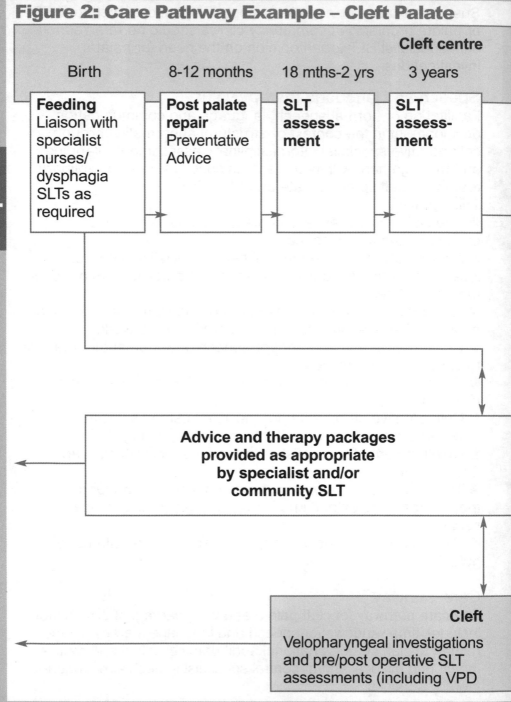

Figure 2: Care Pathway Example – Cleft Palate

Cleft centre

Birth	8-12 months	18 mths-2 yrs	3 years
Feeding Liaison with specialist nurses/ dysphagia SLTs as required	**Post palate repair** Preventative Advice	**SLT assess-ment**	**SLT assess-ment**

Advice and therapy packages provided as appropriate by specialist and/or community SLT

Cleft

Velopharyngeal investigations and pre/post operative SLT assessments (including VPD

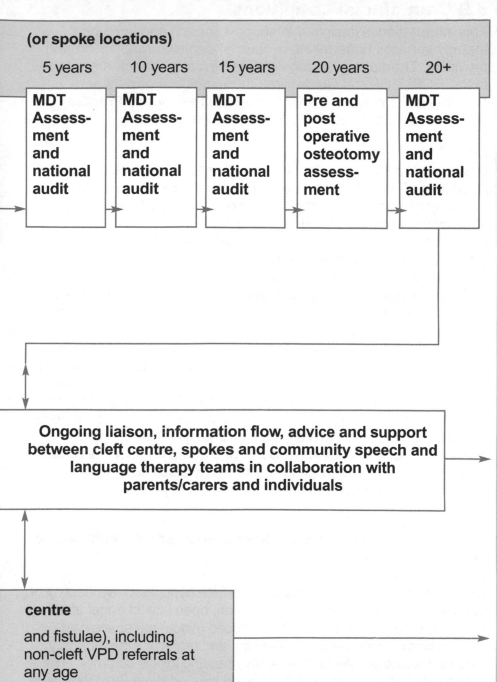

8.9 Craniofacial Conditions

This information is designed to support speech and language therapy services undertaking reviews of service organisation and provision. Therapists seeking detailed clinical guidance are referred to the *RCSLT Clinical Guidelines* (2005), position papers and *Reference Framework: Underpinning Competence to Practise* (2003), available on the RCSLT website: www.rcslt.org

Definition

Craniofacial conditions affect the growth and development of the structures of the face and skull. They may be congenital or acquired. The major categories of craniofacial conditions are listed below:

Craniosynostosis – abnormalities of skull shape and growth associated with premature fusion (synostosis) of the calvarial sutures, occurring before or after birth.

These may affect single or multiple sutures:

(i) **Single suture craniosynostosis** – the most common sutures involved are the sagittal suture (scaphocephalic skull shape) and the metopic suture (trigonocephalic skull shape).

(ii) **Multiple suture craniosynostosis** – usually associated with syndromic conditions. In addition to the calvarial suture, the sutures of the facial skeleton, often the axial or appendicular skeleton are also involved in syndromic craniosynostosis. Deformity of the facial skeleton may result in functional disabilities such as proptosis; upper airway obstruction; speech production difficulties and feeding difficulties (Pereira, 2004; Shipster et al, 2003; Thompson & Britto, 2004). Visceral and CNS abnormalities may also occur in some craniosynostotic syndromes.

Syndromes

(i) The four most common syndromes associated with **multi-suture craniosynostosis** are:

● *Apert syndrome*

Characterised by craniosynostosis, mid face hypoplasia, syndactyly of the hands and feet, class III malocclusion, open bite, choanal atresia or stenosis, fixation of the stapes, reduced middle ear space with chronic serous otitis media. The airway and orofacial structure may result in feeding problems. Conductive hearing loss is common. There may be cleft palate or the palate may be shaped like a Byzantine arch.

● *Crouzon syndrome (craniofacial dysostosis)*
Characterised by craniosynostosis, maxillary hypoplasia, ocular proptosis, class III malocclusion, open bite. There may be feeding problems due to choanal atresia or stenosis. Conductive hearing loss is common resulting from ossicular abnormalities or chronic middle ear disease.

● *Pfeiffer syndrome*
Characterised by craniosynostosis resulting in a clover leaf skull, broad thumbs and broad great toes, shallow orbits and maxillary hypoplasia with class III malocclusion. There is airway compromise caused by choanal atresia or stenosis resulting in feeding difficulties.

● *Saethre-Chotzen syndrome*
Characterised by coronal sutural synostosis, facial asymmetry, ptosis of eyelids, conductive hearing loss, occasional cleft palate.

(ii) *Treacher Collins syndrome*
Treacher Collins syndrome is characterised by bilateral hypoplasia of the cheeks and mandible. The malar and mandibular bones are underdeveloped; the latter resulting in malocclusion of the bite. Additional associations include malformed external ears, down slanting palpebral fissures, coloboma of the eyelids, and hypoplasia of the alae nasae and choanal atresia. Hypoplasia of the pharyngeal muscles may cause feeding problems. Airway obstruction may also result in poor feeding development and reduced growth (Gorlin et al, 1990).

(iii) *Hemifacial microsomia*
This is a large heterogeneous family of disorders and includes several syndromes, (eg Goldenhar syndrome) in which there is asymmetric development of the facial structures, primarily those arising from the first and second branchial arches. Another popular umbrella term used for these disorders is auriculovertebral spectrum. Although the term 'hemifacial' denotes problems on just one side of the face, the majority of individuals actually have abnormalities of both sides of the face, with one side more severely involved than the other (Gorlin et al, 1990).

(iv) *Facial clefts*
These are classified using the Tessier clefting system which describes the clefts situated along definite axes. The Tessier system is anatomic and descriptive. Clefts may be unilateral or bilateral and soft and bony tissue is involved. There are some orofacial clefting syndromes (Gorlin et al, 1990).

(v) *Neurofibromatosis (NF)*
Craniofacial conditions are usually associated with Type 1 neurofibromatosis. Von Recklinghausen (1882) described NF as, "characterised by abnormal cutaneous pigmentation and numerous tumours developing in association with elements of both the central and peripheral nervous system". Functional problems include learning disability, distractibility, impulsiveness, and language and vocabulary deficit (Gorlin et al, 1990).

(vi) *Bony and fibrous overgrowth conditions*
Vascular anomalies are lesions, which can occur anywhere on the body. They are composed of disorganised blood vessels and cause deformity of varying degrees, from mild to severe; the associated functional problems can be minor to life threatening. Management of anomalies affecting the face, base of skull and the brain require the collective expertise of the craniofacial unit.

(vii) *Encephalocele*
This is a protrusion of a part of the cranial contents through a defect in the skull. The mass may contain meninges (meningocele), meninges and brain (meningoencephalocele), or meninges, brain and ventricle (meningocephalocystocele) (Jackson et al, 1983). There are many other craniofacial conditions. Comprehensive texts are referenced at the end of this chapter.

National guidance and sources of further support and information

There are currently four nationally designated craniofacial centres in the UK:
● Birmingham Children's Hospital and University Hospital Birmingham
● Great Ormond Street Hospital, London
● Radcliffe Infirmary, Oxford
● Royal Liverpool Children's Hospital, Alder Hey.

These are funded nationally by the National Specialist Commissioning Advisory Group (NSCAG) to provide tertiary level services for this client group.

Although many craniofacial conditions are rare, relatively large numbers of individuals with craniofacial conditions are seen at these units. Multidisciplinary evaluation and management is essential, due to the complex nature of these conditions.

NSCAG requires that all individuals born with craniofacial conditions have access to multidisciplinary specialist care provided by designated craniofacial units.

- **Changing Faces** www.changingfaces.org.uk
- **Headlines** www.headlines.org.uk

Aetiology

"The origins of craniosynostosis are hereditary, mechanical, teratogenic, and idiopathic" (Aleck-Kirk, 2004).

It is beyond the scope of this document to identify all the factors that may cause craniofacial conditions. The aetiology of single suture synostosis is often unknown but occasionally there may be a genetic basis or teratogenic basis. For example, sodium valproate exposure has been associated with metopic synostosis.

Many syndromic craniofacial conditions have a genetic basis. For example, syndromes associated with multi-suture craniosynostosis are caused by mutations of specific genes.

Cross-referencing with the chapter sections listed below is recommended:

8.8. Cleft palate and Velopharyngeal Disorders
8.11. Deafness
8.14. Dysphagia
8.16. Mental Health
8.18. Pre-school Children
8.20. School-aged Children
8.21. Specific Language Impairment
8.22 Specific Speech Impairment
8.23 Visual Impairment
8.24. Voice
7.2.1 AAC

Incidence

Non-syndromic single suture craniosynostosis

(i) *Metopic synostosis (trigonocephaly)* 1:15,000 live births; male:female, approx 3:1; more common in twins (Lajeune et al, 2001).

(ii) *Sagittal synostosis (scaphocephaly)* 1: 5000 live births; male:female, approx 3:1; Sagittal synostosis accounts for 55% of all cases of synostosis (Lajeune et al, 2001).

(iii)*Unicoronal and bicoronal synostosis* (plagiocephaly and brachycephaly) 1:2, 100-2,500 live births (combined incidence); twice as common in females.
Note: now recognised that a proportion of cases with unicoronal synostosis are the result of FGFR3 mutation, ie *Muenke syndrome*.
(iv) *Lambdoid synostosis* prevalence 2.3 –2.9% of synostoses.

Syndromic multi-suture synostosis fusion of two or more sutures (no formal incidence available)
(i) *Apert syndrome* 1:100,000 live births; 15.5 per million births (Cohen & MacLean, 2000); prevalence 4.5% of all craniosynostosis cases.
(ii) *Crouzon syndrome* 1:25,000 live births; 16.6 per million births (Gorlin et al, 1990).
(iii) *Pfeiffer syndrome* incidence not reported but accounts for approximately 4% of all cases of craniosynostosis (Wilson, 2004).
(iv) Saethre-Chotzen syndrome 1:25,000 to 1:50,000 (Wilson, 2004).
Other syndromes:
Hemifacial microsomia 1:4,000 live births.
Treacher Collins syndrome 1:40,000 to 1:70,000 (often quoted as 1:50,000).
Neurofibromatosis 1:3,000.
Facial Clefts 1:5,000 or 1.4-4.9 per 100,000 live births (Otaki & Kawamoto, 2002).

Vulnerability: risk issues

Communication
Individuals with craniofacial conditions are at high risk for communication difficulties secondary to their oro-facial structures, psychosocial factors, cognitive impairment, hearing and/or visual impairment.
Whilst many children with single suture synostosis are not at risk of speech and language difficulties, there has been an identified increased risk for children with sagittal synostosis (Shipster et al, 2003) and metopic synostosis (Lajeune et al, 2001; Otaki & Kawamoto, 2002; Wilson, 2004).
Aspects of speech and language development that may be affected include:

- Language acquisition – may have developmental language difficulties, also language acquisition may be detrimentally affected by psychosocial, cognitive, hearing and environmental factors.
- Resonance and voice – may be affected by structural abnormalities. Hyponasality is evident in a number of individuals with syndromic conditions due to midface retrusion. Resonance requires monitoring as it may alter following surgical intervention, eg maxillofacial surgery.
- Articulation – errors due to structural problems, eg atypical dentition/dental malocclusion may mean individuals use compensatory movements/postures to improve intelligibility.
- Phonological impairment may co-exist with other articulatory difficulties.

Feeding

Feeding difficulties in children with craniofacial problems are poorly described in the literature. Consequently, accurate prevalence is unknown and the majority of our current knowledge in this area is largely based on clinical experience and local evidence.

The two main predisposing factors in this cohort are abnormal oral facial structure and upper airway obstruction. Other factors include visual impairment, developmental delay, central nervous system malformations, cardiovascular and respiratory anomalies and gastrointestinal anomalies.

Feeding difficulties may be present in the oral stage or pharyngeal stage of swallowing which may arise at any of the main stages of feeding acquisition. There is also a risk of aversive feeding behaviour secondary to frequent hospitalisations and poor/limited feeding experiences. Assessment and management requires a multidisciplinary approach as well as including both the carers and the child themselves (Pereira, 2004).

Other considerations

- Psychosocial factors related to the impact of altered appearance, reduced social opportunity, anxiety, reduced expectations of general ability, academic achievement and communicative ability (Hearst, 2004).
- Frequent hospitalisations and medical appointments may have a negative effect on the opportunities for social interaction and learning

and there may be an increased level of parental stress (Sarimski, 1998).

● Hearing – increased risk for hearing impairment due to persistent otitis media with effusion and/or congenital conductive hearing loss secondary to structural abnormalities of the outer and/or middle ear; particularly in syndromic cases.

Management of risk

A specialist SLT is necessary to provide assessment for specific feeding, speech and language difficulties in relation to the craniofacial condition (often structural) in order for appropriate surgical and/or therapeutic intervention to be planned.

Specialist SLTs closely with both the craniofacial team and local audiology and ENT services to ensure appropriate intervention. There is a need to incorporate principles relating to mild/moderate hearing loss into therapy advice about speech and language development.

Multidisciplinary discussions and decisions within the craniofacial clinic help to ensure the timing for the most appropriate care from all disciplines at all stages of the care pathway.

Speech and language therapy value

Maximisation of the individual's potential for communication and feeding development, in the context of their craniofacial condition, through collaborative specialist inter-disciplinary assessment, planning and management within specialist multidisciplinary craniofacial teams. This entails:

● Specialist clinical assessments and advice throughout childhood, adolescence and adulthood.

● Therapy offered in conjunction with local services with guidance from the specialist clinicians, and when appropriate, therapy offered within specialist centres.

● Appropriate liaison with members of the craniofacial team and local health and educational colleagues.

● Collaborative management of speech and language development in relation to conductive hearing loss.

● When appropriate, collaborative management of resonance problems with appropriate surgical colleagues.

● Collaborative preparation for maxillary osteotomy with maxillofacial

surgeon, orthodontists and psychologists.
● Frequent contact, teaching and CPD for community SLTs to extend knowledge and resources in local services.
● Clinical and audit record keeping in accordance with national guidelines.

8.10 Critical Care

This information is designed to support speech and language therapy services undertaking reviews of service organisation and provision. Therapists seeking detailed clinical guidance are referred to the *RCSLT Clinical Guidelines* (2005), position papers and *Reference Framework: Underpinning Competence to Practise* (2003), available on the RCSLT website: www.rcslt.org

Definition
Critical care refers to the level of care given to a group of individuals who are deemed to be critically ill.
In 2000, a Department of Health report recommended that, "the existing division into high dependency and intensive care [services] based on beds, be replaced by a classification that focuses on the level of care that individual individuals need, regardless of location". The classification system of *Intensive Care Society Standards* (2002) is as follows:

Level 0
Individuals whose needs can be met through normal ward care in an acute hospital.

Level 1
Individuals at risk of their condition deteriorating, or those recently relocated from higher levels of care whose needs can be met on an acute ward with additional advice and support from the critical care team.

Level 2
Individuals requiring detailed observation or intervention including support for a single failing organ system or postoperative care, and those 'stepping down' from higher levels of care.

Level 3

Individuals requiring advanced respiratory support alone or basic respiratory support together with support of at least two organ systems. This level includes all complex individuals requiring support for multi-organ failure.

Many individuals who are critically ill have requirements for the support for their neurological, respiratory and digestive systems all of which can impact on their ability to communicate and swallow independently. Presence of technologies to prolong life/enable clinical management of the individuals with critical illness such mechanical ventilation, tracheostomy tubes, naso-gastric tubes and naso-pharyngeal airways as may also impact on communication and oro-pharyngeal swallowing abilities.

Cross-referencing with the chapter sections listed below is recommended:

8.3. Aphasia
8.6. Brain Injury
8.14. Dysphagia
8.15. Head and Neck Cancer
8.19. Progressive Neurological Disorders
7.2.1 AAC

National guidance

A Department of Health report (2000) recommended that "an appropriately balanced team of staff including therapy professions and support staff is essential to the effective delivery of critical care services. The nature of the critical care service and its need to operate on a 24 hour, seven day a week service, requires that support staff must be available on a similar basis to professional staff, according to workload and individual need."

In June 2002, the Modernisation Agency produced a document detailing multi-professional AHP roles, which "offer unique value to individual care in the critical care setting". This document was produced because "historically, the roles and value of AHP and HCS have been under acknowledged".

Both documents state the benefits of the SLT within the critical care setting and advocate that an SLT should be an integral member of the team.

In addition, studies have shown that weaning is most successful when a multidisciplinary team collaborates (Henneman et al, 2001). This intervention decreased medical ICU lengths of stay (3.6 days) and ventilator lengths of stay (2.7 days).

Aetiology

There are three main causes of communication and/or oro-pharyngeal swallowing disorders in the critical care setting:
● Organic communication/oro-pharyngeal swallowing disorders such as those caused by stroke, head injury, Guillian-Barré Syndrome, post surgical to oral cavity, pharynx or larynx, COPD (Martin-Harris, 2000), ARDS, spinal cord injury, etc.
● Concomitant communication/oro-pharyngeal swallowing disorders such as the effects of critical care neuropathy (due to the disuse atrophy of striated muscle) or the effects of technologies to prolong life/enable clinical management of the individuals' illness, such mechanical ventilation, tracheostomy tubes, naso-gastric tubes and naso-pharyngeal airways (Conlan & Kopec, 2000; Pannunzio, 1996).
● Functional communication/oro-pharyngeal swallowing disorders such as resulting from critical care psychosis or clinical depression. In addition, within the ICU environment an undervaluing of communication can occur due to the level of arousal/medications (Hemsley et al, 2001). Mechanically ventilated individuals report high levels of frustration when communicating their needs (Patak et al, 2004).

Prevalence

Approximately 18.5% of hospitalised individuals require intervention in a critical care environment, level 1-3 (North West London Critical Care Network, 2003).
The literature reports a high range (50-70%) of aspiration reported in this population (Elpern et al, 1987, 1994; DeVita & Spierer-Rundback, 1990; Tolep et al, 1996; Leder, 2002; Gross et al, 2003). Aspiration can frequently be seen in individuals requiring prolonged ventilation of three or more weeks (Elpern et al, 1994; Tolep et al, 1996; Leder, 2002).
However, there have been numerous difficulties in trying to establish the true prevalence and incidence of aspiration in the mechanically ventilated population. The main reason for this is that aspiration is

Chapter 8

identified in different ways in different studies. Thus some studies employ bedside assessments (Elpern et al, 1987) and others use instrumental techniques (Gross et al, 2003; Elpern et al, 1994; Leder, 2002).

In the studies that have employed instrumental techniques it is reported that aspiration can be 'silent' or covert. This questions the veracity of those studies that have relied on overt aspiration detection; indeed, the true incidence of aspiration could be higher than is reported.

There are no studies to date that have examined the prevalence of communication difficulties in this population. However, the inability to speak and the associated communication difficulties that result are a major source of stress for intubated individuals (Menzel, 1998). An exit interview conducted in Derby Royal Infirmary found that 93% of individuals complain of communication problems on ITU.

Vulnerability: Risk issues

The compromised communication and swallowing difficulties experienced by individuals in critical care leads to a number of clinical risks.

Communication disorders

Clinical risk: Inability to communicate effectively, (eg around a clinical need such as pain).

Clinical risk: Compromised psychosocial wellbeing.

Clinical risk: Lack of reliable outcome measures.

Establishing communication for critically ill individuals is largely overlooked in many critical care settings. At best, units may provide communication boards or rely upon attempting to lip read. Both of these options can be time consuming and frustrating for the individuals and staff, leading to significant fatigue for the already fatigued individual (Albarran, 1991).

Nurses often report feeling frustrated and incompetent when they are unable to understand and meet their patients' needs (Engberg-Bergbom et al, 1989). Studies that look at the impact of being communication difficulties in a critical care environment report that "Anxiety, fear, insecurity and inability to sleep are all associated with being unable to speak" (Menzel, 1994). Furthermore, being ventilated and unable to communicate can lead to difficulties with weaning (Arbour, 2000).

Many individuals in ICU describe feelings of disempowerment and social isolation due to their inability to communicate effectively and because they are unable to express how they feel (Hemsley et al 2001). Individuals' inability to talk and communicate was the dominant reason for anxiety during treatment with a respirator (Engberg-Bergbom et al, 1989).

It is assumed that communication problems only affect the individual during the intubation period. However, there is evidence that, even after discharge from hospital the psychological well being of many individuals is affected. This often relates to communication difficulties experienced during their stay in critical care (Hemsley et al, 2001). Menzel (1997; 1998) demonstrated that self esteem and difficulties with communication of individuals in an ITU unit who were unable to speak were significantly associated with individual's emotional responses. Lack of communication can have a significant impact on psychosocial and emotional well being of the individual and effect reliable measurement of outcomes. These types of measures, especially those looking at psychosocial factors, tend to be verbally dependant. If the individual is unable to communicate results will be skewed.

See the following sections regarding vulnerability in specific diagnostic groups:

● Aphasia
● Acquired Brain Injury
● Progressive Neurological Disorders.

Swallowing disorders

Clinical risk: Aspiration pneumonia.

Clinical risk: Compromised nutrition and hydration.

Clinical risk: Increased length of stay due to weaning difficulties.

It is recognised that if the complex interrelationship between eating swallowing and breathing is disrupted then impairment in swallowing can result (Dikeman & Kazandijan, 1995).

Presence of aspiration pneumonia may result in:

● Increased length of stay in critical care (Carter Young & Durrant Jones, 1990).

- Delayed rehabilitation or transfer to a ward.
- Need for prolonged alternative or supplementary feeding.
- Need for drug interventions.
- Increased time from other AHP's such as chest physio.
- Increased stay in hospital: on average 5.5 days longer than other individuals (Carter Young & Durrant Jones, 1990; Odderson et al 1995).

Nasal mask CPAP inhibits the swallow reflex by:
- Increasing the latency of response.
- Decreasing the total number of swallows (Nishino, 1989).

See section regarding Vulnerability in Dysphagia

Speech and language therapy value

Risks can effectively be managed by having an SLT as an integrated member of the team. The SLT works with the team to establish methods of communication at an early stage and advise on the safe introduction of oral intake for those presenting with oro-pharyngeal dysphagia.

Where an organic communication/oro-pharyngeal swallowing disorder exists, eg caused by stroke, head injury, progressive neurological disease, a specialist SLT assessment of individuals in the critical care setting may enable early identification of communication and swallowing deficits and prompt commencement on the appropriate pathways of care which might otherwise be deferred until after transfer out of critical care.

Communication

SLTs can facilitate individual's participation in intervention and recovery within the critical care setting by providing:
- A differential diagnosis of communication difficulties caused by or co-existing with the use of tracheostomy or mechanical ventilation.
- Specialist, individualised intervention/advice/strategies for the individual to maximise communication ability.
- Specialist advice/strategies to family members and multidisciplinary staff to minimise communication difficulties between individual and others.
- Alternative communication devices both low and hi-tech, where appropriate, to augment communication.

By providing timely and ongoing assessment and intervention and providing effective communication strategies and/or aids there may be a reduction in the negative emotional responses (such as fear, anxiety, frustration) and an improvement in the psychological wellbeing of the individual, family and staff (Dikeman & Kazandjian, 2003; Manzano et al, 1993).

By restoring or facilitating communication the individual may participate more readily in intervention and provide valuable feedback on clinical issues such as work of breathing which can often be the clinician's greatest diagnostic tool (Isaki & Hoit, 1997; Spremulli, 2005).

See the following sections regarding speech and language therapy value in specific diagnostic groups:

● Aphasia
● Acquired Brain Injury
● Progressive Neurological Disorders.

Swallowing

SLTs can minimise preventable secondary respiratory complications of swallowing difficulties, which arise from or co-exist with use of tracheostomy/ventilator, by providing:

● Specialist evaluation of swallow function which may include instrumental assessment using Videofluoroscopy or Fibreoptic Endoscopic Evaluation of Swallowing (FEES).

● Information to the MDT on swallow status, to enable informed decision making regarding tracheotomy or ventilator weaning and commencement of oral intake including timing and types of food and liquids.

● Specialist individualised intervention, advice and strategies to maximise swallowing abilities.

By providing the above service the time taken to wean from the tracheostomy/ventilator can be reduced and potentially reduce the length of stay in critical care.

It is recognised that prompt intervention in the management of dysphagia can prevent costly and life threatening complications, such as aspiration pneumonia. Research has shown that the incidence of aspiration pneumonia due to dysphagia can be reduced from 6.7% to 0% through effective management (Odderson et al, 1995).

8.11 Deafness

This information is designed to support speech and language therapy services undertaking reviews of service organisation and provision. Therapists seeking detailed clinical guidance are referred to the *RCSLT Clinical Guidelines* (2005), position papers and *Reference Framework: Underpinning Competence to Practise* (2003), available on the RCSLT website: www.rcslt.org

Terminology

It is acknowledged that individuals may prefer alternative terms, (eg partially hearing, hearing impaired, hard of hearing, deaf) but for the sake of uniformity the term 'deaf' has been used throughout these guidelines.

Where the word 'deaf' is used with lower case 'd', this usually refers to a person with any degree of hearing loss who communicates orally, using aids to maximise residual hearing. Deafness with upper case 'D' is used to describe someone who identifies him/herself as belonging to a cultural community.

Definition

Deafness can include children and adults with a congenital or acquired bilateral permanent deafness that has a significant impact on communication, educational attainment, employment and quality of life. It is usually considered to be those with hearing losses of >40 dB HL (Fortnum et al, 2001; Gibbin, 2003).

Many people who are born deaf or are deafened early in life use British Sign Language (BSL) to communicate. Many people in this group consider themselves part of the Deaf community, which is defined by the use of BSL. Current estimates suggest 50,000 people in the UK use BSL as their first or preferred language.

An increasing proportion of people with severe and profound deafness will receive cochlear implants and may continue to use BSL. This group remains severely or profoundly deaf, but because of increased access to sound, will require different input around their communication needs to those without implants (Archbold, 2004).

A large number of children suffer from a temporary deafness caused by Otitis Media with Effusion (or 'glue ear'). For a proportion of children, the educational difficulties caused will be significant. Many of these children will be dealt with as part of other groups of communication impaired people, for example they may form part of the **pre-school** caseload or the **cleft palate** caseload.

Most of the deaf and hard of hearing people in the UK have developed a hearing loss as they got older (RNID, 2006).

Deafness can also be defined by degree of hearing loss. The Royal National Institute for Deaf People (RNID) defines the following categories:

● Mild deafness
Can cause some difficulty following speech, mainly in noisy situations. The quietest sounds that can be heard are 25-39 decibels.

● Moderate deafness
People with moderate deafness may have difficulty following speech without a hearing aid. The quietest sounds they can hear are 40-69 decibels.

● Severe deafness
People with severe deafness rely a lot on lip-reading, even with a hearing aid, as the quietest sounds they can hear are 70-94 decibels. BSL may be their first or preferred language.

● Profound deafness
The quietest sounds that profoundly deaf people can hear average 95 decibels or more. BSL may be their first or preferred language, but some prefer to lip-read.

Different individuals and their families respond differently to the same degree of hearing loss. The effect of deafness on the individual causes varying degrees of disability between one individual and another, and depends on a large number of influencing factors.

Cross-referencing with further chapter sections as highlighted below is recommended:

8.2. Adult Learning Disability
8.6. Brain Injury
8.8. Cleft Palate and Velopharyngeal Disorders
8.9. Craniofacial Conditions
8.16. Mental Health
8.18. Pre-school Children
8.20. School-aged Children
8.22 Specific Speech Impairment
8.23. Visual Impairment
8.24. Voice
7.2.1 AAC

This guidance does not currently include individuals with an **auditory processing disorder**.

(Central) auditory processing disorder ([C]APD) refers to difficulties in the processing of auditory information in the central nervous system (CNS) as demonstrated by poor performance in one or more of the following skills: sound localisation and lateralisation; auditory discrimination; auditory pattern recognition; temporal aspects of audition, including temporal integration, temporal discrimination, (eg temporal gap detection), temporal ordering, and temporal masking; auditory performance in competing acoustic signals (including dichotic listening); and auditory performance with degraded acoustic signals.

Non-modality-specific cognitive processing and language problems may manifest themselves in auditory tasks, (ie as listening problems); however, diagnosis of (C)APD requires demonstration of a deficit in the neural processing of auditory stimuli that is not due to higher order language, cognitive, or related factors (ASHA, 2005).

Further information on APD may be accessed through the American Speech-Language-Hearing Association's (ASHA) website at: www.asha.org; the British Society of Audiologists (BSA) website at: www.thebsa.org.uk; the Auditory Processing Disorder in the UK (APDUK) website at: www.apduk.org and the Defeating Deafness information service, email: info@defeatingdeafness.org

National guidance and sources of further information and support

● National Deaf Children's Society (NDCS)/RNID guidelines relating to *Working with children under 2* (2004); *Early years* (2004); *In Education* (2003); *Transition from Child to Adult Services* (2005); *For Cochlear Implant* (2005) www.ndcs.org

● *RCSLT Clinical Guidelines,* section on *Deafness*, 2005. www.rcslt.org

● *Social Care for Deafblind Children and Adults.* Department of Health, 2001.

● *Quality standards in education support services for children who are deafblind/multi-sensory impaired.* Sense, 2002 www.sense.org.uk

● RNID www.rnid.org.uk

● The British Association of Teachers of the Deaf www.batod.org.uk

● SENSE www.sense.org.uk

- MRC Institute of Hearing Research
- British Deaf Association www.bda.org.uk
www.britishdeafassociation.org.uk
- British Cochlear Implant Group www.bcig.co.uk

Aetiology

Deafness can be either **conductive** (caused by a problem in the sound-conducting mechanism of the external ear or middle ear) or **sensori-neural** (caused by a problem in the inner ear resulting in a failure of the process of converting sound signals into nerve impulses). Deafness can be further categorised as **congenital** or **acquired**. Acquired deafness can be progressive or of sudden onset.

Aside from the most common causes of deafness, which are ageing and Otitis Media in children, deafness can be caused by a variety of factors, including:

- prematurity
- genetic
- infection
- trauma
- ototoxicity.

Of severe/profound congenital and early onset deafness, 50% has a genetic origin.

A large proportion of cases of deafness are associated with other difficulties. For example, Archbold et al (2004) found that 40% of children receiving cochlear implants had difficulties in addition to deafness.

Incidence and prevalence

The RNID estimates that there are 8.7 million deaf and hard of hearing people in the UK, with 698,000 of these being severely and profoundly deaf.

Approximately one in 1000 babies is born with a significant hearing loss (Fortnum et al, 2001). This incidence of deafness rises over time, so that by the age of nine years at least 1.65 in 1000 children are diagnosed with significant deafness. This figure may be as high as 2.05 in 1000.

The RNID estimates that there are 20,000 children in the UK with deafness in excess of 40dB HL. It is thought that between 4% and 9% of these cases are acquired hearing losses.

Of children with sensori-neural hearing loss, 40% also have visual problems, some very severe (Hall & Elliman, 2002).

23,000 people are classified as deafblind. SENSE estimates that a further 250,000 people experience some degree of combined sight and hearing loss, many in older age.

90% of deaf children are born to hearing parents, and 90% of children born to two deaf parents are hearing. Both these facts have implications for speech and language therapy management.

Estimates for deafness caused by glue ear are in the region of 20% at the age of two years old, and 17% at the age of five.

The RNID estimates that there are 123,000 deafened people over 16 within the UK. The incidence of deafness increases with age, so that 2% of young adults (16-60) are deaf, compared with 55% of people over 60 years-old and 60% of people 71-80 years-old. Of these, 5000 per year will experience sudden deafness.

There are increased incidences of deafness in some ethnic minority groups. For example, the NDCS states that research carried out by Bradford Social Services (1999/2000), indicates that children of Asian origin are four times more likely to suffer from deafness. Almost five in 1,000 Asian children in Bradford are deaf compared with just over one in 1,000 among the non-Asian community.

Vulnerability: risk issues

● Increased risk of speech, language and communication difficulties. Many deaf people rely upon spoken English as their primary means of communication. However, they may be unable to acquire the same level of competence as their hearing peers.

● BSL users rarely meet professionals who share their language. This means communication is often compromised, which has implications for the D/deaf person accessing all areas of healthcare, public services, education and employment (RNID, 2006). This has particular implications for those deaf people who need to access speech and language therapy services.

● Increased risk of child protection and vulnerable adult issues.

● Increased risk of limited educational achievement in children with significant degrees of deafness.

● Increased risk of limited employment opportunities (1999 figures indicate 15% of deaf people unemployed, compared with 6% of hearing people; 33% of deaf people earning less than £10,000, compared with 11.8% of hearing people).

● Increased risk of mental health problems, behavioural, adjustment and emotional issues (Hindley et al, 1994). In addition, there is a scarcity of psychiatric and counselling services specifically for deaf people.

These risks will become greater in situations where:
● deafness is suddenly acquired
● diagnosis of deafness is delayed
● diagnosis of progressive hearing loss, particularly in young children, is delayed
● the deaf individual has additional difficulties.

Speech and language therapy value

In the context of an integrated service with all other agencies:
● Identification of any specific language difficulties existing over and above the impact of deafness.
● Supporting parents in their ability to communicate with and to parent their newly-diagnosed deaf child. The sensitive and considerate handling of early diagnosis of deafness is particularly important (Hind & Davis, 2000).
● Facilitating language acquisition.
● Supporting the decision-making process of the family of a newly-diagnosed deaf child, particularly when 90% of deaf children are born to hearing families with no previous experience of deafness. Issues to be considered include:
● mode of communication
● decisions about cochlear implantation
● nature of schooling.
● Providing assessment, diagnosis, and appropriate intervention to deaf people with communication difficulties. Targeting the impact of deafness on the individual, rather than the diagnosis and the degree of deafness. Main focus on:
● functional communication
● improving speech intelligibility
● access to environmental sounds
● increased speech perception.
● Reducing the negative impact of difficulties with communication caused by deafness.

8.12 Dysfluency

This information is designed to support speech and language therapy services undertaking reviews of service organisation and provision. Therapists seeking detailed clinical guidance are referred to the *RCSLT Clinical Guidelines* (2005), position papers and *Reference Framework: Underpinning Competence to Practise* (2003), available on the RCSLT website: www.rcslt.org

Definition

Developmental stammering occurs initially during childhood. The overt speech symptoms will include some or all of the following: part word repetitions, prolongations, and/or blocking. Coping strategies, for example substituting difficult words, situation avoidance, or changes in nonverbal behaviour may occur early or develop over time. In addition, fear of stammering may cause psychological or emotional distress (RCSLT, 2005).

Acquired stammering usually has a later onset but may also include children and may be associated with a significant event, eg it may be neurogenic, physiological, eg post viral fatigue syndrome; pharmacological; psychogenic; or may be of idiopathic origin (RCSLT, 2005).

Cluttering is usually characterised by perceptually fast/irregular speech rate, poor intelligibility, repetition or cessation of sounds, dysrhythmia, omission or elision of syllables. It may or may not include stammering. Cluttering may co-exist with stammering, language, literacy and/or motoric difficulties (RCSLT, 2005).

Cross-referencing with the chapter sections listed below is recommended:

8.6. Brain Injury
8.16. Mental Health
8.18. Pre-school Children
8.20. School-aged Children

National guidance and sources of further information and support

● *RCSLT Clinical Guidelines*, 2005, section on *Dysfluency*. www.rcslt.org
● British Stammering Association www.stammering.org

Aetiology

Reflects large differences in theoretical orientation. The 'balanced view', includes organic, psychogenic and learning aetiologies. Genetics in 50% of cases (Yairi, 2005).

Stuttering is a multidimensional neuromotor disruption resulting in asynchronous timing of the simultaneous and successive motor movements necessary for relatively effortless, continuous and rapid speech.

Stuttering is caused by the interaction of individually determined, yet unknown, predisposing constitutional factors with precipitating developmental and environmental factors (Shapiro, 1999). Neurophysiological, psychological, social and linguistic factors all probably contribute to its onset and persistence (Guitar, 1998).

Prevalence

The usually accepted figure is 1% (Bloodstein, 1987; Andrews et al, 1983). The magnitude of the problem is felt to be much larger amongst young children: an estimated 5% of children under the age of 5-6 years (Yairi et al, 2005).

There are no reliable figures for adults, but it is suggested that prevalence figures show a decline in stuttering after puberty to less than 1% (Bloodstein, 1987; Andrews et al, 1983).

Vulnerability: risk issues

Individuals with dysfluency may be particularly vulnerable in the following areas:

● **Mental health**

Indicators of difficulty may include:
● Depression, self harm, substance abuse, suicide
● Anxiety, social isolation
● Early childhood mutism (occasional).

● **Social Interaction**

Indicators of difficulty may include:
● Interpersonal difficulties
● Social skills deficits
● Behavioural problems
● Isolation
● Consequences on ability and skill in making friends, forming relationships.

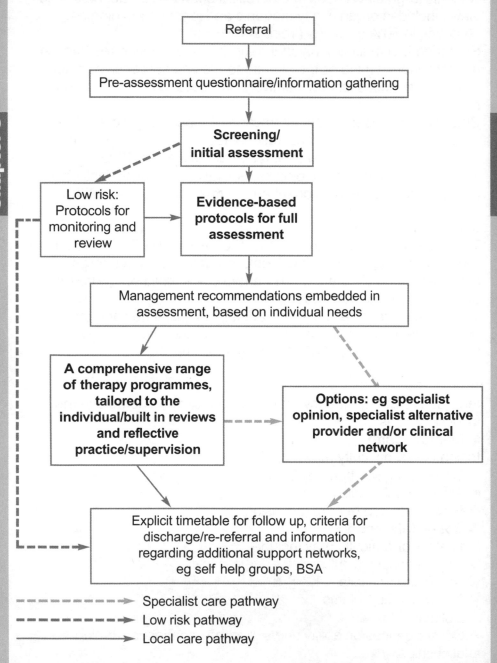

Figure 3: Care Pathway Example: Dysfluency

Referral

Pre-assessment questionnaire/information gathering

Screening/ initial assessment

Low risk: Protocols for monitoring and review

Evidence-based protocols for full assessment

Management recommendations embedded in assessment, based on individual needs

A comprehensive range of therapy programmes, tailored to the individual/built in reviews and reflective practice/supervision

Options: eg specialist opinion, specialist alternative provider and/or clinical network

Explicit timetable for follow up, criteria for discharge/re-referral and information regarding additional support networks, eg self help groups, BSA

- - - → Specialist care pathway
- - - → Low risk pathway
———→ Local care pathway

● Employment/education

Indicators of difficulty may include:

- School refusal, truancy
- Reduced higher educational choices
- Exam selection, (eg avoiding subjects with oral components)
- Academic disadvantage
- Reduced career opportunities
- Discrimination within the workplace.

Speech and language therapy value

● Maximising the potential of children and adults with a disorder of fluency to communicate effectively in the environments and languages in which they need to function.

● Enabling families, carers and professionals to facilitate effective communication in appropriate languages will be fundamental to service delivery.

● Helping people who stammer understand their stammering behaviour and enable them to make changes to their stammer, to facilitate a reduction in avoidance of words, situations and people and encourage easy, less effortful and more effective communication, through both one to one sessions and group therapy.

Prototype care pathway

Each step in the care pathway (see figure 3, opposite) requires explicit criteria/protocols which are in line with RCSLT policy and HPC requirements.

8.13 Dyslexia

The RCSLT is exploring the possibility of a multi-professional policy review forum (to include SLTs, assistants, teachers and the National Autistic Association) to produce a position paper in relation to services to individuals with dyslexia.

8.14 Dysphagia

This information is designed to support speech and language therapy services undertaking reviews of service organisation and provision. Therapists seeking detailed clinical guidance are referred to the *RCSLT Clinical Guidelines* (2005), position papers and *Reference Framework: Underpinning Competence to Practise* (2003), available on the RCSLT website: www.rcslt.org

Definition

The term dysphagia describes eating and drinking disorders which may occur in the oral, pharyngeal and oesophageal stages of deglutition.

Subsumed in this definition are problems positioning food in the mouth and in oral movements, including sucking, mastication and the process of swallowing.

Eating and drinking is a highly complex, multi-system skill involving anatomic stability, neuromuscular control and coordination, sensory perception, gastrointestinal function, cardio-respiratory support and integration from the autonomic nervous system.

Difficulties in sensory perception may create sensitivities and may also lead to psycho-behavioural difficulties in relation to food and drink (Wolf and Glass, 1996).

Cross-referencing with the chapter sections listed below is recommended:

8.1. Acquired Motor Speech Disorders
8.2. Adult Learning Disability
8.3. Aphasia
8.6. Brain Injury
8.7. Cerebral Palsy
8.8. Cleft Palate and Velopharyngeal Disorders
8.9. Craniofacial Conditions
8.15. Head and Neck Cancer
8.17. Palliative Care
8.18. Pre-school Children
8.19. Progressive Neurological Disorders
8.20. School-aged Children
8.24. Voice

National guidance and sources of further information and support

● NSF Guidelines for *Children and Young People* (2004)
● *RCSLT Clinical Guidelines* (2005), section on *Dysphagia*
www.rcslt.org

- The Association for Children with Terminal or Life-threatening Conditions (ACT) www.act.org.uk/act
- BLISS, the premature baby charity www.bliss.org.uk/
- Cleft Lip and Palate Association (CLAPA) www.clapa.com
- Contact a Family www.cafamily.org.uk
- SCOPE www.scope.org.uk
- Muscular Dystrophy Campaign www.muscular-dystrophy.org
- Down's Syndrome Association www.downs-syndrome.org.uk
- British Dietetics Association www.bda.uk.com

8.14.1 Children with Dysphagia

Definition
The client group includes babies, pre-school and school-aged children as well as young people who have difficulties with eating and drinking.

They may have additional anatomical, learning, communication, and sensory, behavioural and physical needs. The nature of their difficulties may be acquired or congenital.

Aetiology
Eating and drinking difficulties can be associated with a number of different conditions:
- Prematurity.
- Neurological deficits, eg cerebral palsy, acquired traumatic brain injury, Rett syndrome.
- Infectious diseases, eg meningitis.
- Neuromuscular disorders, eg muscular dystrophy.
- Respiratory difficulties, eg chronic lung disease, structural abnormalities of the upper respiratory tract, tracheostomy.
- Cardiovascular disorders, eg congenital heart disease.
- Gastrointestinal difficulties, eg gastro-oesophageal reflux, oesophagitis, oesophageal atresia.
- Craniofacial conditions eg cleft palate, Pierre Robin sequence.
- Congenital syndromes, eg Prader-Willi, Down's syndrome.
- Learning disability, (see section 8.14.3).

Some children have isolated eating and drinking difficulties that may be related to sensory difficulties and sensitivities. This is particularly so for children with autism and those with a traumatic feeding history.

Incidence and prevalence
The number of babies, children and young people with eating and drinking difficulties is not clearly classified and therefore are not clearly identified in the literature. However, consideration of data related to specific conditions allows for some estimate to be made.

Cerebral palsy
The prevalence figures for dysphagia within the population of people with cerebral palsy (CP) vary from 27% (Waterman et al, 1992) to 81%.

The association between the severity of CP and eating and drinking difficulties and oral-motor impairment has been demonstrated (Krick & van Duyn, 1984).

Children with CP take up to fifteen times longer to complete a meal (Gisel & Patrick, 1988).

A video fluoroscopy study demonstrated that 33% of the children with CP were aspirating (Reilly et al, 1996).

Cardiac disorders
Approximately one in a hundred children with a cardiac disorder has a risk of concomitant feeding difficulties (Children's Heart Foundation, 2006).

18% of children have been found to be dysphagic after cardiac surgery (Khol et al, 2000).

Gastro-oesophageal reflux (GOR)
Feeding problems affecting behavior, swallowing, and food intake and mother child interaction have been found to be common in infants with GOR (Mathisen et al, 1999; Hyman 1994).

Oesophageal atresia
May affect one in every 4000 live births. Long-term follow up of infants who have had an oesophageal atresia repair has shown that between 60% and 70% experience problems with dysphagia (Munro, 2003).

Cleft lip and palate
Cleft lip and palate affects approximately one in every 600-700 births, (WHO Expert Committee, 2002; Craniofacial Anomalies Network, 2003). Effective feeding is compromised by the inability to achieve negative pressure, to draw fluid from the teat or breast (Bannister, 2001).

More complex feeding difficulties are common in the syndromic cleft population, eg Pierre Robin sequence (Van den Elzen et al, 2001).

Craniofacial conditions

Feeding difficulties in children with craniofacial conditions are poorly described in the literature. Consequently, accurate prevalence is unknown and the majority of current knowledge in this area is largely based on clinical experience and local evidence.

The two main predisposing factors in this cohort are abnormal oral facial structure and upper airway obstruction. Other factors include visual impairment, developmental delay, CNS malformations, cardiovascular and respiratory or gastrointestinal anomalies.

The major craniofacial syndromes that may include feeding difficulties are: Apert; Crouzon; Pfeiffer; Treacher Collins; Nager and Goldenhar (Pereira, 2004).

Learning disabilities

In a recent study, 57% of a group of people with learning disabilities had some level of nutritional difficulties (Kerr et al, 2003) (see 8.14.3).

Autism

Some children with autism may have difficulties with food due to sensory disturbances with smell and texture (Bogdashina, 2004).

Trauma

There is a high incidence of behavioral feeding difficulties associated with children who have had a traumatic medical history, eg tube feeding, surgery, tracheostomy etc (Douglas & Harris, 2001).

Vulnerability: risk issues

Children who do not have appropriate dysphagia management are at increased risk of:

- aspiration
- respiratory infection
- choking
- poor nutrition and weight loss
- poor health
- hospital admission due to respiratory illness
- anxiety and distress within the family
- reduced quality of life

"Whilst the main purpose of eating is to achieve an adequate intake of food in order to sustain growth, the process of eating is not just one of sustaining life: in human societies it is a social event. Infants undergo their earliest communication experiences during feeding" (Reilly, 1993).

It is recognised that any difficulties during mealtimes impact "not only on the physical but also the emotional and well being of the individual" (Arvedson & Brodsky, 1993).

Risk management at the level of service organisation and provision

Competence: Therapists working in this field should have a basic expertise and competence to practice independently at a post registration training level. An SLT at graduate level will have basic management skills for eating and drinking difficulties, but will require supervision and support to develop advanced specialist knowledge and skills related to certain areas such as craniofacial conditions, prematurity and tracheostomy.

A therapist involved in videofluoroscopy assessment must be trained to evaluate the risk of radiation involved in the procedure.

MDT working: A multidisciplinary approach is essential within paediatric eating and drinking management. It will ensure efficient management, joint goal setting, and minimise confusion for the parents (McCurtin, 1998).

The feeding management of children with cleft lip and palate is primarily under the role of the clinical nurse specialist within the cleft lip and palate team.

Location of therapy: Input should occur in the most natural and comfortable setting for the child/young person – at home and at school. Children may also be seen in hospital as part of the evaluation process.

Speech and language therapy value

● Specialised assessment including objective assessment methods.

● Safe maximisation of the child's eating and drinking potential, using appropriate strategies that promote safe and adequate nutritional intake within a setting which supports and enhances the child/young person's wellbeing.

● Supporting the child and significant others in choosing between a number of feeding options and strategies where oral feeding will not be possible.

● Supporting parents/significant others in the process of making mealtimes pleasurable.

● Identification and management of risks to the child as a result of dysphagia.

8.14.2 Adults with Dysphagia

Definition
The term swallowing "refers to the entire act of deglutition from placement of food in the mouth through the oral and pharyngeal stages of the swallow until the material enters the oesophagus through the cricopharyngeal juncture" (Logemann, 2001). "The term dysphagia refers to an impaired swallow. The impairment can occur anywhere from the mouth to the stomach" (Perlman & Schulze-Delrieu, 1997).

Aetiology
Dysphagia can occur as a result of any of the following medical disorders:
● Neuromuscular disorders, eg stroke, PD, MND, MS, PSP, GB, brain tumour, subarachnoid haemorrhage, Wilson's disease, dementia, polyneuropathy, head injury.
● Head and neck cancer, eg laryngeal cancer.
● Oncology, eg lung cancer.
● Cardiopulmonary disorders, eg chronic obstructive pulmonary disease
● Autoimmune disorders, eg HIV, lupus, rheumatoid arthritis.
● Connective tissue disorders, eg scleroderma.
● General medical disorders eg UTI.
● Disorders associated with the elderly, eg cervical osteophytes.
● Disorders caused by trauma, eg smoke inhalation.
● Vascular disorders, eg Bechet's disease.
● Swallow disorders as a result of surgery, eg base of skull surgery, thyroid surgery.
● Tracheostomy.
● Ventilator dependent individuals, eg post-extubation related dysphagia
● Drug related causes, eg long-term use of some anti-psychotic medications.
● Psychogenic causes.

Prevalence and incidence

Stroke

Stroke is the most common cause of adult disability in the UK.
Stroke affects approximately 200 people per 100,000 UK population
every year (National Clinical Guidelines for Stroke, 2004).
Observational studies have shown that 30-40%of conscious
individuals who have experienced stroke have significant dysphagia
on the day of stroke and 15-20% at one week post stroke (RCSLT,
2005; Smithard et al, 1996).
At one month post stroke, 2% of stroke survivors will have swallowing
problems (RCSLT, 2005).

Other neurological deficits

Dysphagia is also commonly associated with other neurological
deficits, eg Multiple Sclerosis; Parkinson's disease; traumatic brain
Injury; motor neurone disease; head and neck injury or carcinoma
(RCSLT, 2005).

Parkinson's disease

Incidence: 17 per 100,000 UK population each year, ie 10,000
new cases per year.
Prevalence: 200 per 100,000 UK population, ie 120,000 cases in
the UK. 41% of individuals with Parkinson's indicated impairment
of chewing and swallowing abilities (Hartelius & Svensson, 1994).

Multiple Sclerosis (MS)

Incidence: MS is diagnosed in 3.5 to 6.6 people per 100 000 each
year (NICE, 2004).
Prevalence: 144 per 100,000 UK population (MS Society, 2006).
There have been few studies on the prevalence of dysphagia in MS
(NICE, 2004).
33% of the MS individuals in one study indicated impairment of
chewing and swallowing abilities (Hartelius & Svensson, 1994).

Dementia

Prevalence: Dementia currently affects over 750,000 people in the UK
Dementia affects one person in 20 aged over 70 years and one
person in five over 80 years of age.

The number of people with dementia in the UK has been estimated as follows using population figures for 2001 (RCSLT, 2005):
- England: 652,600
- Scotland: 63,700
- Northern Ireland: 17,100
- Wales: 41,800.

Studies that look at the incidence of swallowing difficulty in dementia show a high rate of dysphagia:
- 68% of those in a home for the aged (Steele, 1997).
- Bronchopneumonia was the leading cause of death in Alzheimer's disease; 28.6% in this study were found to be aspirating (Horner et al, 1994).
- Swallowing problems are also a concern in other types of dementia, eg vascular dementia (Stach, 2000) and those conditions where neurological signs are present alongside cognitive impairment, eg Huntington's disease; progressive supranuclear palsy; Parkinson's disease and dementia with Lewy bodies (Logemann, 1998).

There are no prevalence figures for dysphagia in some neurological populations.

Vulnerability: risk issues

Individuals who do not have appropriate dysphagia management are at high risk of:
- aspiration (Smithard et al, 1996)
- developing respiratory infection (Doggett et al, 2001)
- choking and death (Marik & Kaplan, 2003)
- poor nutrition and weight loss (Wright et al, 2005)
- poor health (Hudson et al, 2000)
- anxiety and distress within the family (Choi-Kwon et al, 2005)
- hospital admission or extended hospital stay (Low et al, 2001)
- reduced quality of life (Nguyen et al, 2005).

Risk management at the level of service organisation and provision

Competence: SLTs working with individuals with dysphagia should meet the RCSLT dysphagic competencies.

Managing risks associated with videofluoroscopy

Competence: SLTs who participate in videofluoroscopy should have the appropriate training, be competent and meet the RCSLT competencies and guidelines. Considerable clinical judgement is required when conducting this procedure as the study may have to be further modified or terminated if the individual appears unable to protect the airway even after use of intervention techniques (ASHA, 2002).

Safety: Local radiation safety procedures should be adhered to. Care should be taken to limit the field and duration of the exposure, while at the same time, gaining sufficient clinical information to address the purpose of the study. Local infection control procedures should be adhered to.

MDT working: Based upon the results of the study, the SLT should interact as a member of a team to plan safe swallowing strategies to insure proper nutrition and to make recommendations regarding oral versus non-oral feeding safety (ASHA, 2002).

Managing risks associated with FEES

Competence: Post-graduate training and clinical experience in the use and interpretation of FEES has two main components:

1. Hands on training in handling an endoscope safely and effectively

2. Knowledge-based training in indications for the examination, how to perform the examination, how to interpret abnormal findings, and how to use FEES in dysphagia management (Langmore, 2002).

SLTs performing FEES examinations or participating in FEES examination should be competent in this procedure and meet the RCSLT competencies and guidelines.

SLTs performing FEES or participating in FEES examination should have knowledge of the contraindications for the procedure, eg individuals with a history of broncospasm or laryngospasm, extreme movement disorders, those who cannot tolerate the endoscope (Aviv et al, 2000; Murray & Carrau, 1999).

Managing risks associated with scintigraphy

Competence: SLTs who participate in scintigraphy should have the appropriate training.

MDT working: Scintigraphy should be carried out with the appropriate medical and imaging staff, as well as speech and language therapy.

Safety: Individuals should not be 'over exposed' to aspiration during the procedure. Risks associated with manometry/ electromyography/ultrasound/MRI (Murray & Carrau, 1999).

Speech and language therapy value
Provision of an efficient, effective and comprehensive assessment and management service tailored to individual needs and delivered within the context of multidisciplinary working.

8.14.3 Adults with Learning Disability and Dysphagia

Definition
Adults with a learning disability (ALD) who have developmental or acquired dysphagia.

National guidance
● Department of Health, *Valuing People,* 2001.
● National Patient Safety Agency, 2004. *Understanding Patient safety issues for people with learning disabilities*
● *RCSLT ALD Position Paper.* RCSLT, 2003 www.rcslt.org

Aetiology
It has long been accepted that ALD have a higher incidence of additional health problems than the general population. These problems include increased respiratory difficulties, poor nutrition and hydration, and choking (Aziz & Cambell-Taylor, 1999).
Dysphagia has been identified as a key risk area for people with learning disabilities (NPSA, 2004).
In recent reports by Watson (2004) and Crawford (2005), SLTs working in the UK identified the following as primary causes of dysphagia in the people they were working with. Featuring most highly were:
● Neurological causes of dysphagia including CP and particular syndromes, for example Rett's syndrome, Down's syndrome, and Down's syndrome with dementia.
● Profound and multiple/complex learning disability.

- Dysphagia associated with behavioural difficulties
- Dysphagia without a specific causal factor

The following were also identified as causes of dysphagia:

- autism
- head injury
- psychiatric illness
- stroke
- cerebral tumour
- neurological degenerative conditions such as, MND, MS and Parkinson's disease.

In addition:

- Anatomical problems can cause sensory and motor problems which make eating and drinking more difficult or uncomfortable.
- Gastro-oesphageal reflux is common in people with learning disabilities and physical difficulties and is associated with a higher level of eating and drinking difficulties. Management of reflux may not be routine and can complicate a dysphagia (Koufman, 2002).
- Medication use (especially Clozapine) and medication complications can cause or exacerbate dysphagia (Schechter, 1998; Sokoloff & Pavlakovic, 1997).

Prevalence

There is still limited research in the area of dysphagia in adults with a learning disability. The research that exists confirms that it is a significant difficulty, resulting in serious health consequences for adults with learning disability.

- Swallowing difficulties are more common in people with learning disabilities (NPSA, 2004).
- A US study (Rogers et al, 1994) found 33% of individuals in a long stay institution were referred for advice on feeding disorders.
- 5.3% of community-based individuals and 36% of hospital based individuals displayed dysphagia (Hickman & Jenner, 1997).
- Over a period of six years, 5.27% of all ALD in the Manchester area were referred for advice regarding dysphagia (Chadwick et al, 2003).
- An audit in 2004 (Watson, 2004) found that 54.6% of people on adult learning disability dysphagia caseloads had CP or severe and complex needs.
- Dysphagia increases with the degree of physical difficulty (Hardwick, 1993) and is complicated by conditions such as epilepsy.

Different types of dysphagia in ALD

A US study found that 70% of individuals had oral stage dysphagia, 82% had pharyngeal, and 55% had oesophageal stage dysphagia (Hardwick, 1993).

A UK study found that 97.5% of individuals studied had oral stage dysphagia, 65% had pharyngeal stage dysphagia, 17.5% had oesophageal dysphagia. 65% of those studied had problems at more than one stage (Chadwick et al, 2003).

Vulnerability: risk issues

For exploration of general vulnerabilities of adults with learning disability, see 8.2 on **Adult Learning Disability**.

Adults with learning disability are more at risk of having dysphagic difficulties that go unrecognised (Dobson, 2003).

Admittance to hospital with an acute condition and a vulnerability around swallowing may leave the adult with learning disability very vulnerable to inappropriate types of food and drink being offered, as well as to these being offered in an inappropriate way.

Adults with learning disability who do not have appropriate dysphagia assessment and management are at high risk of:

● aspiration
● dehydration
● developing respiratory infection a leading cause of early death for people with learning disabilities' (Hollins et al, 1998; NPSA, 2004)
● choking and death
● poor nutrition and weight loss
● poor health
● anxiety and distress within the family
● hospital admission or extended hospital stay
● reduced quality of life
● poor oral health (Aziz & Cambell-Taylor, 1999; Beange et al, 1995; Cook & Kahrilas, 1999; Eyman et al, 1990; Rogers et al, 1994).

Because of the presence of a learning disability, individuals may be unable to follow the guidance given without high levels of support and supervision.

A lack of compliance with eating and drinking guidelines, particularly if the person self feeds, will heighten the risks listed above (Chadwick et al, 2003).

Managing the risks at the level of service organisation

Competence: SLTs working in this area, as a minimum, should have training to a post basic level. This training can be gained either by attending an accredited training course, or via work based and supervised competency development programs. SLTs at all levels should have adequate clinical and professional supervision when working in this area.

Therapists need to be fully aware of all the risks that are specific to dysphagia (see section 8.14.2).

SLTs working with ALD should have an awareness of the issue of 'safeguarding adults' and know why and how to make a referral to the appropriate agencies if they feel an adult with a learning disability is unsafe.

MDT working: Individualised treatment programmes based on interdisciplinary working are widely recognised to be the most effective way of managing dysphagia in this client group (Arvedson, 1993). The SLT working with ALD and dysphagia should be working within a multidisciplinary framework.

Therapy context: The SLT will be required to visit a variety of environments, dependent on the person they are working with. It is important that the SLT sees people eating and drinking in their most naturalistic environments. It may be necessary for the SLT to liaise between a number of environments for any one individual, to ensure equity of service in all.

See also the section on Risk Management in Adults with Dysphagia.

Speech and language therapy value

● Provision of timely and effective assessment and intervention. This includes management of the risks of dysphagia to the individual; development of strategies to enable appropriate nutrition and hydration, through maximisation and/or development of the eating and drinking skills of the individual, and carer support strategies.

● Provision of services that aim to develop and maintain mealtimes as pleasant occasions, including appropriate meals, pleasant environment and sensitive support from carers.

● Training and supporting carers to meet the needs of the person with learning disabilities and dysphagia on a daily basis. Training is also aimed to empower carers to identify people with dysphagia; to identify changes in individuals they care for, and to make appropriate referrals to speech and language therapy.

● Engagement in preventative health planning through the development of person-centred health action plans. The SLT, alongside the multidisciplinary team, the health action plan facilitators and the individual concerned, works to ensure the process used to develop health action plans and the plans themselves are accessible to the individual (DH, 2001).

● Contribution to and involvement in service-user consultations.

8.15 Head and Neck Cancer

This information is designed to support speech and language therapy services undertaking reviews of service organisation and provision. Therapists seeking detailed clinical guidance are referred to the *RCSLT Clinical Guidelines* (2005), position papers and *Reference Framework: Underpinning Competence to Practise* (2003), available on the RCSLT website: www.rcslt.org

Definition

Head and neck cancer is the general name that encompasses many different forms of cancer.

There are over 30 specific sites in the head and neck cancer group. The majority of these cancers arise from the surface layers of the aerodigestive tract (UAT): the lips, mouth, tongue, pharynx and larynx.

Other UAT sites include the salivary glands, nose, sinuses and middle ear, but these cancers are relatively rare.

Cancers that originate in the nerves and bone of the head and neck are even more rare.

Cancer of the thyroid is unlike UAT cancers, apart from being uncommon, but the services required for individuals overlap and it is therefore included in this group.

Head and neck cancer, although relatively uncommon, carries a high level of morbidity and mortality.

Cross-referencing with the chapter sections listed below is recommended:

8.14. Dysphagia
8.17. Palliative Care
7.2.1 AAC

National guidance and sources of further information and support

● National Association Laryngectomy Clubs (NALC) guidelines
● British Association of Head and Neck Oncologists (BAHNO) consensus document
● NICE guidelines for head and neck and supportive palliative care
● Scottish Intercollegiate Guideline on Head and Neck cancer, 2005 www.sign.ac.uk
● *RCSLT Clinical Guidelines* (2005), section on *Head and neck cancer* www.rcslt.org
● *RCSLT Invasive Procedures Guidance,* 2004 www.rcslt.org

Aetiology

The aetiology of head and neck cancer is complex.
Epidemiological studies have implicated tobacco smoking and alcohol consumption as the major determinants of the disease in westernised countries. Individually these two factors increase the risk of oral cancer, but if combined, alcohol and smoking show a multiplicative risk.

● **Tobacco** The main risk factor for head and neck cancer is cigarette smoking. Pipe smoking also leads to an increased incidence of the disease. In some population groups there is a strong association with tobacco chewing and 'snuff dipping'. Combinations of tobacco, slaked lime, betel nuts, and spices are responsible for high regional and ethnic variations in head and neck cancer worldwide.

● **Alcohol** Increased risk of head and neck cancer has been associated with heavy consumption of spirits, beer or wine. Alcohol itself has not been implicated directly as an oral carcinogen, but it is thought to promote carcinogenesis by a number of mechanisms, eg topical carcinogens, such as those found in tobacco, become more potent when accompanied by alcohol.

Many modern mouthwashes sold for oral hygiene purposes contain alcohol in significant concentration. The long-term effects of these preparations on oral mucosa, has not yet been established.

● **Nutrition** Nutritional deficiencies (in particular, iron) produce atrophy of the oral mucosa, and may allow ingress of various carcinogenic substances.

Diets high in anti-oxidant vitamins (vitamins A, C and E) appear to offer protection. Therefore a diet high in fruit and vegetables is recommended.

● **Sunlight** Ultra-violet light is important in the aetiology of lip cancer, due to actinic radiation damage. It is not important in other head and neck cancers.

● **Infective causes** Human papilloma viruses have been postulated as causative factors in the aetiology of head and neck cancer and precancer, but the research is inconclusive at present.

Potentially malignant lesions of the mucosa, showing evidence of candidal infection have a higher risk of malignant transformation. However the role of chronic candidosis in the development of cancer is complex.

● **Oncogenes** The role of cancer promoting genes (oncogenes) and tumour suppressor genes, in relation to head and neck cancer is a complex and rapidly developing field. Gene therapy for 'at risk' individuals and families may hold possibilities for the future.

● **Pre-existing mucosal abnormalities** Some carcinomas are preceded by premalignant changes. Identification of such changes gives a warning of risk and presents an opportunity for close follow up and provision of preventive measures.

Although leukoplakia is commoner, erythroplakia and speckled leukoplakia should be viewed with greater suspicion. These lesions have a much higher potential than leukoplakia for malignant transformation. Indeed many of these lesions may already be squamous cell carcinomas, or carcinomas in situ, or show severe epithelial dysplasia.

Oral lichen planus is thought by some to be a pre-malignant lesion in around 1% of individuals. The erosive and plaque-like forms may be more prone to malignant transformation.

● **Social Deprivation** Although head and neck cancer occurs in all strata of society, social deprivation is identified as a specific risk.

● **Other** Of growing concern is the cohort of individuals who, with no obvious risk factors, are developing head and neck cancer. These individuals are often young and have aggressive tumours with poor prognosis.

Prevalence and incidence

Laryngeal cancer
Each year in the UK around 2300 people are diagnosed with cancer of the larynx.

Four out of five laryngeal cancers are diagnosed in men. 70% are diagnosed in people over 60 years-old.

Incidence

Incidence varies throughout the UK, eg rates in Scotland are significantly higher than in other parts of the UK, which correlates with the higher rates of tobacco and alcohol consumption.

Table 2: Number of new cases of laryngeal cancer in 2001

	England	Wales	Scotland	N. Ireland	UK
Males	1,477	99	255	53	1884
Females	328	23	52	13	416
Total	**1,805**	**122**	**307**	**66**	**2,300**

Table 3: Crude rate per 100,000 of population, of new cases of laryngeal cancer in 2001

	England	Wales	Scotland	N. Ireland	UK
Males	6.2	7.1	10.5	6.4	6.6
Females	1.3	1.5	2.0	1.5	1.4
Persons	3.7	4.2	6.1	3.9	3.9

Oral cancer

In the UK, around 4,400 people each year are diagnosed with oral cancer.

Oral cancer is more common in men than in women, however in the UK the sex ratio has decreased from around 5:1, to less than 2:1 in fifty years.

In the UK the risk of developing oral cancer increases with age, 86% of cases are aged 50 or over.

Oral cancer is strongly related to social and economic deprivation, with the highest rates occurring in the most disadvantaged sections of the community.

The association is particularly strong for men. In Scotland, for individuals diagnosed between 1991-1995, incidence rates were twice as high for those in the most disadvantaged category compared with the least disadvantaged. This reflects the higher tobacco consumption in the more disadvantaged groups.

Table 4: Numbers of new oral cancer individuals UK 2001

	England	Wales	Scotland	N. Ireland	UK
Males	2,245	166	376	81	2,868
Females	1,202	92	204	34	1,532
Total	**3,447**	**258**	**580**	**115**	**4,440**

Table 5: Crude rate of new oral cancer individuals per 100,000 of population UK 2001

	England	Wales	Scotland	N. Ireland	UK
Males	9.4	11.8	15.4	9.8	10.0
Females	4.8	6.1	7.8	3.9	5.1
Persons	7.0	8.9	11.5	6.8	7.5

Table 6: Number of new cases of oral cancer (site specific) in UK 2001

Site	Males	Females	Persons	M:F ratio
Mouth	843	561	1404	1.5:1
Tongue	784	455	1239	1.7:1
Oropharynx	532	185	717	2.9:1
Piriform sinus	207	44	251	4.7:1
Hypopharynx	112	88	200	1.3:1
Lip	245	114	359	2:1
Other and ill defined	145	85	230	1.7:1
Oral cancer	2,868	1,532	4,400	1.9:1

Incidence

As with laryngeal cancer, incidence varies throughout the UK. Incidence in Scotland is higher, and studies of the disease in minority ethnic populations in Britain have reported high rates in south Asian and Chinese populations, in which the habit of areca nut or betal quid chewing is still prevalent.

The incidence of oral cancer varies strikingly around the world. The highest age standardised rates (over 20 per 100,000 population) are reported in parts of Europe and south central Asia. In high risk countries such as Sri Lanka, India, Pakistan and Bangladesh, oral cancer is the most common cancer in men and may account for up to 30% of all new cases of cancer, compared to 2% in the UK and 8% in France.

Incidence of oral cancer also varies by tumour site.

Vulnerability: risk issues

Specific to laryngectomy
Management of TE Puncture and/or prosthesis
Inappropriate management can lead to:
- aspiration
- closure of puncture
- respiratory complications
- loss of or failure to acquire voice.

Prosthesis replacement
Inappropriate management can lead to:
- tissue trauma
- creation of false tract, during prosthesis change
- aspiration of gastric contents via TEP during valve change due to vomiting
- unsuccessful replacement
- unsafe environment for carrying out procedure
- inappropriate skill mix of staff carrying out procedure
- vasovagal attack.

Aspiration
- centrally through voice prosthesis
- peripherally around voice prosthesis
- of the prosthesis
- of water while bathing, etc.

Allergic reaction
- to stoma products and skin preparations.

Respiratory distress
- stoma shrinkage
- stoma blockage.

Fire/electrocution
- electrolarynx not checked or serviced regularly
- storage of electrolaryx close to metal objects.

Head and neck cancer in general

Dysphagia

- aspiration during speech and language therapy intervention leading to possible litigation
- dehydration
- malnutrition
- aspiration and possible subsequent pneumonia
- reduced oral intake
- alternative feeding
- distress
- loss of confidence
- embarrassment
- impact on quality of life.

Decreased communication skills

- isolation
- distress
- loss of confidence
- breakdown in family support
- ostracised by public/family
- embarrassment
- impact on quality of life.

Altered body image

- social isolation
- depression.

Radiotherapy

- reduced function
- xerostomia
- mucositus.

Poor oral hygiene

- pain
- infection.

Reduced sensation

- altered function
- drooling
- embarrassment.

Contamination and infection

- MRSA
- Hepatitis B.

Late presentation
● tumour stage will affect survival rate.
Compliance
● poor compliance can affect intervention outcomes.
Invasive procedures
● associated risks of FEES and videofluoroscopy as per Invasive Procedures Guideline, RCSLT, 2004.
Recurrence
● Client group at high risk of recurrence, or developing new cancers in the head and neck region and other parts of the body such as lung.

Speech and language therapy value

Multidisciplinary teams (MDT), with a wide range of specialties, will be central to the service. They will be responsible for assessment, intervention planning and management of every individual.

SLTs will play a crucial role in the above from the pre intervention assessment period until rehabilitation is completed and speech and swallowing function has been maximised within the constraints of the planned intervention/management.

SLTs will also be part of coordinated local support teams in order to provide long-term support and rehabilitation for individuals in the community. These teams will work closely with every level of the service from primary care teams to the specialist MDT.

Specific resources required

● SVR equipment and stoma accessories plus inflation related budget.
● Voice recording equipment.
● Acoustic analysis equipment.
● Fibreoptic endoscopy facilities for voice and FEES and access to disinfection facilities for SCOPE.
● Local and national information on support groups/places where information, financial advice, details of complementary intervention can be accessed.
● Electrolarynx, voice amplifiers, communication aids.
● Access to specialised services and equipment if not available on site, eg V/F FEES, stroboscopy.

8.16 Mental Health

This information is designed to support speech and language therapy services undertaking reviews of service organisation and provision. Therapists seeking detailed clinical guidance are referred to the *RCSLT Clinical Guidelines* (2005), position papers and *Reference Framework: Underpinning Competence to Practise* (2003), available on the RCSLT website: www.rcslt.org

Definition

Mental health is the capacity of each and all of us to feel, think and act in ways that enhance our ability to enjoy life and deal with the challenges we face. It is a positive sense of emotional and spiritual well-being that respects the importance of culture, equity, social justice, interconnected and personal dignity (Meltzer et al, 2000). Mental health problems can be described as:

● Difficulties and/or disabilities in the realm of personal relationships, psychological development, the capacity for play and learning and in distress and maladaptive behaviours. They are relatively common and may or may not be persistent (PHIS, 2006).

Furthermore:

● When mental health problems are persistent, severe or complex, and interfere with a person's day-to-day functioning, they are often defined as mental disorders. In some severe cases, the term psychiatric or mental illness is used (PHIS, 2003).

Cross-referencing with all the chapter 8 client-group sections is recommended.

8.16.1 Mental Health: Paediatric

Definition

The full scope of this group is difficult to define as it is an emerging area of speech and language therapy involvement.

One of the increasing areas of involvement is with children with **selective mutism**, formerly known as elective mutism. This is a disorder of childhood that is characterized by the persistent lack of speech in at least one social situation, despite the ability to speak in other situations.

Onset of selective mutism typically occurs before a child is five years old. However, it is usually first noticed when the child enters school. Specific features of this disorder are described in the Diagnostic and Statistical Manual of Mental Disorders (DSM-IV-TR) (2000, pp125-127) as follows:

● Consistent failure to speak in specific social situations (in which there is an expectation for speaking, eg at school) despite speaking in other situations.
● The disturbance interferes with educational or occupational achievement or with social communication.
● The duration of the disturbance is at least one month (not limited to the first month of school).
● The failure to speak is not due to a lack of knowledge of, or comfort with, the spoken language required in the social situation.
● The disturbance is not better accounted for by a communication disorder, (eg stuttering) and does not occur exclusively during the course of a pervasive developmental disorder, schizophrenia, or other psychotic disorder.

National guidance and sources of further support and information

● *NSF on Mental Health* – Standard 9, *The mental health and psychological wellbeing of children,* 2004. Department of Health
● *Together We Stand: a thematic review of the commissioning role and management of children and adolescent mental health services,* 1995. HMSO.
● Selective Mutism www.asha.org/public/speech/disorders/Selective-Mutism.htm
● MIND, the mental health charity www.mind.org.uk
● Rethink www.rethink.org
● Scottish Association for Mental Health www.samh.org.uk

Aetiology

Risk/vulnerability factors include learning disability or any kind of enduring physical ill health, eg epilepsy, physical or sexual abuse, witnessing domestic violence, parent with mental health difficulty, being looked after and accommodated.
Risk accumulates, in that the presence of more than one risk factor substantially increases the risk of developing mental health problems.

Incidence and prevalence

9.5% (Meltzer et al, 2000) overall prevalence of 'mental health disorder', ie a problem of sufficient severity and persistence to have a significant impact on the child's functioning and relationships.
Evidence from around the world indicates higher prevalence rates and we may need to reflect a range ie up to 14% in a Canadian study (Waddel et al, 2002).
Incidence/prevalence of speech and language difficulties in psychiatric population: 62% (Goodyer, 2000) of children had a speech and language impairment, 28% previously identified and 34% unsuspected.
Selective mutism is a rare disorder that affects less than 1% of individuals in mental health settings. It is slightly more common in girls than in boys (ASHA, 2006).

Vulnerability: risk issues

Children with communication difficulties and mental health problems are at high educational and psychosocial risk, including suicide and self harm.

Speech and language therapy value

● Identification of communication difficulties.
● Provision of appropriate intervention in order to reduce risk, develop resilience and promote wellbeing.
SLTs are best placed to be key workers in the MDT for children with selective mutism (ASHA, 2006).

8.16.2 Mental Health: Adult Dementia

Definition

Dementia is a clinical syndrome characterised by widespread loss of function (DH, 2001).
Features include impairment of memory, thinking, orientation, comprehension, calculation, learning capacity, language and judgement (WHO, 1992).
Communication disorder becomes apparent during the course of all types of dementia varying according to disease type, duration and other factors including pre-morbid skills and environment (Bryan & Maxim, 1996). It may be an initial presenting feature of the disease.

Studies that look at the incidence of swallowing difficulty in dementia show a high rate of dysphagia.

National guidance and sources of further information and support
● *National Service Framework for older people* (England) (2001) www.dh.gov.uk/PolicyandGuidance
● *NSF for mental health,* 1999 www.dh.gov.uk/PolicyandGuidance
● RCSLT Position Paper on Dementia, 2005 www.rcslt.org
● MIND www.mind.org.uk/
● Alzheimer's Society UK www.alzheimers.org.uk

Aetiology
There are over 100 different causes of dementia. The most common are Alzheimer's disease, vascular dementia and dementia with Lewy bodies. Every person who experiences dementia does so in their own individual way, but there is usually a decline in memory, reasoning and communication skills and a gradual loss of the skills needed to carry out daily activities (Alzheimer's Society UK, 2004).

Prevalence
Dementia currently affects over 750,000 people in the UK.
The number of people with dementia in the UK has been estimated as follows, using population figures for 2001:
● England: 652,600
● Scotland: 63,700
● Northern Ireland: 17,100
● Wales: 41,800.
The well-established prevalence rates for dementia in the UK are:

Age (years)	Prevalence
40-65	1 in 1000
65-70	1 in 50
70-80	1 in 20
80+	1 in 5

Vulnerability: Risk issues
● Misdiagnosis of condition.
● Individuals do not have access to most clinically effective

intervention (Department for Health *Standards for Better Health* (SBH) standard 2).
● Other aspects of intervention are delayed (SBH standard 5):
● Communication impairments are commonly found in individuals with a range of dementia syndromes (Snowden & Griffiths, 2000; Bayles et al, 1993). Detailed analysis of language can contribute to accurate diagnosis (Bucks et al, 2000) and management of conditions. Language assessment contributes to differential diagnosis between different types of dementia (Snowden & Griffiths, 2000) and make a vital contribution to early diagnosis (Garrard & Hodges, 1999).
● Individuals and carers do not receive specialist advice with regard maximising their existing skills (SBH standard 2).
● Challenging behaviour increases staff and carer burden (Haley et al, 1994):
● Inability to communicate effectively may be the cause of many challenging behaviours (Bryan & Maxim, 2003; Stokes, 2004).
● Individual safety, in some cases may be compromised due to social exclusion or isolation (SBH standard 1 and NSF standard 1):
● Individuals may experience social exclusion (Hagberg, 1997).
● Communication impairment can cause a lack of confidence that impacts on feelings of self worth and hinders an individual's ability to assert their views and wishes.
● Eating and drinking problems have well documented effects on physical health but also have adverse effects on self-esteem, socialisation and enjoyment of life including anxiety and panic during mealtimes (RCSLT, 2005).
● Costs are incurred due to carer ill health.
● Hospital admission/day services may be needed to support individual if carer is unable to cope:
● There is evidence that carers find behavioural and communication problems more stressful than aspects of Activities of Daily Living (ADL) and self care impairments (Haley et al, 1994).
● Caring for people with dementia costs over £1 billion per year in the UK (not including loss of carers earnings or cost of carers stress induced ill health) (Alzheimer's Society UK, 2004).
● Carer burden has been shown to improve with intervention (Barnes, 2003).

● Individuals will have inadequate access to services and choice (SBH standard 5; NSF standard 3):
● Many individuals with communication impairment are unable to access services due to poor language skills. SLTs are uniquely qualified to assess an individuals capacity to communicate and understand information and to advise on the most effective means of presenting information and choices to the individual, maximising their opportunity to exert free choice (RCSLT, 2005).
● Increased risk of aspiration pneumonia (incurring additional resource).
● Increased risk of nutritional compromise (incurring additional resource).
● Avoidable death due to malnutrition, choking and aspiration pneumonia (RCSLT, 2005):
● Studies that look at the incidence of swallowing difficulty in dementia show a high rate of dysphagia:
● 68% of those in a home for the aged (Steele et al, 1997).
● Bronchopneumonia was the leading cause of death in Alzheimer's disease in another study (Horner et al, 1994); 28.6% in this study were found to be aspirating.
● Swallowing problems are also a concern in other types of dementia, eg vascular dementia (Stach, 2000) and those conditions where neurological signs are present alongside cognitive impairment, eg Huntington's disease, progressive supranuclear palsy, Parkinson's disease and dementia with Lewy bodies (Logemann, 1998).

Risk management at the level of service organisation

MDT working: Individuals with suspected dementia should have access to SLT assessment and management as part of a multidisciplinary team with specialist mental health skills (Heritage & Farrow, 1994).

Competence: Advanced dysphagia training is required. Junior therapists working within mental health services must have access to specialist SLT supervision.

Speech and language therapy value

● Providing detailed assessment of communication skills that contributes to the diagnosis process, provides a baseline to monitor change and evaluates ongoing intervention.

- Assisting in differential diagnosis through detailed assessment.
- Providing support to carers based on assessment findings.
- Providing for reassessment to monitor change.
- Providing individual communication programmes to benefit individuals.
- Helping the individual to achieve greater insight into their communication difficulties (where appropriate); in turn to reduce frustration caused by communication impairment and improve confidence.
- Supporting and training carers with regard general communication strategies as well as individual specific advice.
- Assessment of eating and drinking difficulties.
- Providing advice and strategies with regard to eating and drinking difficulties.
- Helping the MDT understand the individual's communication difficulties.

8.17 Palliative Care

This information is designed to support speech and language therapy services undertaking reviews of service organisation and provision. Therapists seeking detailed clinical guidance are referred to the *RCSLT Clinical Guidelines* (2005), position papers and *Reference Framework: Underpinning Competence to Practise* (2003), available on the RCSLT website: www.rcslt.org

Definition
WHO definition of palliative care for adults
Palliative care is an approach that improves the quality of life of individuals and their families facing the problem associated with life-threatening illness, through prevention and relief of suffering by means of early identification and impeccable assessment and treatment of pain and other problems (WHO, 2006).
Physical, psychosocial and spiritual palliative care:
- provides relief from pain and other distressing symptoms
- affirms life and regards dying as a normal process
- intends neither to hasten or postpone death
- integrates the psychological and spiritual aspects of individual care
- offers a support system to help individuals live as actively as possible until death
- offers a support system to help the family cope during the individuals illness and in their own bereavement

● uses a team approach to address the needs of individuals and their families, including bereavement counselling, if indicated

● will enhance quality of life, and may also positively influence the course of illness

● is applicable early in the course of illness, in conjunction with other therapies that are intended to prolong life, such as chemotherapy or radiation therapy, and includes those investigations needed to better understand and manage distressing clinical complications.

WHO definition of palliative care for children

Palliative care for children represents a special, albeit closely related field to adult palliative care. WHO's definition of palliative care appropriate for children and their families is as follows; the principles apply to other paediatric chronic disorders (WHO, 1998a):

● palliative care for children is the active total care of the child's body, mind and spirit, and also involves giving support to the family

● it begins when illness is diagnosed, and continues regardless of whether or not a child receives treatment directed at the disease

● health providers must evaluate and alleviate a child's physical, psychological, and social distress

● effective palliative care requires a broad multidisciplinary approach that includes the family and makes use of available community resources; it can be successfully implemented even if resources are limited

● it can be provided in tertiary care facilities, in community health centres and even in children's homes.

For further general information see ACT's website, at: www.act.org.uk/act, which works to improve care and services for all children in the UK with life-threatening or terminal conditions.

The palliative care approach aims to promote both physical and psychosocial wellbeing and is an integral part of all clinical practice, whatever the illness or its' stage, informed by knowledge and practice with palliative care principles (NCHSPCS, 1995).

The following sections refer specifically to **palliative care for adults**.

National guidance and sources of further information and support

● NICE *Palliative and Supportive Care Guidance* (2004), in particular Chapter 10 – **Rehabilitation** *for guidance on national standards for speech and language therapy provision.*

- *Fulfilling Lives.* Rehabilitation in Palliative Care NCHSPCS, 2000.
- *National Service Framework for long-term conditions,* 2005. Department of Health.
- The Hospice Information Service www.hospiceinformation.info
- The National Council for Palliative Care www.ncpc.org.uk

Aetiology

The hospice movement was founded by Dame Cecily Saunders in 1967 to provide care to people suffering symptoms resulting from advanced life-threatening disease.

The majority of people receiving palliative care continue to be those individuals who are suffering from advanced cancer (see section 15 on Head and Neck Cancer).

In recent years, it has been recognised that the palliative care approach to disease management can be applied to a number of non-malignant, life-threatening diseases. These conditions include:

- HIV/AIDS
- renal disease
- heart failure
- respiratory disease
- neurological disease
- vascular disease
- co-morbidity associated with learning disabilities.

Incidence and prevalence

Between year 2003-2004, 85,211 new individuals with cancer, and 3,115 new individuals with a non-cancer diagnosis (see below) accessed specialist palliative care services in England, Wales and Northern Ireland (NCPC, 2005).

Diagnosis	% of 3,115
HIV/AIDS	7%
MND/MS/spinal disease	34%
Heart/stroke	35%
Respiratory	24%

There is limited research into the prevalence of communication or swallowing problems in the palliative population. The Allied Health

Professions Palliative Care Project Team in Glasgow (2004) found in their survey found that out of 150 palliative individuals interviewed, 68 individuals reported communication or swallowing problems, but only 10 were referred to speech and language therapy.

Further research is required to contribute to the evidence base, particularly with reference to advanced, life-threatening disease and communication and swallowing disorders.

Vulnerability: risk issues

There is little doubt that difficulties in communication and/or swallowing can impact significantly on quality of life.

● Communication problems can interfere with the ability to express needs or desires to family, friends and carers or to understand essential information related to care.

● Swallowing problems can deny the social, cultural, religious and personal pleasures associated with eating. Without access to specialist care, individuals may suffer from distressing symptoms associated with oropharyngeal dysphagia.

Many types of cancer, in various sites in the body, can result in communication and/or swallowing difficulties, but they are most common in tumours of the brain, head and neck or upper digestive tract.

Research also suggests that individuals with lung cancer may be a particularly vulnerable group who may experience voice and swallowing disorders.

These problems can also be caused, or compounded by, by different intervention approaches, eg medication, surgery, radiotherapy, chemotherapy.

Speech and language therapy value

Individuals with life-threatening disease require responsive and flexible speech and language therapy services to ensure that they can access them when and where they need them without undue delay.

Assessment, intervention and management of communication and swallowing difficulties are a key part of an holistic approach to individual care. Where the problem cannot be fully resolved, the SLT can advise on strategies to ensure the best possible function.

Individuals with communication disorders may require increased support in communicating wishes regarding complex intervention and management decisions, eg symptom management, consent to intervention, and preferred place of care.

From a swallowing perspective, the focus of intervention may shift from the prevention of complications and include risk management of dysphagia, thus minimizing symptoms and maximising individual comfort (Eckman & Roe, 2005).

As educators, SLTs have a critical role in providing information to individuals and carers on communication and swallowing impairments and management options.

The principles of intervention with individuals in this client group are outlined below:

● assess only as required to provide the answers to plan management
● minimal intervention for maximum gain
● maintain function where possible
● improve function if appropriate and realistic
● utilise compensatory strategies, diet modifications and safe swallow strategies
● work as member of MDT
● provide holistic, individual centred care
● facilitate communication between individual and team
● provide education and information
● advise on risk-benefit evaluation.

8.18 Pre-school Children

This information is designed to support speech and language therapy services undertaking reviews of service organisation and provision. Therapists seeking detailed clinical guidance are referred to the *RCSLT Clinical Guidelines* (2005), position papers and *Reference Framework: Underpinning Competence to Practise* (2003), available on the RCSLT website: www.rcslt.org

Definition

Speech, language and communication needs in pre-school children refers to all children prior to entry to primary level education (typically under five years old) who present with, or are at risk of, failure to make age appropriate progress in speech, language and communication. Children who have speech, language and communication needs have inadequate communication for their circumstances and relative to other children of their age.

It refers to all forms of communication, including spoken and non-verbal, and incorporates both the understanding and use of these in achieving functional communication.

Pre-school children may present with difficulties in their speech, language and communication development and/or ability in relation to their peers. These difficulties may be identified as being delayed or disordered.

The speech, language and communication difficulty may arise independently, (ie primary) or as a consequence of other identified difficulties, (ie secondary) such as learning, physical, sensory, attention or behavioural difficulty. It may or may not have an identifiable aetiology.

Children may have difficulty with one or more aspects of speech, language and communication. In addition, difficulties with eating and drinking may arise at this age (see section 8.14 on Dysphagia).

Difficulties may arise with receptive language, expressive language, social communication, speech, fluency or voice.

Cross-referencing with the chapter sections listed below is recommended:

8.4. Autism Spectrum Disorder
8.5. Bilingualism
8.6. Brain Injury
8.7. Cerebral Palsy
8.8. Cleft Palate and Velopharyngeal Disorders
8.9. Craniofacial Conditions
8.11. Deafness
8.12. Dysfluency
8.14. Dysphagia
8.16. Mental Health
8.17. Palliative Care
8.20. School-aged Children
8.21. Specific Language Impairment
8.22 Specific Speech Impairment
8.23. Visual Impairment
8.24. Voice
7.2.1. AAC

National guidance and sources of further information and support

● *Every Child Matters* Children's services strategy, 2005
www.everychildmatters.gov.uk

- *RCSLT Clinical Guidelines* (2005), section on *Pre-school Children* www.rcslt.org
- AFASIC www.afasic.org.uk
- I CAN www.ican.org.uk
- CaF www.cafamily.org.uk
- Council for Disabled Children www.ncb.org.uk/cdc
- Dyspraxia Foundation www.dyspraxiafoundation.org.uk
- NAPLIC www.naplic.org.uk
- NASEN www.nasen.org.uk
- NAS www.nas.org.uk
- National Parent Partnership Network www.parentpartnership.org.uk
- OAASIS www.oaasis.co.uk

Aetiology

In many cases there is no known cause of the speech, language and communication needs and these may be the child's primary difficulty. However, speech, language and communication needs may arise as a consequence of other factors including:
- hearing impairment/deafness, including persistent intermittent hearing loss
- learning disability from:
- an identified genetic aetiology, eg Down's syndrome
- pre, peri or postnatal trauma
- an unidentified aetiology.
- global developmental delay
- prematurity
- acute or chronic medical conditions
- cleft lip and palate
- physical disability
- mental health and/or emotional and behavioural factors
- other genetic factors or
- environmental influences including:
- child protection issues
- family history of speech, language and communication needs, mental health, learning difficulty, hearing impairment or other special needs.

Prevalence and incidence

Prevalence: Speech, language and communication needs may be the most common disability presenting in early childhood (Law, 1992). Estimates of the proportion of pre-school children with speech, language and communication needs vary according to the nature of the study data collection, classification and identification of speech, language and communication needs and the population studied.

For example, the range of estimates of prevalence of speech, language and communication needs across the UK population is between 2% and 25%, varying due to different data collection methods and criteria (Law, 1992).

In the US, a language screening failure rate in kindergarten children of 26.2% was found (Tomblin et al, 1997), but this dropped to 7.4% with detailed assessment. However, another study (Locke et al, 2002) investigated four year olds in areas of deprivation and found prevalence of speech, language and communication needs as high as 55%.

Incidence

Little has been written about incidence of speech, language and communication needs in children.

Broomfield & Dodd (2004) found an overall incidence (of speech, language and communication needs for children who have no additional disability who were referred and attended paediatric speech and language therapy assessment) of 16.3% in a single year. Almost 75% of these cases were under five years old. The extrapolated incidence rate for preschool children (constraints as above) is over 12%.

The actual incidence of speech, language and communication needs in a pre-school population will be greater than this, given that not all cases are referred and attend local speech and language therapy services.

Recent estimates of speech, language and communication needs both with and without additional disability within Sure Start populations (the 25% most deprived areas across the UK) are as high as 35% new cases being identified each year.

Vulnerability: risk issues

Speech, language and communication difficulty may impact on future learning and achievement, literacy, behaviour and social-emotional functioning and independence.

Speech and language therapy value

● Promoting the development of speech, language, communication and eating/drinking in targeted at-risk groups.
● Maximising the development of referred children's speech, language, communication and eating/drinking skills.
● Educating and empowering parents, carers, educational/social services staff and significant others in the support and development of children's speech, language and communication skills.
● Establishing effective, functional communication skills through the development of understanding, listening and auditory processing, play, non-verbal communication, interaction, expression and speech. This involves:
● providing advice, information and training to other professionals in the team
● providing an integrated service with parents/carers, other agencies and professions
● assessment, diagnosis and appropriate intervention

8.19 Progressive Neurological Disorders

This information is designed to support speech and language therapy services undertaking reviews of service organisation and provision. Therapists seeking detailed clinical guidance are referred to the *RCSLT Clinical Guidelines* (2005), position papers and *Reference Framework: Underpinning Competence to Practise* (2003), available on the RCSLT website: www.rcslt.org

Definition

A neurological disorder is a condition affecting any part of the central or peripheral nervous system. Progressive neurological disorders refer to those conditions where there is a progressive deterioration in functioning. These disorders are likely to affect the individual for the rest of his/her life.
Some of the disorders progress more rapidly than others, (eg motor neurone disease) and some follow a more unpredictable course with relapses and remissions, (eg Multiple Sclerosis). Examples of progressive neurological disorders include multiple sclerosis, motor neurone disease, Parkinson's disease, Huntington's disease, Friedreich's ataxia, multiple system atrophy and progressive supranuclear palsy.

Cross-referencing with the chapter sections listed below is recommended:
8.1. Acquired Motor Speech Disorders
8.2. Adult Learning Disability
8.3. Aphasia
8.6. Brain Injury
8.14. Dysphagia
8.16. Mental Health
8.17. Palliative Care
8.24. Voice
7.2.1 AAC

National guidance and sources of further information and support

- King's MND care pathway www.mndassociation.org
- Epilepsy pathway – Action on Neurology www.dh.gov.uk
- NICE Guidelines for MS www.nice.org.uk
- *NSF for long-term conditions* www.dh.gov.uk
- *NSF older people* www.dh.gov.uk/PolicyandGuidance
- *NSF for mental health* www.dh.gov.uk
- PSP Association www.pspeur.org/association
- Sarah Matheson Trust www.msaweb.co.uk/
- Huntington's Disease Association www.hda.org.uk
- Motor Neurone Disease Association www.mndassociation.org
- Multiple Sclerosis Society www.mssociety.org.uk
- Parkinson's Disease Society www.parkinsons.org.uk

Types of disorder

In the UK there are 10 million people living with a neurological condition. Each year 600,000 people (1% of the UK population) are newly diagnosed with a neurological condition (Neurological Alliance, 2003).

However, these figures are not specific to progressive neurological disorders – they include all neurological disorders, progressive and non-progressive (including stroke, dementia, cerebral palsy and brain injury).

It is predicted that the numbers of people with neurological disorders will continue to increase as a result of people living longer, advances in health care and the ongoing development of diagnostic techniques.

Incidence and prevalence of some progressive neurological conditions:

● Motor neurone disease (MNDA, 2004): Incidence; 2 per 100,000 Prevalence; 7 per 100,000

● Multiple Sclerosis (MS Society, 2006): Incidence; 4 per 100,000 Prevalence; 144 per 100,000

● Parkinson's disease (Parkinson's Disease Society, 2006): Incidence; 17 per 100,000 Prevalence; 200 per 100,000

● Friedreich's ataxia (Ataxia UK, 2006): Prevalence; 1-2 per 50,000

● Progressive supranuclear palsy (PSP Association, 2006): Prevalence; 5-6 per 100,000 (Or up to 15 per 100,000 considering non diagnosis and mis-diagnosis)

● Multiple-system atrophy (Sarah Matheson Trust, 2006): Prevalence: 1 per 100,000

● Huntington's disease (HDA, 2006): Prevalence: 13.5 per 100,000 (approximately).

Incidence and prevalence

There are studies looking at prevalence of communication and swallowing problems in the various different disorders. The figures in these studies are very wide-ranging and look at different aspects and variables and it is therefore difficult to be accurate about prevalence. However, all progressive disorders, at various times and usually in the later stages, have potential to cause major communication and swallowing problems. The figures for prevalence range between 30%-80%.

For further information, please refer to the national organisation associated with the specific conditions.

See also the section on Adult Acquired Dysphagia.

Vulnerability: risk issues

The nature of progressive neurological disorders is such that there are generic risks inherent in the disease process. Some individuals are referred to speech and language therapy services before diagnosis, yet others may not be referred for many months post diagnosis.

Some of the issues and resulting risks involved in progressive neurological disorders are outlined in the following table.

	Communication	Swallowing
1. Fatigue	• Deteriorates with fatigue • Reduced ability to use AAC	• Deteriorates with fatigue • Can alter hourly/ daily
2. Impaired cognition	• Difficulty utilising therapeutic strategies/ techniques • Often subtle changes and can go undetected • Reduced participation in activities/ social communication • May need different strategies to ensure communication is as effective as possible	• Lack of insight into difficulties can lead to non-acceptance/ utilisation of recommendations • May need different egstrategies to ensure safety
3. Rapid or unexpected deterioration	• May need AAC equipment at short notice • Therapy response time may be inadequate and lead to frustration/ isolation	• Chest infection • Dehydration • Malnutrition • Respiratory difficulties • Fear/ anxiety around choking
4. Unmanaged chronic problems	• Frustration/ isolation	• As 3 • Poor oral hygiene can cause mouth infection with increased risk of chest infection
5. Variability/ unpredictability	• Frustration/ isolation • Can be hour to hour or day to day	• As 3 • Can be hour to hour or day to day

	Communication	Swallowing
6. Friend/ family carer strain	• Lack of adequate support for carer can cause breakdown of relationships • May become 'translator' for the person when communication becomes too difficult	• Fear/ anxiety around choking • For those unable to feed themselves, feeding competencies of carers can be variable and can impact on person's safety
7. Social Services/ agency carers	• May be inconsistency of personnel which may result in breakdown of communication	• Carers will need very specific and detailed recommendations of dietary modifications and feeding systems • Unable to deviate from the recommendations if person refuses to accept them, leading to conflict
8. Acceptance of diagnosis	• Denial of problems and reluctance to accept help • The individual may experience an ongoing sense of bereavement as skills and abilities are gradually lost. The individual may not automatically utilise adaptation and coping strategies. This often depends on personality and support received.	• Denial of problems and reluctance to accept help leading to 3

Chapter 8

	Communication	Swallowing
8 continued. Acceptance of diagnosis	• Discussion around diagnosis may be ongoing for months/years. Where communication is an issue, the ability to communicate about emotional and psychological issues may deteriorate, causing further difficulties in being able to 'talk through' acceptance	
9. Acute admissions	• Too ill to use AAC • Environment not communication-friendly • Unable to verbalise wishes	• Poor knowledge of person's abilities/wishes by ward staff • Risk of being kept nil by mouth until hospital SLT assessment • If condition is medication-dependant, e.g Parkinson's, alternative methods of giving medication may not be in place early enough
10. Palliative care	• Discussions around end of life issues may be left too late, resulting in the person being unable to take part in full discussions about their care plan	• May be allowed oral nutrition for quality of life, accepting the risks of aspiration

	Communication	Swallowing
11. Co-morbidity	• Factors other than the original diagnosis may exacerbate communication difficulties and may not be diagnosed and managed	• Factors other than the original diagnosis may exacerbate swallowing difficulties and may not be diagnosed and managed
12. Medication	• There may be specific on/off times in level of communication abilities due to medication	• There may be specific on/off times in level of swallowing abilities due to medication

Managing the risk at the level of service organisation

The following are key issues in working with these client groups:

● Early intervention is vital to ensure the person, and their carer/s, understand the condition and are educated and supported in their ability to deal with ongoing and deteriorating communication and swallowing issues (DH, 2005).

● A flexible and responsive approach is often required as the needs of people with rapidly progressing conditions can change overnight (Worthington, 1996).

● Forward discussion while the person is able to communicate effectively is important in preparing for alternative methods of communication and nutrition where these are likely to deteriorate significantly.

Speech and language therapy value

SLTs use their knowledge and skills of communication and swallowing within the context of both the core multidisciplinary team, and the wider team including, social services and palliative care, to ensure:

● promotion and maintenance of independence as far as possible

● promotion and maintenance of an acceptable quality of life

● individual self-management with or without the support of carers, family and friends

- facilitation of individual choice and decision making around lifestyle and end of life issues
- provision of information and support at the appropriate times
- provision of equipment to support communication where necessary.

8.20 School-aged Children

This information is designed to support speech and language therapy services undertaking reviews of service organisation and provision. Therapists seeking detailed clinical guidance are referred to the *RCSLT Clinical Guidelines* (2005), position papers and *Reference Framework: Underpinning Competence to Practise* (2003), available on the RCSLT website: www.rcslt.org

Definition

School-aged children, irrespective of where they are being educated, who are failing to make typical progress in speech, language and/or communication.

This may include children with voice, articulation, speech intelligibility, dysfluency, language, interaction or general communication difficulties.

The children may have difficulties in one or more of these areas, as well as concomitant eating/drinking difficulties.

Cross-referencing with the chapter sections listed below is recommended:

8.4. Autism Spectrum Disorder
8.5. Bilingualism
8.6. Brain Injury
8.7. Cerebral Palsy
8.8. Cleft Palate and Velopharyngeal Disorders
8.9. Craniofacial Conditions
8.11. Deafness
8.12. Dysfluency
8.13. Dyslexia
8.14. Dysphagia
8.16. Mental Health
8.18. Pre-school Children
8.21. Specific Language Impairment
8.22 Specific Speech Impairment

8.23. Visual Impairment
8.24. Voice
7.2.1 AAC

National guidance and sources of further information and support

- *Every Child Matters,* 2005 www.everychildmatters.gov.uk
- *RCSLT Clinical Guidelines* (2005), section on *School-aged Children* www.rcslt.org
- RCSLT Position Paper, 2006, *Supporting Children with Speech and Communication Needs within Integrated Children's Services*

See also chapter 3, section on Children's services/education strategy

- AFASIC www.afasic.org.uk
- ICAN www.ican.org.uk
- CaF www.cafamily.org.uk
- Council for Disabled Children www.ncb.org.uk/cdc
- Dyspraxia Foundation www.dyspraxiafoundation.org.uk
- NAPLIC www.naplic.org.uk
- NASEN www.nasen.org.uk
- NAS www.nas.org.uk
- National Parent Partnership Network www.parentpartnership.org.uk
- OAASIS www.oaasis.co.uk

Aetiology

In many cases there is no known cause of the speech, language and communication needs and these may be the child's primary difficulty. However, speech, language and communication disorders (SLCD) may arise as a consequence of other conditions including:

- cleft palate
- genetic syndromes
- cerebral palsy and other physical impairment
- ear, nose and throat issues
- neurological conditions
- developmental coordination disorder (DCD)
- autism spectrum disorders (ASD)
- cognitive impairment

- psychiatric or mental health issues
- specific language impairment
- auditory processing disorders.

Prevalence

The prevalence of SLCD in the school population is very difficult to estimate. Estimates of the prevalence of SLCD by speech and language therapy services vary widely because of the many variations in service profile which have the potential to impact on SLCD. Relevant dimensions include:
- urban or rural distribution
- areas of social deprivation
- high incidence of 'looked after' children
- vulnerable populations, eg drug and alcohol abuse or parents with learning disability
- pre-school preventative services, eg Sure Start.

However, the accepted level of prevalence is that 10% of school aged children have a SLCD which could potentially affect their educational attainment.

See also the sections related to Specific Language Impairment and Specific Speech impairment.

Vulnerability: risk issues

SLTs work with children with any SLCD that has an effect on their social or educational development or on their mental health and wellbeing. The risk of impact on wellbeing should be of paramount importance in the clinical decision around whether intervention should take place. Child protection issues must also be taken into account at this point.

Educational transition needs to be recognised as a time of heightened risk.

SLTs should consider the risk to the child if intervention does not take place. This judgement should include consideration of whether the SLT is the appropriate person to reduce the risk, given that professionals from other disciplines may have more understanding of the issue, (eg mental health risks) or those in the child's environment may be in a better position to handle the risk, with guidance from the SLT.

Risk to health and wellbeing for children with eating, drinking and swallowing disorders, including saliva control issues may be reduced by a specially trained and qualified SLT. See section on Paediatric Dysphagia.

Speech and language therapy value
● Diagnosis of SLCD
● Profiling of SLCD impact and child's skills and needs
● Intervention for SLCD will only be appropriate if there is an identifiable impact from the SLCD and if there is an identifiable outcome from the intervention. When this is the case, speech and language therapy value is:
● to develop and maximise communication skills in all environments
● to promote inclusion into school and social contexts
● to promote access to curriculum
● to minimise secondary difficulties arising out of communication impairments such as emotional and behavioural difficulties and literacy difficulties
● to support parents as child's communication needs change and develop throughout childhood and adolescence
Specifically for school-aged children with **language impairments**, the main aim is to maximise their comprehension and production of language in both oral and written forms and also maximise their use of those abilities so that they can reach their full potential both educationally (including literacy) and socially.
For those with **speech impairments**, the main aim is to maximise intelligibility to reach full potential educationally and socially. Children's support needs will vary throughout childhood and adolescence.
The modalities of SLCD requiring intervention may include:
● spoken language
● alternative and/or augmentative communication
● facial expression, body language and social interaction
● written language.

8.21 Specific Language Impairment
This information is designed to support speech and language therapy services undertaking reviews of service organisation and provision. Therapists seeking detailed clinical guidance are referred

to the *RCSLT Clinical Guidelines* (2005), position papers and *Reference Framework: Underpinning Competence to Practise* (2003), available on the RCSLT website: www.rcslt.org

Definition
International Classifications of Diseases (WHO, 1993):
● Language skills, as assessed on standardised tests, are below the two standard deviations limit for the child's age.
● Language skills are at least one standard deviation below non-verbal IQ assessed on standardised tests.
● There are no neurological, sensory or physical impairments that directly affect the use of spoken language, nor is there a pervasive developmental disorder.
A distinction is made between receptive language disorder, where comprehension is more than two standard deviations below age level and expressive language disorder, where only expressive language is severely affected, and where understanding and use of non-verbal communication and imaginative language functions are within the normal range.
The American Psychiatric Association's Diagnostic and Statistical Manual (1994) definition is similar to the above and also includes mention that the language difficulties interfere with academic or occupational achievement or with social communication).
Specific language impairment (SLI) is not a homogenous disorder. It can affect the various subcomponents of language to varying degrees, resulting in each child presenting with a different profile of difficulty. The subcomponents affected can be:
● receptive language
● expressive language
● word finding
● speech/phonology
● pragmatics
● attention and listening
● auditory memory.
Cross-referencing with the chapter sections listed below is recommended:
8.4. Autism Spectrum Disorder
8.5. Bilingualism
8.6. Brain Injury

Sources of further information and support

- AFASIC www.afasic.org.uk
- ICAN www.ican.org.uk
- CaF www.cafamily.org.uk
- Council for Disabled Children www.ncb.org.uk/cdc
- Dyspraxia Foundation www.dyspraxiafoundation.org.uk
- NAPLIC www.naplic.org.uk
- NASEN www.nasen.org.uk
- NAS www.nas.org.uk
- National Parent Partnership Network
www.parentpartnership.org.uk
- OAASIS www.oaasis.co.uk

Aetiology

SLI is a developmental condition and changes over time. The causes of SLI are likely to be multifactorial (Bishop, 1992) with both extrinsic and intrinsic factors influencing the child's development.

The classical definitions above have been arrived at by a process of exclusion. The following definition of SLI takes into account both intrinsic and extrinsic factors (Lees & Urwin, 1991).

A language disorder is that language profile which, although it may be associated with a history of hearing, learning, environmental and emotional difficulties, cannot be attributed to any one of these alone or even just the sum of these effects, and in which one or more of

the following is also seen:
1. A close positive family history of specific difficulty in language development.
2. Evidence of cerebral dysfunction, either during development or by the presence of neurological signs.
3. A mismatch between the various subsystems of language in relation to other aspects of cognitive development.
4. A failure to catch these differences up with 'generalised' language help.
(The most common presentation is a combination of the above factors 1,3 and 4. factor 2 is rare).

Prevalence and incidence
Varied reports of frequency are documented according to definition:
● 5% of children in the UK, eg 36,000 in year 2 have SLI (Law et al, 2000).
● Estimated ratios of approximately 2.8 males to every female (Robinson, 1987).
● Many children with SLI experience severe long-term difficulties. More than 72% of children who had SLI at age five remained impaired at age 12 (Beitchman et al, 1994).

Vulnerability: risk issues
SLI can have a profound and lasting effect on children's lives. The impact of these difficulties will vary according to the severity of the problem, early identification, the support the child receives, the child's confidence and the demands of the child's environment.
Learning:
SSLI can affect all areas of learning and access to all areas of the National Curriculum.
● Early language impairment is clearly associated with continued academic difficulties into adulthood (Young et al, 2002).
● Comprehension difficulties make children very vulnerable in relation to education (Hooper at al, 2003).
● Children with specific speech and language difficulties often have associated literacy problems with persistent difficulties in the areas of phonological awareness and spelling (Stackhouse, 2000).
● SLI can significantly affect maths learning (Donlan, 1998).

Social and Behavioural problems:
● Children with SLI can experience social and behavioural problems and these problems increase over time (Redmond and Rice, 1998).
● Many children with SLI appear to be withdrawn socially (Coster et al, 1999).
● Poor interaction and increased withdrawal leads to poor self esteem (Jerome et al, 2002).
● Aggressive behavioural difficulties are reported in young children with SLI (Carson et al, 1998).
● Children with SLI are at risk of being bullied at school (Conti-Ramsden & Botting, 2004).
● There is a higher incidence of behavioural and psychiatric problems in children with SLI (approximately 50%) compared to non-impaired children (approximately 12%) (Goodyer, 2000).
● Young offenders are found to have high levels of speech and language communication difficulties (Bryan, 2004).
● Some children continue to show severe difficulties into adult life. These difficulties can include problems with theory of mind, verbal short term memory and phonological processing and an increased risk of psychiatric difficulties (Clegg et al, 2005).

Speech and language therapy value
● Identification and diagnosis of this disorder.
● To devise pathways and programmes of therapy.
● To integrate therapy targets into the educational curriculum through collaborative practice.
● To maximise communication potential by skilling others in their use of facilitative strategies and/or use of augmentative communication systems.
● To raise awareness, support and train professionals in identifying and working with children with SLI.
● To support parents and facilitate communication in functional settings.

8.22 Specific Speech Impairment

This information is designed to support speech and language therapy services undertaking reviews of service organisation and provision. Therapists seeking detailed clinical guidance are referred to the *RCSLT Clinical Guidelines* (2005), position papers and *Reference Framework: Underpinning Competence to Practise* (2003), available on the RCSLT website: www.rcslt.org

Definition

Child speech disorders may be developmental or acquired. Developmental speech disorders are distinguishable from speech delays by unusual patterns of speech development, as evidenced in speech data analysis.

The term 'developmental disorder' specifies a difference from 'normal' patterns of development in relation to chronological age (Grunwell, 1995). Characteristics of normal developmental phonological processes, such as 'stopping, fronting, cluster reduction' would not normally be categorised as characteristic of a speech disorder but as normal immaturities. However where immature patterns persist after expected norms for maturation they might contribute to a diagnosis of speech disorder under the definition of persisting speech difficulties (Pascoe et al, in print). Where characteristics of both delay and disorder co-exist a diagnosis of mixed developmental speech delay/disorder may be appropriate.

This section describes a profile of moderate/severe speech disorders where descriptors and needs are more specific than those outlined in sections on pre-school, school-age and SLI. However a degree of overlap is inevitable.

The term 'speech disorders' implies a more severe disturbance than most cases of developmental delay. The severity of the disorder might be clearly evident at first assessment or it might become evident in the early stages of therapy, when conventional therapy approaches prove ineffective or when more evidence emerges, such as disturbances in connected speech, auditory processing disturbances, vowel distortions, inconsistencies in speech production or possible structural factors (tonsils/adenoids/palate function). In such cases more detailed speech analyses and medical/ psychological investigations are likely to be necessary and the level of SLT input may need to be reviewed. Additional needs might include increased speech and language therapy provision: a second opinion from a specialist therapist, more frequent therapy, regular liaison with teaching assistants or classroom assistants, or daily therapy in speech and language unit provision.

Degree of severity in speech disorders cannot be defined in terms of delay because, unlike language disorders, the most severe speech disorders are so unusual that they cannot be described in relation to age or stage of development.

Subjective, non-specific descriptors such as unintelligible speech may be applied to a spontaneous speech sample but appropriate intervention would necessarily require specific assessments to differentiate between the many factors contributing to unintelligibility. Speech disorders are more precisely described in relation to a range of theoretical perspectives: phonetic/articulatory disorder (Gibbon, 2002), articulation disorder with phonological consequences (Grundy and Harding, 1995), phonological disorder (Dodd, 1995; Grunwell, 1995), psycholinguistic (Dodd, 1995; Stackhouse & Wells, 1997).

Specific speech impairment is a term that encompasses specific difficulty at any level of input or output processing. Severity of speech impairment can also be defined by the pattern of progress. An absence of progress in response to extended therapy is indicative of more severe difficulties.

Cross-referencing with the chapter sections listed below is recommended:

8.4. Autism Spectrum Disorder
8.5. Bilingualism
8.6. Brain Injury
8.7. Cerebral Palsy
8.8. Cleft Palate and Velopharyngeal Disorders
8.9. Craniofacial Conditions
8.11. Deafness
8.12. Dysfluency
8.13. Dyslexia
8.14. Dysphagia
8.16. Mental Health
8.18. Pre-school Children
8.20. School-aged Children
8.21. Specific Language Impairment
8.24. Voice
7.2.1 AAC

Sources of further information and support
● AFASIC www.afasic.org.uk
● I CAN www.ican.org.uk
● CaF www.cafamily.org.uk
● Council for Disabled Children www.ncb.org.uk/cdc
● Dyspraxia Foundation www.dyspraxiafoundation.org.uk

- NAPLIC www.naplic.org.uk
- NASEN www.nasen.org.uk
- NAS www.nas.org.uk
- National Parent Partnership Network
www.parentpartnership.org.uk
- OAASIS www.oaasis.co.uk

Aetiology

Although many speech disorders can be hypothetically attributed to physical constraints such as oro/nasal structure, fluctuating hearing loss, restricted language use, dyspraxia, etc (Shriberg, 1995), it is not uncommon for speech disorders to be diagnosed without any identifiable aetiology.

Recent studies have explored the association between speech difficulties with a range of variables: pre- and peri-natal problems; ear, nose and throat (ENT) problems; unusual sucking habits and positive family history (Broomfield and Dodd, 2004; Fox et al, 2002). Fox et al (2002) were unable to find a direct link between precipitating factors and type of speech disorder whereas a further study evolved a complex system of diagnostic markers for directly linking speech findings to aetiology (Shriberg, 2003).

Incidence

Few statistics exist which distinguish between speech disability and speech and language disability. Estimated number of referrals for speech and language disability in the UK is 85,000-90,000. Broomfield and Dodd (2004) reported their survey of 1100 referrals to Middlesbrough PCT, in which 29% of those attending for speech and language therapy assessment were found to have speech difficulties and 40% of these children had a primary speech disorder. Within that study, 35% of the phonological disorders were severe or profound and would have been classified as 'specific speech impairments'.

Vulnerability: risk issues

- Speech processing problems can have psychosocial consequences in school: bullying, low self-esteem and lack of motivation (Nash and Stengelhofen, 2002).
- Specific speech impairments change very little without intervention (Broomfield & Dodd, in print).

● Atypical speech processes may stabilise without early intervention.

● Socialisation and literacy skills, ie reading, writing and spelling, may be compromised without active therapy prior to school entry (Nathan et al, 2004).

Managing the Risk at the Level of Service Organisation

Children with speech disorder need direct input from speech and language therapy in order to progress (Law et al, 2000).

This is best provided by a specialist service that enables:

● Early differential diagnosis (Williams & Stackhouse, 2000). Speech assessments that screen primarily for symptoms of developmental delay, may fail to identify specific speech impairment.

● Early intensive and differential intervention:

● to prevent stabilisation of/to destabilise atypical simplification processes and their phonological sequelae especially where a history of hearing impairment is a contributing factor.

● The provision of therapy programmes that are tailored to the unique needs of the individual with a complex and severe speech disorder. Intervention may be provided individually, in pairs or in small groups. General fronting/stopping speech-group approaches to intervention are highly unlikely to be effective in treating severe speech impairments.

● Focus on speech impairment. Neglect of specific speech impairment in favour of treating co-existing language disorders as the first priority may precipitate a progressive phonological disorder affecting all phonological development from time of diagnosis to time of intervention.

● Separate reporting of intervention outcomes for SSI as opposed to intervention outcomes for delayed speech development.

● Intervention to be provided primarily by an SLT with developed expertise in complex and severe speech disorder. Follow-up activities may be continued by an SLT assistant or a teaching assistant in school but demonstration of specific techniques with frequent reminders of the technique by the SLT or the use of video therapy, is essential.

Travel to specialist centres may be necessary for some technically supported interventions such as electro-palatography (EPG).

Severe persisting speech disorders may require language unit placement.

Speech and language therapy value

● To distinguish between characteristics and types of speech delay and specific speech disorders.

● To identify, assess, diagnose and to investigate and/or treat all aspects of complex speech disorders: consonant production, vowels, voice, nasality, prosody, rate, volume, inconsistency connected speech and intelligibility (Howard, 2004).

● To adopt a hypothesis testing approach to accurately diagnose the nature of particularly complex/severe speech disorders and contributory factors.

● To differentiate between the additional burden of care for SSI versus speech delay.

● To ensure that therapy approaches are appropriate and targeted to the nature of the underlying deficits and strengths.

● To inform and advise parents and educators of the nature of each specific disorder and to introduce problem specific advice.

● To ensure that intervention for speech disorders is based on appropriate theoretical models and current evidence (Baker & McLeod, 2004).

● To promote auditory attention in children with a history of recurrent otitis media and/or hearing loss as early as possible.

● To maximise communicative competence thus promoting social integration, emotional behavioural competence and educational attainment including literacy.

Acquired child speech disorders

Acquired child speech disorders most commonly result in motor speech disorders such as dysarthria or apraxia and their clinical description and profile of vulnerability is covered in the section on cerebral palsy.

In children therapy for acquired head injury is particularly complex because pre-morbid stages of linguistic and speech processing skills would not be known. Therapy involves stimulating retrieval of lost function and facilitating resumption of speech development. Profiles of other acquired speech disorders such as late onset selective mutism; voice disorders; injury related speech impairments; sudden onset of hypo- or hypernasality; late diagnosis of tongue tie and growth related articulatory disorders, cannot be described as a group and hence guidance will be derived from other sections of this book.

8.23 Visual Impairment

This information is designed to support speech and language therapy services undertaking reviews of service organisation and provision. Therapists seeking detailed clinical guidance are referred to the *RCSLT Clinical Guidelines* (2005), position papers and *Reference Framework: Underpinning Competence to Practise* (2003), available on the RCSLT website: www.rcslt.org

Definition

Visual impairment may be congenital or acquired. Several causes of visual impairment are age-related, eg cataract, glaucoma and macular degeneration so it is more common in the elderly than in children.

The term visual impairment is not a single entity. A number of ocular and systemic conditions can result in a continuum of visual loss, which can range from blurring of vision, visual field loss to a complete lack of vision. Severe short sightedness or a refractive error can be a cause of visual impairment, despite some improvement if spectacles are worn. Very few people are totally blind.

Visual impairment should not be confused with simple refractive error such as low levels of short sightedness, which can be corrected by spectacles or contact lenses.

Some people who have a visual impairment are registered with social services. There are two categories: severely sight impaired/blind and sight impaired/partially sighted. It is important to note that many people who have a visual impairment are not registered. Registration depends on legal rather than functional definitions. Therefore, it is not possible to know how well a person who is registered actually sees in everyday situations.

Visual impairment may include:

● **Reduction of clarity of vision**: poor visual acuity, or the blurring of vision. It may affect close vision, distance vision, or both.

● **Disturbances of visual field**: a loss or disturbance of part of the field of vision: this may involve central vision, peripheral vision, or the left, right, upper, and lower fields of vision. Some people experience a random loss or disturbance of their visual field.

- **Difficulties affecting eye movements**: including difficulties in maintaining steady gaze and smooth and co-ordinated eye movements.
- **Light sensitivity**: problems associated with glare, sunlight, etc.
- **Cortical difficulties**: problems with interpreting, integrating and understanding visual stimuli.
- **Colour blindness**: unusual in females, but affects about 8% of males.

An individual may be affected by more than one of the above, sometimes on a permanent basis, sometimes on a changing or transitory basis.

Some people who have visual impairment have additional disabilities. Terminology is confused, inconsistently applied and subject to fashion, so it is often unclear what any one term (such as *visually impaired with additional disabilities* or *multiply disabled and visually impaired*) is intended to mean.

What is important is that visual impairment can co-occur with a range of other disabilities, including for example, severe or profound learning difficulties (SLD or PMLD), and physical disabilities such as cerebral palsy, epilepsy, hearing impairment, a progressive neurological condition and autism.

Some people who have a visual impairment have more than one additional disability. These different disabilities interact in complex ways, such that the overall impact is much greater than the simple sum of the various disabilities. People who have an acquired neurological event such as stroke or traumatic brain injury can also experience visual difficulties as a result of the brain damage.

The term *deafblind* is increasingly being replaced by *dual* (or even *multi-*) *sensory impairment*. There is no widely accepted definition. For some education professionals, deafblind is applied to a child who has both a visual and a hearing impairment of sufficient severity to warrant substantial curriculum intervention or differentiation. This excludes children with severe or profound learning difficulties and those with a mild to moderate dual sensory impairment who function primarily as having either visual or hearing impairment, and who are broadly within the typical developmental range for their age.

Currently, a significant number of children who have visual impairment and additional disabilities are from ethnic minority groups, so bilingualism is sometimes a factor.

There are grounds for believing that visual defects can play a significant role in dyslexia, and there is increasing evidence of visual dysfunction in some people with autism spectrum disorder. Cross-referencing with all the chapter sections is recommended.

National guidance and sources of further information and support

● The Royal National Institute of the Blind www.rnib.org.uk
● RNIB *See Change* booklet on visual impairment and stroke in older people www.rnib.org.uk
● The National Federation of Families with Visually Impaired Children. www.db2design.co.uk/look/userupdate/default.asp
● Scottish Sensory Centre www.ssc.mhie.ac.uk
● National Blind Children's Society www.nbcs.org.uk
● Sense, for children and adults who are deafblind or have associated disabilities www.sense.org.uk
● *Hearing and sight loss: A handbook for professional carers.* Butler (2004). Age Concern

Aetiology

Perfect vision requires that three components work perfectly: the eyes, including their muscular control system, the optic nerve, and the visual cortex of the brain.

A visual impairment may arise if there is something faulty with any of these three components. In some people there are problems with two components; in some, with all three.

● **Ocular defects**: damage to, or disease of, the eye, which may be of accidental, genetic or unknown origin, or associated with disease, eg diabetes.

● **Cortical visual impairment (or cerebral visual dysfunction)**: affecting vision at some stage after the light energy received by the eye is converted into electrical energy. It is likely to be associated with brain damage or compression, (congenital or acquired), such as a stroke, tumour or head injury. Cortical visual impairment can include blurred vision, double vision (diplopia), visual field loss (homonymous hemianopia) and perceptual difficulties such as visual agnosia where face and object recognition are problematic.

A study carried out on a general population of elderly people in Rotterdam in The Netherlands, concluded that, "...after glaucoma, stroke was the second most common cause of visual field loss in persons younger than 75 years" (Skenduli-Bala et al, 2005).

● **Squints (strabismus)**: generally, onset is in infancy, although it can be associated with neurological problems in older people.

There are many causes of visual impairment, which cannot all be listed here.

See Bowman et al (2001) for the causes of visual impairment in children.

The website of the Royal National Institute of the Blind (RNIB) provides further information about numerous conditions.

Visual impairment should not be confused with *reduced vision* which includes:

● **Refractive errors**, which result from the failure of the eye to bend rays of light appropriately. Refractive errors can be corrected with spectacles.

● **Cataracts**, resulting in gradual blurring of vision, which can be operated on in a simple day case procedure, dramatically improving the vision, after which a sight test is necessary.

Prevalence

Department of Health (DH) survey data suggests that there may be as many as two million people in the UK with sight problems, the majority being over 60 years of age. This is exemplified in the DH figures for England (2003).

22% of people registered as blind had additional disabilities (34,145 people).

Table 7: Number of people on the register of blind people by age group

0–4	5–17	18–49	50–64	65–74	75+	All ages
725	3,230	17,090	14,520	15,460	105,655	156,675

Table 8: Number of people on the register of partially sighted people by age group

0–4	5–17	18–49	50–64	65–74	75+	All ages
585	4,230	15,315	12,935	16,640	105,525	155,230

25% of all registered blind people who had an additional disability were also recorded as deaf or having a hearing impairment.
20% of people registered as partially sighted had additional disabilities (31,135 people).
23% of all registered partially sighted people who had an additional disability were also deaf or had a hearing impairment (1,830 Deaf, 5,025 HI).

Children

An RNIB survey (2003) estimated that two children in every 1000 in the UK are blind or partially sighted. 50% of the population surveyed were shown to have additional disabilities: 30% with severe or profound and multiple learning difficulties (Skenduli-Bala et al, 2005).

Vulnerability: risk issues

● Children who have a visual impairment are at risk with regard to acquiring the basic skills of interacting with other people, and thus may experience significant delays in the development of communication. They may follow a developmental path that is different from that in sighted children. Paradoxically, once language skills are well developed, children who have a visual impairment rely even more on language for learning about the world than sighted children do.

● Children who have visual impairment with additional disabilities are at even greater risk with regard to acquiring interaction and communication skills. For many, AAC will be necessary.

● There is a risk that individuals who have visual impairment lack social awareness and develop inappropriate behaviors; there may thus be a greater risk of children being teased, bullied or isolated at school or adults experiencing difficulties at work.

● There is an increased risk of child protection and vulnerable adult issues.

● Individuals with a visual impairment are at risk of social exclusion and isolation.

● There may be reduced employment opportunities for people who have a visual impairment.

● There is a reduced awareness of risk to own safety caused by visual impairment.

● Acquired visual impairment can limit rehabilitation opportunities

and return to activities of daily living, including driving.
- Visual impairment can lead to increased anxiety about situations.
- There is a risk that visual impairment can mask other difficulties, such as language difficulties, cognitive function and perceptual awareness.

Speech and language therapy value
- Assisting in the assessment of visual impairment of individuals with speech and/or language difficulties.
- Profiling the communication strengths and difficulties of an individual with visual impairment.
- Supporting carers and other professionals in promoting the acquisition of early interaction and communication skills in young children and those who have visual impairment with additional disabilities.
- Supporting carers and other professionals in promoting the acquisition of language skills and social skills.
- Supporting carers, friends and other professionals in promoting the rehabilitation of interaction, communication and social skills in those with an acquired visual impairment.
- Advising carers and other professionals with regard to AAC and supporting and promoting its use.

8.24 Voice

This information is designed to support speech and language therapy services undertaking reviews of service organisation and provision. Therapists seeking detailed clinical guidance are referred to the *RCSLT Clinical Guidelines* (2005), position papers and *Reference Framework: Underpinning Competence to Practise* (2003), available on the RCSLT website: www.rcslt.org

Definition
Voice disorders classification (Mathieson, 2001):
1) Organic
a) Structural abnormalities: congenital, eg laryngeal web; acquired, eg trauma.
b) Neurogenic, eg RLN paralysis.

c) Endocrinological, eg myxoedema
d) Laryngeal disease, eg neoplasms
2) Behavioural
Hyperfunctional
a) Muscle tension Dysphonia (MTD) without observable changes in the vocal fold mucosa (vocal strain/vocal misuse).
b) MTD leading to changes in the vocal fold mucosa (vocal abuse), eg vocal fold nodules.
Psychogenic
eg conversion symptom/dysphonia.
Voice disorders range from complete absence of the voice (aphonia) to varying degrees of vocal impairment (dysphonia). Abnormalities can involve one or more of the vocal parameters: habitual pitch, pitch range, loudness, vocal note quality, resonance, flexibility and stamina.
Cross-referencing with the chapter sections listed below is recommended:
8.1.Acquired Motor Speech Disorders
8.7. Cerebral Palsy
8.12. Dysfluency
8.14. Dysphagia
8.16. Mental Health
8.17. Palliative Care
8.19. Progressive Neurological disorders
7.2.1 AAC

National guidance and sources of further information and support
● The Centre for Change and Innovation (CCI) at the Scottish Executive individual pathways for ENT, including a pathway for hoarseness www.cci.scot.nhs.uk
● *RCSLT Clinical Guidelines* (2005), section on *Voice* www.rsclt.org
● *RCSLT Clinical Guidelines* (2005), section on *Use of Nasendoscopy* www.rcslt.org
● British Voice Association www.british-voice-association.com
● The General Teaching Council for Scotland (2002) Voice and the Teaching Profession www.data.teachers.org.uk/resources
● Voice Care Network www.voicecare.org.uk

Aetiology

Whatever the underlying aetiology, vocal changes are the manifestation of disordered laryngeal, respiratory and vocal tract function, that might reflect structural, neurological, psychological and behavioural problems as well as systemic conditions (Mathieson, 2001).

The aetiology of many voice disorders is multifactorial with behavioural, emotional and lifestyle factors either influencing the individual's management of the problem or being the primary cause of the problem. The outcome of intervention can only be successful if the aetiological features are accurately identified and acted upon by the clinician and individual (Stemple, Glaze and Gerdman, 1995).

Prevalence and incidence

One study in England revealed a prevalence of 121 cases of voice disorder per 100,000 population (Mathieson, 2001).

It has been suggested that up to 40,000 new individuals with dysphonia are referred to and treated by SLTs annually in Britain (Carding, 2000).

There is much more awareness of voice problems as an occupational health risk, so more people are coming forward for help with their vocal problems.

'Professional voice user' is often applied to those individuals whose professional role and employment are dependent on effective and efficient voice use, eg actors, politicians, radio announcers, barristers, the clergy, singers, teachers and lecturers (Martin & Darnley, 2004). People who use their voice professionally are at risk of occupational voice disorders.

A large-scale survey found that 20% of teachers reported voice problems during the teaching year (Russell et al, 1998). Approximately 15% of individuals attending voice clinics are teachers (Morton & Watson, 1998; Bufton, 2000).

Vulnerability: risk issues

Health

● Dysphonia may be the first symptom of laryngeal pathology, which if left untreated, can progress into a more serious medical condition and require surgery.

● Untreated voice disorders can develop into more complex disorders, which may have serious economic, psychosocial and personal consequences.

● The treatment of a voice problem is likely to reduce its severity and the time needed for recovery (Russell et al, 1998; Lehto et al, 2003).

Economic/employment consequences

● Dysphonia is an occupational health illness affecting workers in a wide range of jobs, such as teaching, call centre workers and aerobics instructors (Heidel & Torgerson, 1993; Pearson, 2001).

● Professional voice users may have careers disrupted by voice rest, surgery or diminished vocal power associated with a disordered or diseased larynx (Rulnick et al, 1998).

● Studies have demonstrated the effects of teaching on voice problems and the adverse impact on professional careers is well documented. In the 1990s, the courts found in favour of two teachers whose voice loss, which effectively forced them into early retirement, was agreed to be the result of their teaching roles (Martin & Darnley, 2004).

● In a study of 100 teachers with dysphonia, 96% complained of vocal fatigue (Calas et al, 1998).

● 20% of teachers may miss work because of voice problems (Smith et al, 1998).

Psychosocial effects/family and social relationships

All voice disorders reduce the speaker's communication effectiveness in various ways, such as impaired intelligibility, self image difficulties, family and social relationship problems and emotional issues. Psychosocial effects such as anxiety and depression may also occur (Mathieson, 2001; Scott et al, 1997).

Speech and language therapy value

To provide a combination of clinical expertise, multidisciplinary working, research and technology so that this client group can have the highest standard of voice care from referral to discharge.

As a result of the service, a large percentage of individuals will be enabled to achieve a voice which falls within an accepted range whereas for others, the goal may be optimum voice. In addition to this service being individual orientated, it must also inform commissioners about the needs of the client group and the impact of vocal problems.

Key aims (Mathieson, 2001).
● To assess individuals referred to the service with voice disorders and provide appropriate intervention and management after diagnosis, formulating an hypothesis and setting goals to improve vocal functioning.
● To reduce or eliminate vocal tract discomfort.
● To improve laryngeal function.
● To eliminate/reduce potentially damaging vocal tract manoeuvres.
● To reduce distress related to the voice disorder.
● To restore the vocal skills necessary for the individual's occupational and social needs.

References

Acquire after Brain Injury www.acquire.org.uk
Albarran, JW. A review of communication with intubated patients and those with tracheostomies within an intensive care environment in *Intensive Care Nursing*, 1991:7; pp179-186.
Allied Health Professional Services. The Allied Health Professions Palliative Care Team – an assessment of need, 2004. www.palliativecareglasgow.info
Alzheimer's Society UK. *Policy Position Paper on Demography*, 2004.
Andrews, G, Craig, A, Feyer, A-M, Hoddinott, S, Howie, P, Neilson, M. Stuttering. A Review of Research findings and theories circa 1982 in (Review) *Journal Speech and Hearing Disorders,* 1983:48: pp226-46.
American Psychiatric Association. *DSM-IV Diagnostic and Statistical Manual iv – 4th edition*, 2000.
American Speech-Language-Hearing Association (ASHA). *Communication Bill of Rights: The National Joint Committee for the Communication Needs of Persons with Severe Disabilities*, 1992.
ASHA. *Guidance on selective mutism*. www.asha.org
ASHA. Instrumental diagnostic procedures for swallowing in *Desk top reference*, 2002:3; pp17-27.
Arbour, R. Sedation and pain management in critically ill adults in *Critical Care Nurse*, 2000:20(5); pp 39-56.

Archbold, S. Cochlear implantation: challenges for the education of the deaf: paper presented at the 7th European Symposium on Paediatric Cochlear Implantation, Geneva, Switzerland, 2004.

Arvedson, JC & Brodsky L (Eds). *Paediatric Swallowing & Feeding: Assessment and Management*. Whurr Publishers, 1993.

Arvedson, JC. Management of Swallowing Problems in Arvedson, JC & Brosky, L (ed) *Paediatric Swallowing and Feeding Assessment and Management*. Singular, pp 327-387.

Ataxia UK, 2006. www.ataxia.org.uk

Attwood, T. *Help for the Child with Asperger's Syndrome: A Parent's Guide to Negotiating the Social Service Maze*. Jessica Kingsley Publishers, 2004.

Aviv, JE, Kaplan, ST, Thomson, JE, Spitzer, J, Diamond, B, Close, LG. *The safety of flexible endoscopic evaluation of swallowing with sensory testing (FEESST): An analysis of 500 consecutive evaluations*, 2000.

Aziz, SL & Cambell-Taylor, I. Neglect and abuse associated with under nutrition in long-term care in North America: causes and solutions in *Journal of Elder Abuse and neglect,* 1999:10, pp91-117.

Bannister, P. Early feeding management in Watson ACH, Sell, DA, Grunwell, P (Eds). *Management of Cleft Lip and Palate*. Whurr, 2001.

Baker, E, Croot, K, McLeod, S, Paul, R. Tutorial paper: Psycholinguistic models of speech development and their application to clinical practice in *Journal of Speech, Language, and Hearing Research,* 2001:44; pp685-702.

Baker, E. & McLeod, S. *Evidence-based management of phonological impairment in children in Child Language Teaching and Therapy*, 2004:20(3); pp261-285(25).

Barnes, CJ. *Chatter Matters. A presentation for Carers of People with Communication and Memory Difficulties*. Alzheimer's Society UK, 2003.

Battle, D. *Communication Disorders in Multicultural Populations.* Butterworth-Heinemann,1998.

Beange, H, McElduff, A, & Baker, W. Medical Disorders of Adults with Mental Retardation: A Population Study in *American Journal on Mental Retardation,* 1995:99; pp 595-604.

Beitchman, JH, Brownlie, EB, Inglis, A, Wild, J et al. Seven year follow up of speech/language impaired and control children:

Speech/language stability and outcome in *Journal of the American Academy of Child and Adolescent Psychiatry,* 1994:33; pp1322-1330.

Bergbom-Engberg, I & Haljamae, H. Assessment of patients' experience of discomforts during respiratory therapy in *Critical Care Medicine*, 1989:17(10); pp1068-1072.

Bethseda, MD. *Disorders of vocal abuse and misuse*. National Institute on Deafness and Other Communication Disorders, 1999.

Beukelman, DR & Yorkston, KM (Eds). *Communication disorders following traumatic brain injury*. Pro-Ed, 1991.

Bishop, DVM in Fletcher, P. and Hall, D (Eds). *Specific Speech and Language Disorders in Children.* Whurr Publishers, 1992.

Bloodstein, O. *A Handbook on Stuttering*, 1987.

Bogdashina, O. *Sensory Perceptual Issues in Autism and Asperger Syndrome.* Jessica Kingsley Publishers, 2004.

Bott et al. Behaviour problems associated with lack of speech in people with learning disabilities in *Journal of Intellectual Disability Research*, 1997:41; pp3-7.

Bowman, R, Bowman, R & Dutton, G. *Disorders of Vision in Children*. RNIB, 2001.

Bradley, H. Assessing and Developing Successful Communication in Lacey, P & Ouvry, C (Eds). *People with Profound and Multiple Learning Disabilities.* David Fulton, 1998.

British Society of Medicine and Royal College of Physicians. *Rehabilitation following an acquired brain injury: National Clinical Guidelines*, 2003.

British Society of Rehabilitation Medicine (BRSM). *Rehabilitation after traumatic brain injury,* 1998.

Brooks, D, Augton, M, Bond, M, Jones, P & Rizui, S. Cognitive sequelae in relationship to early indices of severity of brain damage after severe blunt head injury in *Journal of Neurology and Psychiatry,* 1980:43; pp529-534.

Broomfield, J, Dodd, B. Children with speech and language disability: caseload characteristics in *International Journal of Language & Communication Disorders*, 2004:39(3); pp303-324(22).

Broomfield, J & Dodd, B. Clinical Effectiveness in Dodd, B (Ed), *Differential Diagnosis and Treatment of Children with Speech Disorder*. Whurr, 2005; pp211-229.

Broomfield, J, & Dodd, B. The nature of referred subtypes of primary speech disability in *Child Language Teaching and Therapy,* 2004:20(3); pp135-151.

Brumfitt, S. Losing your sense of self: What aphasia can do in *Aphasiology,* 1993:7; pp569-575.

Bryan, K. Preliminary Study of the prevalence of speech and language difficulties in young offenders in *International Journal of language and Communication Disorders,* 2004:39(3); pp391-400.

Bryan, K & Maxim, J. Managing language and communication difficulties in Alzheimer's dementia: the link to behaviour in Adams & Manthorpe (Eds), *Dementia Care.* Arnold. 2003.

Bucks et al. Linguistic analysis of spontaneous, conversational speech in probable Alzheimer's disease in *Aphasiology,* 2000:14; pp17-91.

Calas, M et al. *Vocal Pathology of Teachers, Revue de Laryngologie, Otologie et Rhinologie,* 1989:110; pp397-406.

Carding, P. *Evaluating Voice Therapy.* Whurr Publishers, 2000.

CARF. *Standards Manual and Interpretive Guidelines for Medical Rehabilitation,*1996.

Carson, DK, et al. Comparisons of children with delayed and normal language at 24 months of age on measures of behavioural difficulties, social and cognitive development in *Infant Mental Health Journal,* 1998:19; pp59-75.

Carter Young, E, Durrant Jones, L. *Developing a Dysphagia Programme in an Acute Care hospital: A Needs Assessment,* 1990.

Ceci, J. *Handbook of cognitive, social-Neuropsychological Aspects of Learning Disabilities.* Erlbaum,1986.

Chadwick, DD, Jolliffe, J & Goldbart, J. Adherence to Eating and Drinking Guidelines for Adults with Intellectual Disabilities and Dysphagia in *American Journal on Mental Retardation,* 2003:108(3); pp202-211.

Chamberlain et al. Preliminary findings on communication and challenging behaviour in *Learning difficulty,*1993:39(2); pp118-125.

Cherney, LR & Halper, AS. Swallowing problems in adults with traumatic brain injury in *Seminars in Neurology,* 1996:16(4); pp 42-50.

Children's Acquired Brain Injury Interest Group. *Must Try Harder? Meeting the educational needs of children after acquired brain injury,* 2003. (The 'Must Try Harder; Project Team, c/o Dr R Forsyth, Children's Out-patients, Newcastle General Hospital, Newcastle upon Tyne).

Child Brain Injury Trust (CBIT) www.cbituk.org

Children's Heart Federation www.childrens-heartfed.org.uk 2005.

Choi-Kwon, S, Kim, HS, Kwon, SU, Kim, JS. Factors affecting the burden on caregivers of stroke survivors in South Korea in *Archives Physical Medical Rehabilitation*, 2005:86(5); pp1043-1048.

Clegg, J, Hollis, C, Mawhood, L,& Rutter, M. Developmental Language Disorders – a follow-up in later adult life. Cognitive, language and psychosocial outcomes in *Journal of Child Psychology and Psychiatry,* 2005:46; pp128-149.

Clinical Standards Advisory Group (CSAG). *Cleft Lip and/or Palate Report of a CSAG Committee,* 1998.

Cohen, MM, MacLean RE. *Craniosynostosis diagnosis,evaluation, and management – 2nd edition*. Oxford University Press, 2000.

Cohen, SR, Cho, DC, Nichols, SL, Simms, C, Cross, KP. American society of maxillofacial surgeons' outcome study: preoperative and postoperative neurodevelopmental findings in single-suture craniosynostosis in *Plastic & Reconstructive Surgery*, 2004:15/114(4); pp841-847; discussion pp848-849.

Conlan, AA, Kopec, SE. Tracheostomy in the ICU: a review in *Intensive Care Med,* 2000:15(1) pp1-13.

Connolly, D. & O'Dowd, T. Impact of different disabilities arising from head injury on the primary care giver in *British Journal of Occupational Therapist,* 2001:64(1); pp41-6.

Conti-Ramsden, G, and Botting, N. Social Difficulties and Victimisation in Children with SLI at 11 years of age in *Journal of Speech, Language and Hearing Research,* 2004:47(1); pp145-172.

Cook, IJ & Kahrilas, PJ. AGA technical review on management of oropharyngeal dysphagia in *Gastroenterology,*1999:116; pp455-478.

Coster, FW et al. Specific Language Impairments and Behavioural Problems in *Folia Phoniatrica et Logopaedica,* 1999:51; pp99-107.

Crawford, H. ALD and dysphagia: the need for evidence based care in *RCSLT Bulletin*, January 2005.

Crutchley, A. Bilingual children with SLI attending language units: getting the bigger picture in *Child Language Teaching and Therapy*, 1999; pp 201-217.

Crutchley, A, Conti-Ramsden, G, and Botting, N. Bilingualism and specific language impairment in children attending language units in *European Journal of Disorders of Communication,* 1997a:32(2); pp 267-276.

Crutchley, A, Conti-Ramsden, G, and Botting, N, Bilingual children with specific language impairment and standardized assessments: preliminary findings from a study of children in language units in *International Journal of Bilingualism,* 1997b:1.

Davis, A, Yoshinaga-Itano, C, & Hind, S. *Commentary: Universal newborn hearing screening: implications for co-ordinating and developing services for deaf and hearing impaired children*, 2001.

Dawodu, ST. Traumatic Brain Injury Definition, Epidemiology, Pathophysiology, 2004. www.emedicine.com

Department of Education & Skills. *Sure Start planning pack for all: Guidance on involving minority ethnic children and families*, 1999. www.dfes.gov.uk

Department of Health. *Better Health in Old Age,* 2004. www.dh.gov.uk

Department of Health. *Bournewood Consultation*, 2005. www.dh.gov.uk

Department of Health. *Comprehensive Critical care: A review of adult critical care services,* 2000. www.dh.gov.uk

Department of Health. *Improvement, expansion and reform ensuring that 'all' means 'all'*, 2004. www.dh.gov.uk

Department of Health. *The NHS Plan: A plan for investment, a plan for reform*, 2000. www.dh.gov.uk

Department of Health. *NSF for long-term conditions*, 2005. www.dh.gov.uk

Department of Health. NSF for mental health, 1999. www.dh.gov.uk

Department of Health. *NSF for older people*, 2001. www.dh.gov.uk

Department of Health. *Quality protects: Black and ethnic minority children and their families*, 1998. www.dh.gov.uk

Department of Health. *Supporting People with Longer-Term Conditions. An NHS and Social Care Model to support local innovation and integration,* 2005. www.dh.gov.uk

Department of Health. *Valuing People: A New Strategy for Learning Disability for the 21st Century,* 2001. www.dh.gov.uk

DePompei, R & Blosser, J. *Communication: How communication changes over time.* Lash & Associates Publishing, 1998.

De Vita, MA & Spierer-Rundback, L. Swallowing disorders in patients with prolonged orotracheal intubation or tracheostomy tubes in *Critical Care Medicine*, 1990:18(2); pp 1328-1330.

Dikeman, KJ & Kazandjian, MS. *Communication and swallowing management of tracheostomised and ventilatordependent adults.* Singular publishing Group, 2003.

Ding, R, Logemann, JA. *Head and neck,* 2005:27/9; pp809-813.

Dodd, B. *A problem solving approach to clinical management differential diagnosis and treatment of children with phonological disorders.* Whurr, 1995; p149.

Doggett, DL, Tappe, KA, Mitchell, MD, Chapell, R, Coates, V, Turkelson, CM. Prevention of pneumonia in elderly stroke patients by systematic diagnosis and treatment of dysphagia: An evidence-based comprehensive analysis of the literature in *Dysphagia,* 2001:*16;* pp279-295.

Donlan, C (Ed). *The Development of Mathematical Skills.* Psychology Press, 1998.

Douglas, J & Harris, B. Description and Evaluation of a Day-Centre-Based Behavioural Feeding Programme for Young Children and their Parents in *Clinical Child Psychology and Psychiatry,* 2001:6(2); pp241-256(16).

Duffy, R. *Motor speech disorders: Substrates, differential diagnosis and management* -2nd edition. Mosby Books, 2005.

Duncan, DM, and Gibbs, DA. Mainstream bilingual school children: A model for remediation in Duncan, D (Ed), *Working with bilingual language disability.* Chapman and Hall, 1989; pp176-197.

Eames, S, McKenna, K, Worrall, L & Read, S. The suitability of written education materials for stroke survivors and their carers in *Topics in Stroke Rehabilitation,* 2003:10(3); pp70-83.

Eckman, S, & Roe, J. Speech and language therapists in palliative care – what do we have to offer? in *International Journal of Palliative Nursing,* 2005:11(4); pp179-181.

Ekberg, O, Hamdy, S, Woisard, V, Wuttge-Hannig, A & Ortega, P. Social and Psychological Burden of Dysphagia: Its Impact on Diagnosis and Treatment in *Dysphagia,* 2002:7(2); pp139-46.

Elpern, EH, Jacobs, ER & Bone, RC. Incidence of aspiration in tracheally intubated adults in *Heart & Lung,* 1987:16(5); pp527-531.

Elpern, EH, Scott, MG, Petro, MA & Ries, MH. Pulmonary Aspiration in Mechanically ventilated patients with tracheostomies in *Chest,* 1994:105(2); pp563-566.

Eyman, R, Grossman, H, Chaney, R & Call, T. The Life Expectancy of Profoundly Handicapped People with Mental Retardation in *The New England Journal of Medicine,* 1990:323; pp 584-589.

Fortnum, HM, et al. *Prevalence of Permanent Childhood Hearing Impairment in the UK* BMJ, 2001 (September).

The Foundation for People with Learning Disabilities. *Learning Disabilities: The Fundamental Facts,* 2000.

Fox, A, Howard, D & Dodd, B. Risk factors in speech disorder in *IJLCD,* 2002:37; pp117-132.

Garrard, P & Hodges, JR. *Semantic dementia: Implications for the neural basis of language and meaning* in Aphasiology 1999:13(8); pp609-623.

Gibbon, FE, Wood, SE. Articulatory drift in the speech of children with articulation and phonological disorders in *Percept Mot Skills,* 2002:(1); pp295-307.

Gillberg, G. *The epidemiology of autism: NAS International Conference Procedings*, 2002.

Gisel, EG & Patrick, J. Identification of children with cerebral palsy unable to maintain a normal nutritional state in *Lancet,* 1988:1; pp283-286.

Goodyer, IM. Language Difficulties and Psychopathology in Bishop, DVM, et al, *Speech and Language impairments in Children. Psychological Press,* 2000.

Gorlin, RJ, Cohen, M, Hennekam, RCM. *Syndromes of the Head and Neck (Oxford Monographs on Medical Genetics) – 4th Edition.* Oxford University Press, 2001.

Gorlin, RJ, Cohen, M & Levin, LS. *Syndromes of the Head and Neck – 3rd edition.* Oxford University Press, 1990.

Gregg et al. The incidence of cleft lip and palate in Northern Ireland in *British Journal of Orthodontics*, 1994:21; pp387-392.

Griffiths M, Clegg, M. (Eds). *Cerebral Palsy: Problems and Practice.* Human Horizons Series, 1988.

Gross, RD, Mahlmann, J & Grayhack JP. Physiologic effects of open and closed tracheostomy tubes on the pharyngeal swallow in *Annals of Otology, Rhinology and Laryngology*, 2003:112(2); pp143-152.

Grundy, K, & Harding, A. Developmental speech disorders in Grundy K, *Linguistics in clinical practice.* Whurr, 1995.

Grunwell. Assessment of phonology in Grundy, K, *Linguistics in clinical practice.* Whurr, 1995.

Guitar, B. *Stuttering: An Integrated Approach to its Nature and Treatment: 2nd edition*, 1998.

Guttierrez-Clellen, VF. Language choice in intervention with bilingual children in *American Journal of Speech-Language Pathology,* 1998; pp 291-302.

Haley, WE, Wadley, VG, West, CAC, & Vetzel, LL. How care-giving stressors change with severity of dementia in *Seminars in speech and language,* 1994:15(3); pp195-205.

Hall, DMB & Elliman, D. Health for All Children. OUP, 2002.

Halper, AS, Cherney, LR, Cichowski, K & Zhang, M. Dysphagia after head trauma: The effect of cognitive-communicative impairments on functional outcomes in *Journal of Head Trauma Rehabilitation,* 1999:14(5).

Hagan, C. Language disorders in head trauma in Holland, A. (Ed.), *Language disorders in adults.* College Hill Press, 1984.

Hagberg, B. The dementias in a psychodynamic perspective in Miesen and Jones (Eds), *Care giving in dementia: Research and Applications.* Routledge, 1997.

Harding, A, Grunwell, P. Cleft palate speech characteristics: A literature review in *European Journal for Disorders of Communication,* 1996 (December).

Harding, A, Sell, D. Cleft Lip and Palate and associated disorders in Wright, J & Kersner, M (Eds), *Speech and Language Therapy: the decision making process,* 2001.

Hardwick, KD. Clinical manifestations of dysphagia in individuals with mental retardation: an exploratory study. Unpublished doctoral dissertation, University of Texas at Austin, 1993.

Harrington, KT et al. Report of Mild Traumatic Brain Injury Committee of the Head Injury Interdisciplinary Special Interest Group of the American Congress of Rehabilitation Medicine of mild traumatic brain injury in *Journal of Head Trauma Rehabilitation,* 1993; p8.

Hartelius and Svensson. Speech and swallowing symptoms associated with Parkinson's Disease and Multiple Sclerosis: a survey in *Folia Phonatrica Logopaedica,* 1994:46(1); pp 9-17.

Headway – the brain injury association www.headway.org.uk

Hearst, D. The Child with Craniosynostosis: Psychological Issues in Hayward R, Jones B, Dunaway D, Evans R (Eds), *The Clinical Management of Craniosynostosis,* 2004.

Heidel, SE, Torgerson, JK. Vocal problems among aerobic instructors and aerobic participants in *Journal of Communication Disorders* 1993:26; pp179-91.

Heilman, KM, Saffran, A & Gerwind, N. Closed Head Trauma and Aphasias in *Journal of Neurology, Neurosurgery and Psychiatry,* 1971:34; pp265-269.

Helfrich-Miller, KR, Rector, KL & Straka, JA. Dysphagia: its treatment in the profoundly retarded patient with cerebral palsy in *Archives of Physical and Medical Rehabilitation*, 1986:67; pp520-525.

Hemsley, B. et al. Nursing the patient with severe communication impairment in *Journal of Advanced Nursing*, 2001(35); pp827-835.

Henneman, E et al. Effect of a collaborative weaning plan on patient outcome in the critical care setting in *Crit Care Med*, 2001:29(2); pp297-303.

Heritage, M, & Farrow, V. Research shows the profession has a valuable role with elderly mentally ill people in *Human Communication*, 1994 (February); pp15-16.

Hickman, J & Jenner, L. ALD and Dysphagia: issues and practice in *Speech and Language Therapy in Practice*, 1997: (Autumn); pp8-11.

Hilari, K et al. Predictors of health-related quality of life in people with chronic aphasia in *Aphasiology*, 2000:17(4); pp365-381.

Hind, S & Davis, A. Social-emotional ramifications for families with deaf infants in *American Annals of the Deaf*, 2000:128; pp407-417.

Hindley, P, Hill, P, McGuigan, S, Kitson, N. *Psychiatric Disorder in Deaf and Hearing Impaired Children and Young People: a prevalence study.* National Deaf Children's Society, 1994.

Hinojosa, J, Esparza, J, Munoz, MJ, Salvan, R, Romance, A, Alen, J, Munoz, A. Surgical Treatment of Trigonocephalies and Associated Hypotelorbitism in *Neurociurgia,* 2002:13(6); pp437-445.

Hollins. S, Attard, T, Von Frounhofer, McGuigan, S, & Sedgewick, P. Mortality in people with learning disability: risks, causes, and death certification findings in London in *Developmental Medicine and Child Neurology,* 1998:40; pp50-56.

Holm, A, and Dodd, B. Comparison of cross-language generalisation following speech therapy in *Folia Phoniatrica et Logopaedica,* 2001:53(3); pp166-172.

Holm, A, Dodd, B, Stow, C, and Pert, S. Identification and differential diagnosis of phonological disorder in bilingual children in *Language Testing,* 1999:16(3); pp271-292.

Hooper, SJ et al. Core language predictors of behavioural functioning in early elementary school children: Concurrent and longitudinal findings in *Behavioural Disorders,* 2003:29(1); pp10-21.

Horner, J, Alberts, MJ, Davison, D, Cook, GM. Swallowing in Alzheimer's disease in *Alzheimer's Disease and Associated Disorders*, 1994:8(3); pp177-189.

Howard, S. Connected speech processes in developmental speech impairment: observations from an electropalatographic perspective in *Clinical Linguistics & Phonetics*, 2004:18(6-8); pp405-417.

Hudson, H, Daubert, C, Mills, R. The interdependency of protein-energy malnutrition, aging and dysphagia in *Dysphagia,* 2000:15; pp31-38.

Humphreys, RP. *Encephalocele and dermal sinuses* in Cheek WR, Marlin AE, McLone DG, Reigel DH & Walker ML (Eds), *Paediatric Neurosurgery: Surgery of the Developing Nervous System – 3rd Edition*. Saunders,1994; p96.

Huntington's Disease Association, 2006. www.hda.org.uk

Isaki, E. & Turkstra, L. Communication abilities and work re-entry following traumatic brain injury in *Brain Injury*, 2000:14; pp441-453.

Isaki, E & Hoit, JD. Ventilator Supported communication: a survey of Speech-Language Pathologists in *Journal of Medical Speech-Language Pathology,* 1997:5(4); pp263- 273.

Jackson, IT, Tanner, NSB, Hide, TAH. Frontonasal encephalocele: 'Long nose hypertelorism' in *Annals of Plastic Surgery,* 1983:11; p490.

Jerome, AC et al. Self-esteem in children with specific language impairment in *Journal of Speech, Language and Hearing Research,* 2002:45(4); pp700-714.

Jung, JH with Gagne, JP, Godden, AL, Leeper, HA, Moon, JB, Seewald, RC, (Eds) *Genetic Syndromes in Communication Disorders.* College Hill Publication, Little Brown and Company, 1989.

Kagan, A. Revealing competence of aphasic adults through conversation: A challenge to health professionals in *Topics in Stroke Rehabilitation,* 1995:2(1); pp15-28.

Kapp, SKA. *Mental Development and Learning Disorders in Children with Single Suture* Craniosynostosis in *Cleft Palate-Craniofacial J,* 1998:35(3); pp197-203.

Keil, S. Survey of educational provision for blind and partially sighted children in England, Scotland and Wales in 2002 in *The British Journal* 2003 *of Visual Impairment*, 2003:21(3); pp93-97.

Kerr, A, et al. Medical needs of people with intellectual disability require regular reassessment and the provision of client-carer held reports in *Journal of Intellectual Disability Research*, 2003:47; pp134-145.

King, NF, et al. Early predictions of assessing post injury symptoms following mild and moderate head injuries in *British Journal of Clinical Psychology,* 1999:38(1); pp15-25.

Kohl, LM,et al. *The incidence of swallowing dysfunction in paediatric patients following open heart surgery.* Circulation, 2000:102,pp469-470

Koufman, JA. Laryngopharyngeal reflux is different from classic gastroesphageal reflux disease in *ENT Journal, 2002:*81 (Supp 2); pp7-13.

Krick, J & van Duyn, MAS. The relationship between oral-motor involvement and growth: a pilot study in a paediatric population with cerebral palsy in *Journal of the American Dietetic Association*, 1984:84; pp555-559.

Lash and Associates Publishing. *Myths & Facts: When your child has a brain-injury*, 1998. www.lapublishing.com

Lajeunie, E, et al. Craniosynostosis and Foetal Exposure to Sodium Valproate in Institute National de la Sante et de la Recherche Medical U 393, Paris in *Journal Neurosurgery,* 2001:95(5); pp778-82.

Lees, J. *Children with Acquired Aphasia.* Whurr Publishers,1993.

Lees, J, and Urwin, S. *Children with Language Disorders*, Whurr Publishers, 1991.

Lefton-Grief, MA. Diagnosis and management of paediatric feeding and swallowing disorders: role of the speech language pathologist in Tuchman, DN, Walter, RS (Eds). *Disorders of Feeding and Swallowing in Infants and Children: Pathophysiology, Diagnosis and Treatment*. Singular Publishing, 1994; pp97-114.

Langmore, SE. *Endoscopic evaluation and treatment of swallowing disorders.* Thieme, 2001.

Law, J (Ed).*The Early Identification of Language Impairment in Children*. Chapman & Hall, 1992.

Law, J, Boyle, J, Harris, F, Harkness, A, & Nye, C. Prevalence and Natural History of speech and language delay: findings from a systematic review of the literature in *International Journal of Language and Communication Disorders*, 2000:35(2); pp165-188.

Law, J, Boyle, J, Harris, F, Harkness, A & Nye, C. Prevalence and Natural History of speech and language delay: findings from a systematic review of the literature in *International Journal of*

Language and Communication Disorders, 2000:35(2); pp165-188.

Leder, S. Incidence and type of aspiration in acute care patients requiring mechanical ventilation via a new tracheostomy in *Chest*, 2002:122(5); pp1721-1725.

Lishman, WA. *Organic Psychiatry: The Psychological Consequences of Cerebral Disorder – 3rd Edition*. Blackwell Science, 1998.

Literacy Trust. *Languages spoken by pupils in London*, 2000. www.literacytrust.org.uk/research/lostop3.html

Locke, A, Ginsborg, J & Peers, I. Development and disadvantage: implications for the early years and beyond in *International Journal of Language and Communication Disorders*, 2002:37; pp3-15.

Logemann, JA. *Evaluation and Treatment of Swallowing Disorders*. College Hill Press, 1983.

Logemann, J. *Evaluation and Treatment of Swallowing Disorders – 2nd Edition*. College Hill Press, 1998.

Low, J, Wyles, C, Wilkinson, T, Sainsbury, R. The effect of compliance on clinical outcomes for patients with dysphagia on videofluoroscopy in *Dysphagia,* 2001:16; pp123-127.

Malia, K & Duckett, S. *Establishing minimum recommended standards for post-acute brain injury* in *Brain Injury*, 2001:15(4); pp357-362.

Manzano, JL, Lubillo, S, Henriquez, D, Martin, JC, Perez, MD, & Wilson, DJ. Verbal Communication with ventilator dependent patients in *Critical Care Medicine*, 1993:21(4); pp512-517.

Marik, PE & Kaplan, D. Aspiration pneumonia in dysphagia in the elderly in *Chest,* 2003:124; pp328-336.

Marsh, NV & Knight, RG. Relationship between cognitive deficits and social skill after head injury in *Neuropsychology*, 1991:5(2); pp107-117.

Martin, S & Darnley, L. *The Teaching Voice – Second Edition*. Whurr Publishers, 2004.

Martin-Harris-B, Optimal patterns of care in patients with COPD in *Semin- Speech-Lang*, 2000: 21(4), pp311-22.

Mathieson, L. *The Voice and Its Disorders – 6th edition*. Whurr Publishers, 2001.

Mathisen, B, Worrall, L, Masel, J, Wall, C, Shepherd, RW. Feeding problems in infants with gastro-oesophageal reflux disease: a controlled study in *Journal of Paediatric Child Health,* 1999:35(2); pp163-169.

McCurtin, A. *The Manual of Feeding Practice*. Winslow Press Ltd, 1998.

McKay, LE, Morgan, AS & Bernstein, BA Swallowing disorders in severe brain injury: Risk factors affecting return to oral intake in *Archives of Physical Medicine and Rehabilitation,* 1999:80; p365.

McLaren, J, Bryson, S. Review of recent epidemiological studies of mental retardation: prevalence, associated disorders and aetiology in *American Journal of Mental Retardation*, 1997:92(3); pp243-54.

McGuire, L, Burright, R, Williams, R & Donovick, P. Prevalence of traumatic brain injury in psychiatric and non psychiatric subjects in *Brain Injury,* 1998:12(3); pp207-214.

Meltzer, H, Gatward, R, Goodman, R, Ford, T. *Mental health of children and adolescents in Great Britain*. Office of National Statistics, 2000.

Menzel, L. Need for communication related research in mechanically ventilated patients in *American Journal of Critical Care*, 1994:3(3); pp165-167.

Menzel, K. A comparison of patients' communication related responses during intubation and after extubation in *Heart and Lung,* 1997.

Menzel, L. Factors related to the emotional responses of intubated patients to being unable to speak in *Heart and Lung*, 1998:27(4); pp245-252.

Mooney, MP, & Siegel, ML. *Understanding Craniofacial Anomalies*. Wiley-Liss, 2002.

Morton,V and Watson,DR. in Martin, S & Darnley, L. *The Teaching Voice – Second Edition*. Whurr Publishers, 2004.

Morton, V & Watson, DR. The Teaching Voice: problems and perceptions in *Logopedics Phoniatrics Vocology,* 1998:23; pp133-9.

Moss, NE & Wade, DT. Admission after head injury: How many occur and how many are recorded? In *Brain Injury,* 1996:27(3); pp159-161.

Munro F.D. *Dysphagia in children: a paediatric surgical perspective* International Congress Series, 2003: 1254; pp135-139

Motor Neurone Disease Association, 2004. www.mndassociation.org

Murray, T & Carrau, RL. Functional Tests of Swallowing in *Comprehensive management of swallowing disorders,* 1999; pp75-79.

Murdoch, BE & Theodoros, DG. *Traumatic Brain Injury: Associated Speech, Language and Swallowing Disorders.* Singular Thompson Learning, 2001.

Murphy et al. *Epidemiology of self injury, Research to Practice*. BILD publications, 1993.

MS Society and MS Research Trust, 2006. www.mssociety.org.uk

Najenson, T, et al, Recovery of communicative functions after prolonged traumatic coma in *Scandinavian Journal of Rehabilitation Medicine,* 1978:10; pp15-21.

Nash, P, Stengelhofen, Brown, J & Toombs, L. *Improving children's communication: managing persistent difficulties.* Whurr, 2002.

Nash, M. Swallowing problems in the tracheostomised patient in *Otolaryngologic Clinics of North America*, 1988:21(4); pp701-709.

Nash, P, Stengelhofen, J. *Improving Children's Communication: Managing Persistent Difficulties,* 2002.

Nathan, E, Stackhouse, J, Goulandris, N, & Snowling, M. Educational consequences of developmental speech disorder: Key Stage 1 National Curriculum assessment results in English and Mathematics in *British Journal of Educational Psychology,* 2004:74; p173-186.

National Autistic Society (NAS). *Good Practice Guidelines – Adults with Asperger's Syndrome*, 2002.

NAS website information, 2005. www.nas.org.uk

NAS.*National Autism Plan for Children*, 2003.

National Council for Hospice and Specialist Palliative Care Services (NCHSPCS). *Fulfilling Lives – Rehabilitation in Palliative Care*, 2000.

The National Council for Palliative Care. *National Survey of Individual Activity Data for Specialist Palliative Care Services for 2003-2004*, April 2005.

National Council for Hospice and Specialist Palliative Care Services, 1995.

National Head Injury Foundation. *An Educator's manual: What educators need to know about students with traumatic brain injury,* 1985.

National Patient Safety Agency (NPSA). *Understanding the Patient Safety Issues for People with Learning Disabilities,* 2004. www.npsa.nhs.uk

Neurological Alliance. *Neuro Numbers*, April 2003.

NICE. *Guidelines for Improving Supportive and Palliative Care for Adults with Cancer,* 2004.

NICE. *Head injury: Triage, assessment, investigation and early management of head injury in infants, children and adults. Clinical guidance 4*, 2003. www.nice.org.uk

Nguyen, NP, Frank, C, Moltz, CC, Vos, P, Smith, HJ, Karlsson, U, Dutta, S, Midyett, A, Barloon, J, Sallah, S. The impact of dysphagia on quality of life after treatment of head and neck cancer in *Int. Journal Radiat Oncol Bio Phys,* 2005:1:61(3); pp772-778.

NICE. Clinical Guideline on Head and Neck Cancer, 2004.

Nishino, T, Sugimori, K, Kohchi, A & Hiraga, K. Nasal constant positive airway pressure inhibits the swallowing reflex in *American Review of Respiratory Disorders,* 1989:140(5); pp1290-3.

NHS Modernisation Agency. Critical Care Programme: The role of healthcare professionals within critical care services, 2002. www.wise.nhs.uk/sites/clinicalimprovcollab

Northern, JL, & Downs, MP. *Hearing in Children – 5th Edition.* Lipincott Williams & Wilkins, 2002.

Northern Ireland Cancer Registry, 2004.

North West London Critical Care Network. *Critical illness Audit,* 2003.

Oates, J. Evidence base for the prevention and treatment of hyperfunctional voice disorders, paper presented at Pevoc, 2005, (in press).

Odderson, R, Keaton, JC, McKenna, BS. Swallowing management in patients on an acute stroke pathway: quality is cost effective in *Archives of Phys Meds Rehabil,* 1995:76; pp1130-1133.

Office of National Statistics (ONS) London, 2004.

O'Flatter CA & Douglas JM. Living with cognitive communication difficulties following TBI: a model of interpersonal communication to categorise subjective experience in *Aphasiology,* 1997:11(9); pp889-911.

Oka, S. *Epidemiology and genetics of clefting: With implications for etiology.* In H.K. Cooper, R.L.Harding, W.M. Krogman, M.Mazaheri, & R.T.Millard, (Eds). *Cleft palate and cleft lip: A team approach to clinical management and rehabilitation of the patient.* Philadelphia: W.B. Saunders. 1981.

Ozaki, W, and Kawamoto, HK Jr. Craniofacial Clefting in Lin, KY, Ogle, RC, and Jane JA (Eds.), *Craniofacial Surgery: Science and Surgical Technique.* Saunders, 2002; pp309-331.

Paediatric Epidemiology Group. *Traumatic Brain Injury Study,* 2005. (c/o 30 Hyde Terrace, Leeds LS2 9LN).

Paediatric Rehabilitation. Editorial: Paediatric rehabilitation; improving recovery and outcome in childhood disorders, 2001:4(1).

Pannunzio, TG. Aspiration of oral feedings in patients with

tracheostomies in *AACN Clin Issues,* 1996:7(4), pp560-9.

Peterson-Falzone, SJ, Hardin-Jones, MA, Karnell, MP, *Cleft palate speech – 3rd edition.* Mosby Inc, 2001.

Parkes, J, Donnelly, M and Hill, AE. *Focusing on Cerebral Palsy: Reviewing and Communicating Needs for Services.* Scope, 2001.

Parkinson's Disease Association, 2005.

Parkinson's Disease Society, 2006. www.parkinsons.org.uk

Parr, S, Duchan, J & Pound, P. *Aphasia Inside Out: Reflections on Communication and Disability.* Open University Press, 2003.

Parr, S, Byng, S, Gilpin, S & Ireland, C. *Talking About Aphasia: Living with Loss of Language After Stroke.* Open University Press, 1997.

Pascoe, M, Stackhouse, J & Wells, B. Children's Speech and Literacy Difficulties 3 in *Persisting Speech Difficulties.* Wiley, (in press).

Patak-L et al. *Heart and Lung:* Journal of Acute and critical care, 2004:33/35; pp308-320.

Perlman, AL & Schulze-Delrieu, K. *Deglutition and its disorders.* Singular Publishing, 1997.

Pereira, V. Feeding in Craniosynostosis in Hayward R, Jones, B, Dunaway, D, Evans, R (Eds). *The Clinical Management of Craniosynostosis,* 2004.

Powell, T. *Head Injury A Practical Guide.* Headway and Winslow Press, 2004.

Powers, S, Gregory, S, Thoutenhoofd, E. The Educational Achievements of Deaf Children: a literature review in *Deafness and Education International,* 1998:1(1); pp1-99.

Prescott,NJ et al. *Identification of susceptibility loci for nonsyndromic cleft lip with or without cleft palate in a two stage genome scan of affected sib pairs,* Human Genetics, 2000:106(3) pp345-350

PSP Association, 2006. www.pspeur.org/association

Public Health Institute of Scotland. National Needs Assessment for Autism Spectrum Disorder, 2001.

Public Health Institute of Scotland. The SNAP consultation with children, young people and parents, 2003. www.phis.org.uk

Quine, L. Behaviour problems in severely mentally handicapped children, *Psychological Medicine,* 1986:16(4); pp895-907.

Ramig, LO & Verdolini, K. Treatment efficacy: Voice Disorders in *Journal of Speech, Language and Hearing Research,* 1998:41; S101-S116.

Redmond, SM, and Rice, ML. The socio-emotional behaviours of children with Speech and Language Impairment: Social Adaptation or social deviance? in *Journal of Speech, Language and Hearing Research,* 1998:41; pp688-700.

Reilly, S. Feeding Problems in Children with Cerebral Palsy in *Current Paediatrics*, 1993.

Reilly, S. & Skuse, D. Characteristics and management of feeding problems of young children with cerebral palsy, *Dev Med Child Neur*, 1992:34; pp379-388.

Reilly, S, Skuse, DH, Poblete, X. The prevalence of feeding problems and oral motor dysfunction in children with cerebral palsy: a community survey in *Journal of Paediatrics*, 1996:129; pp877-82.

Rimmel, RW, Jane, JA & Bond, MR. Characteristics of the head injured patient in Rosenthal, M, Griffith, ER, Bond, MR & Miller, JD (Eds) *Cognitive rehabilitation for persons with traumatic brain injury: A functional approach*, Paul H Brookes, 1990.

RNID. Brief on Deafness, Employment and Discrimination. www.rnid.org.uk

The Royal Society of Medicine Press. Management of Head & Neck Cancers in *Effective Health Care*, 2004:8(5).

Robinson, RJ. The causes of language disorder: introduction and overview in *Proceedings of the First International Synposium on Specific Speech and Language Disorders in Children.* Aphasic, 1987.

Roe, J. Oropharyngeal dysphagia in non-head and neck malignancies: risk factors and quality of life issues in *European Journal of Palliative Care,* 2005:12(6); pp229-232.

Rogers, B, Stratton, P, Msall, M, Andres, M, Champlain, MK, Koerner, P & Piazza, J. Long-term morbidity and management strategies of tracheal aspiration in adults with severe developmental disabilities in *American Journal on Mental Retardation*, 1994:4; pp490-498.

Rose, FD, Johnson, DA, Attree, EA. Rehabilitation of the head-injured child: basic research and new technology in *Paediatric Rehabilitation,* 1997:1(1).

Rose, TA, Worral, LE, and McKenna, KT. The effectiveness of aphasia-friendly principles for printed health education materials for people with aphasia following stroke in *Aphasiology,* 2003:17(10); pp947-963.

Rokade, A, Rosser, M, Pearman, K, Kuo, M. *Airway management in children with craniofacial anomalies.* IFOS Rome, 2005 (unpublished).

Chapter 8

Rosser, M. *Feeding problems in less severe hemifacial microsomia.* *Craniofacial Society* GB & Ireland, 2004 (unpublished).

Rosser, M, Proops, D. *Management of single sided deafness in children with hemifacial microsomia – an evidence based approach.* Craniofacial Society of GB and Ireland, 2005.

Rosser, M. Feeding problems in *Treacher Collins Syndrome.* Craniofacial Society GB & Ireland, 2004.

Rosser, M, Pearman, K. *The dilemmas of managing persistent otitis media in children with craniofacial syndromes.* Conference Otitis Media, Amsterdam, 2005 (unpublished).

Royal College of Physicians (RCP) *National Clinical Guidelines for Diagnosis and Management of Stroke in Childhood,* 2004.

RCP. *National Clinical Guidelines for Stroke – 2nd Edition,* 2004.

RCP. *Vocational assessment and rehabilitation after acquired brain injury. Inter-agency guidelines, 2004.*

Royal College of Speech and Language Therapists (RCSLT). Adult Learning Disabilities Position Paper, 2003.

RCSLT. *RCSLT Clinical Guidelines,* 2005. www.rcslt.org

RCSLT. *Communicating Quality 2,* 1996.

RCSLT. Invasive Procedures Guideline, 2000.

RCSLT. *Position paper on Dementia,* 2005.

RCSLT. *Reference Framework: Underpinning Competence to Practise,* 2003.

RCSLT. *RCSLT SIG Bilingualism Good Practice Guidelines,* (to be revised, 2005).

RCSLT. *Speech and Language Therapy provision for people with dementia: RCSLT position paper,* 2005.

Royal Hospital of Neuro-disability. Submission to Health Select Committee Inquiry into Head Injury: Rehabilitation. 2001.

Royal National Institute for the Blind (RNIB). *See Change,* booklet. www.rnib.org.uk

Rumsey, N, Bull, R. The effects of facial disfigurement on social interaction in *Human Learning,* 1986:5; pp203-208.

Russell, A. et al. Prevalence of voice problems in teachers in *Journal of Voice,* 1998:12(4); pp467-479.

Russell, JR & Harding, A. Speech development and early intervention in Watson, ACH, Grunwell, P and Sell, D (Eds) *Management of Cleft Lip and Palate,* 2001.

Salt, N. et al. The contribution of speech and language therapy to palliative care in *European Journal of Palliative Care,* 1999:6(4); pp126-129.

Sandy, JR. Journal of the Royal College of Surgeons, 2003:1; pp9-16.

Sapir, S & Aronson, A. Aphonia after closed head injury: aetiologic considerations in *British Journal of Disorders of Communication,* 1985:20; pp289-296.

Sarah Matheson Trust, 2006. www.msaweb.co.uk

Sarimski, K. Children with Apert Syndrome: behavioural problems and family stress in *Developmental Medicine and Child neurology,* 1998:40; pp44-49.

Sarno, MT & Levita, E. Characteristics of verbal impairment in closed head injury in *Archives of Physical Medicine Rehabilitation,* 1986:67; pp400-405.

Sel, ID, Harding, A. and Grunwell, P. An assessment for speech disorders associated with cleft palate and/velopharyngeal dysfunction (revised) in *International Journal of Language and Communication Disorders,* 1998:33.

Schechter, G. Systemic causes of dysphagia in adults in *Otolaryngologic clinics of North America,* 1998:31(3); pp525-535.

Scholefield, JA. Aetiologies of aphonia following closed head injury in *British Journal of Disorders of Communication,* 1987: 22; pp167-172.

Schott, J, and Henley, A. *Culture, religion and childbearing in a multiracial society: A handbook for health professionals.* Butterworth Heinemann, 1996.

Scope, 2006. www.scope.org.uk

Scott, S. et al. Functional dysphonia: a role for psychologists in *Psychology, Health & Medicine,* 1997:2(2).

Scottish Cancer Registry ISD, 2004.

Scottish Executive. *The same as you? A review of services for people with learning disabilities, 2000.* www.scotland.gov.uk

Scottish Intercollegiate Network. *Management of individuals with stroke: Rehabilitation, Prevention, Management of Complications and Discharge Planning.* SIGN 64, 2002. www.sign.ac.uk

Scottish Intercollegiate Guidelines Network. *Assessment, Diagnosis, and Clinical Intervention for Children and Young People with ASD,* (in press).

Scottish Intercollegiate Guidelines Network. Head and Neck Cancer, 2005.

Scottish Intercollegiate Guidelines Network. *Management of patients with stroke: Identification and management of dysphagia*. SIGN 78, 2004. www.sign.ac.uk

Scottish Intercollegiate Guidelines Network. *Management of patients with stroke part I: Assessment, investigation, immediate management and secondary Prevention*. Guideline 13, 1997. www.sign.ac.uk

Sell, D. Issues in perceptual speech analysis in cleft palate and related disorders: a review in *International Journal of Language & Communication Disorders*, 2005: 40(2); pp103-121.

Sell, D. Ma, L. A model of practice for the management of velopharyngeal dysfunction in *British Journal of Oral and Maxillofacial Surgery*, 1996:34: pp357-363.

Shapiro, DA. *Stuttering Intervention: A Collaborative Journey to Fluency Freedom,* 1999.

Shimoji, T, Shimabukuro, S, Sugama, S, Ochiai, Y. Mild Trigonocephaly with Clinical Symptoms: Analysis of Surgical Results in 65 Patients in *Child's Nervous System,* 2002:18(5); pp215-24.

Shipster, C. Speech and Language Characteristics of Craniosynostosis in Hayward R, Jones B, Dunaway D, Evans R (Eds),*The Clinical Management of Craniosynostosis,* 2004.

Shipster, C, Hearst, D, Somerville, A, Stackhouse, J, Hayward, R, Wade, A. Speech, language, and cognitive development in children with isolated sagittal synostosis in *Dev Med Child Neurol*, 2003:45; pp34-43.

Shipster, C, Hearst, D, Dockrell, JE, Kilby, E, Hayward, R. Speech and language skills and cognitive functioning in children with Apert Syndrome: a pilot study in *International Journal of Communication Disorders,* 2002:37(3); pp325-343.

Shprintzen, RJ. *Syndrome Identification for speech therapists an illustrated pocket guide.* Singular Thomsen Learning, 2001.

Shprintzen, RJ. *Genetics, Syndromes and Communication Disorders.* Singular Publishing Group, 1997.

Shprintzen, RJ. *Syndrome Identification for Speech-Language Pathology.* An Illustrated Pocket Guide. Singular Publishing Group, 2000.

Sidoti, EJ Jr, Eugene, J, Marsh, JL, Marty-Grames, L, Noetzel, MJ. Long-term Studies of Metopic Synostosis: Frequency of Cognitive Impairment and Behavioural Disturbances in *Plastic & Reconstructive Surgery* February, 1996:97(2); pp276-281.

Shriberg, LD. Diagnostic markers for child speech-sound disorders: introductory comments in *Clin Linguist Phon,* 2003:17(7); pp501-5.

Shriberg, LD. Five subtypes of developmental phonological disorders in *Clin Commun Disord,* 1994:4(1); pp38-53.

Sinha, G, Corry, P, Subesinghe, D, Wild, J and Levene, MI. Prevalence and type of Cerebral Palsy in a British ethnic community: the role of consanguinity in *Developmental Medicine and Child Neurology,* 1997:39; pp259-262.

Shipster, C, Sirimanna, T, Hearst, D, Yap, SL, Gillespie, B, Evans, R, Hayward, R. Speech and language characteristics and feeding issues in children with Pfeiffer Syndrome type 2 and 3 in *Proceedings of the 10th International Congress of the International Craniofacial Society of Craniofacial Surgery*. Monduzzi Editore, 2003.

Skenduli-Bala, E. et al. Causes of incident visual field loss in a general elderly population. The Rotterdam Study in *Arch Ophthalmol,* 2005:123; pp233-238.

Sokoloff ,LG & Pavlakovic, R. Neuroleptic-induced dysphagia in *Dysphagia,* 1997:12; pp177-179.

Smith, A, Khoo, AK, Jackson, ITM. A Modification of the Kernahan "Y" Classification in Cleft Lip and Palate Deformities in *Plastic & Reconstructive Surgery,* 1998:102(6); pp1842-1847.

Smith, E. et al. Frequency of voice problems among teachers and other occupations in *Journal of Voice,*1998:12(4).

Smithard, DG, O'Neill, PA, Park, C, Morris, J, Wyatt, R, England, R, Martin, DF. Complications and outcome after acute stroke: does dysphagia matter in *Stroke* 1996:27; pp 1200-1204.

Snow, P, Douglas, J & Ponsford, J. Discourse assessment following traumatic brain injury: a pilot study examining some demographic and methodological issues in *Aphasiology*, 1995: 9; pp365-380.

Snowden, JS, & Griffiths, H. Semantic dementia: assessment and management in Best, Bryan & Maxim. *Semantic Processing: Theory and Practice*. Whurr, 2000.

Sperber, GH. *Craniofacial Development*. B C Decker Inc, 2001.

Stackhouse, J & Wells, B (Eds). *Children's Speech and Literacy Difficulties 1: A Psycholinguistic Framework.* Whurr Publishers, 1997.

Spriesterbach D.C. *Psychological Aspects of the Cleft Palate Problem*. Iowa City: University of Iowa Press,1973.

Stackhouse, J & Wells, B (Eds). *Children's Speech and Literacy Difficulties 2: Identification and Intervention.* Whurr Publishers, 2001.

Winter, K. Speech and language therapy provision for bilingual children: aspects of the current service in *International Journal of Language and Communication Disorders*, 1999:34(1); pp85-98.

Spremulli, M. Restoring speech and swallow control in Advance for Speech and Language Pathologists and Audiologists, 2005.

Stach, CB. Vascular Dementia and Dysphagia in *Topics in Stroke Rehabilitation;* 2000:7(3) pp1-10.

Stackhouse, RJ in Bishop, DVM & Leonard, L, *Speech and Language Impairments in Children.* Psychology Press, 2000.

Steele, CM, Greenwood, C, Ens, I, Robertson, C & Seidman-Carlson, R. Mealtime Difficulties in a Home for Aged in *Dysphagia*, 1997:12(1); pp43-50.

Stemple, JC. *Voice Therapy-Clinical Studies*. Mosby Year Book,1983.

Wilson, JA, Deary, IJ, Scott, S, MacKenzie, K. Functional Dysphonia in *BMJ* 1995:311; pp1039-40.

Stokes, G. *Challenging behaviour in dementia. A person centered approach.* Bicester. Winslow Press, 2000.

Stow, C, and Dodd, B. A survey of bilingual children referred for investigation of communication disorders: a comparison with monolingual children referred in one area in England in *Journal of Multilingual Communication Disorders,* 2005:3(1); pp1-23.

Sullivan, PB, & Rosenbloom L. (Eds). *Feeding the Disabled Child*. Mac Keith Press, 1996.

Swift, TL & Wilson, SL. Misconceptions about brain injury among the general public and non expert health professionals: an exploratory study in *Brain Injury,* 2001:15(2); pp149-165.

Thompson, DNB & Britto, J. Classification and Clinical Diagnosis in Hayward, R, Jones, B, Dunaway, D, Evans, R (Eds), *The Clinical Management of Craniosynostosis,* 2004.

Tolep, K, Getch, CL & Criner, GJ. Swallowing dysfunction in patients receiving prolonged mechanical ventilation in *Chest*, 1996:109(1); pp167-172.

Tomblin, JB, Smith, E & Zhang, X. Epidemiology of Specific Language Impairment: prenatal & perinatal factors in *Journal of Communication Disorders* 1997:54; pp167-173.

United Cerebral Palsy. *Cerebral Palsy Facts and Figures*, 2001. www.ucp.org/ucp_generaldoc.cfm/1/9/37/37-37/447

University of Glasgow. *Oral Cancer Prevention & Detection*, 2003.

Van den Elzen, APM, Semmekrot, BA, Bongers, EMHF, Huygen,

PLM, Marres HAM. Diagnosis and treatment of the Pierre Robin Sequence: results of a study and review of the literature in *European Journal of Pediatrics,* 2001:160; pp47-53.

Von Recklinghausen, F. Ueber die multiplen fibroma der haut und ihre Beziehung zu den multiplen neuromen. A Hirschwald, 1882.

Waddel, C, Offord, D, Shepherd, C, Hua, J & Mcewan, K. Child psychiatry epidemiology and Canadian public policy making: the state of the science and the art of the possible, *Canadian Journal of Psychiatry,* 2000:47; pp825-832.

Waterman, ET, Koltai, PJ, Downey, JC, Cacace, AT. Swallowing disorders in a population of children with cerebral palsy in *International Journal of Paediatric Otorhinolaryngology,* 1992:24: pp63-71.

Watson, F. Learning disabilities and dysphagia: the patient safety agenda in *RCSLT Bulletin,* 2004 (December).

Watson, N, Lucas, C, Hoy, A & Back, I. *Oxford Handbook of Palliative Care.* Oxford University Press, 2005.

Welsh Cancer and Intelligence and Surveillance Unit, 2004.

Welsh Health Planning Forum, 1992.

Williams P, Stackhouse, J. Rate, accuracy and consistency: diadochokinetic performance of young, normally developing children in *Clinical Linguistics & Phonetics,* 2000:14(4); pp267-293(27).

Wilson, L. Incidence and Epidemiology of Craniosynostosis in Hayward, R, Jones, B, Dunaway, D, Evans, R. (Eds) *The Clinical Management of Craniosynostosis,* 2004.

Winter, K. Numbers of bilingual children in speech and language therapy: Theory and practise of measuring their representation in *International Journal of Bilingualism,* 2001:5(4), pp465-495.

Wing, L & Gould, J. Severe impairments of social interaction and associated abnormalities in children: epidemiology & classification in *Journal of Autism & Developmental Disorders*, 1979:9; pp11-29.

Wolf, LS, & Glass, RP. Feeding & Swallowing Disorders in Infancy in *Therapy Skill Builders*, 1992.

Wood R. Understanding Neurobehavioural disability in Rodger Ll, Wood R & McMillan, TM (Eds), *Neurobehavioural Disability and Social Handicap Following Traumatic Brain Injury,* Psychology Press, 2001.

Worthington, A. Psychological aspects of motor neurone disease: a review in *Clinical Rehabilitation,* 1996:10; pp185-222.

Chapter 8

World Health Organisation (WHO). *ICD-10 Criteria for Dementia*, 1992. www.who.int

WHO. *ICIDH-2*, 1999. www.who.int

WHO. The International Classification of Diseases: classification of mental and behavioural disorders in *Diagnostic criteria for research (ICD 10) – 10th edition*, 1993.

WHO. *Palliative care*, 1996. www.who.int/cancer/palliative

Wright, L, Cotter, D, Hickson, M, Frost, G. Comparison of energy and protein intakes of older people consuming a texture modified diet with a normal hospital diet in *Journal Human Nutrition Dietetics,* 2005:18; pp213-219.

Yairi, E, Cox, N, Roe, C, Suresh, R, Cook, E. *Chromosomal Signals for Genes underlying Stuttering: A Preliminary Report at 7th Oxford Dysfluency Conference*, 2005.

Ylvisaker, M, & Feeney, T. Reconstruction identity after brain injury in *Brain Impairment,* 2000:1; pp12-28.

Young, AR, et al. Young adult academic outcomes in a longitudinal sample of early identified language impaired and control children in *Journal of Child Psychology and Psychiatry,* 2002:43(5); pp635-645.

Acts of Parliament

All available at: www.opsi.gov.uk

The Children's Act 1989

The Children Act 2004

Disability Discrimination Act 1995

Human Rights Act 2000

Mental Health Capacity Act 2005

Race Relations Amendment Act 2000

Chapter 9

Service Monitoring, Improvement, Evaluation and Development

9.1 Quality Framework for Clinical Services

The new NHS will have quality at its heart. Without it there is unfairness. Every patient who is treated in the NHS wants to know that they can rely on receiving high quality care when they need it. Every part of the NHS, and everyone who works in it, should take responsibility for working to improve quality (DH, 1997).

The governments across the four UK countries are committed to improving the quality of services within the independent sectors and the public sectors of health, education and social care.

9.1.1 What is quality?

Any assessment of quality will depend on the particular values and perspective of the person making the assessment.

In recognition of this, regulatory and inspection bodies are now taking a multiple perspective view of services provided. This includes identifying how to assess quality from the perspective of all stakeholders including the commissioners of services, managers, professionals and, with patient choice at the heart of policy developments, individual service users and carers (Huycke et al, 2000; Maxwell, 1984; Ovretveit, 1998).

Key dimensions of quality services:

● **Accessibility** (ease of access for individuals. Includes tackling such factors as distance, time and linguistic or cultural barriers).

● **Equity** (equal services for individuals with equal needs; reducing health variations by targeting need).

● **Effectiveness** (the intervention achieves the desired effects).

● **Relevance** (services are appropriate to need).

● **Efficiency** (services achieve the desired effects most economically).

● **Responsiveness** (meets individual/carer needs whilst being responsive to changes in circumstances and knowledge).

- **Safety** (services minimise the risk of harm and actual harm).
- **Appropriateness of resources, services and information** in order to achieve the above. This includes:
- **skilled staff in sufficient numbers** (appropriate skill-mix of staff; knowledgeable and skilled in using evidence-based practice)
- **networks across services and agencies**
- **information systems collecting and providing relevant information**
- **Governance** (leadership and accountability for all activity).

Making a commitment to quality a reality involves establishing and maintaining a system of national and local accountability and monitoring, and developing programmes of quality improvement. The system, implemented within the NHS in order to engineer a quality service in which the public would have confidence, involves:
- **clear national standards**
- **provision of services that comply with the standards**
- **service monitoring and evaluation.**

9.1.2 Clear national standards

National service standards
National service standards are available through the relevant sector Inspectorates:

England
- Health: Healthcare Commission. www.healthcarecommission.org.uk
- Social Care: Commission for Social Care Inspection (CSCI) www.csci.org.uk
- Education: OfSTED www.ofsted.gov.uk

The Healthcare Commission is working closely with the CSCI and OfSTED to develop a joint inspection framework and will be merging with the CSCI by 2008.

Northern Ireland
- Education: Education and Training Inspectorate www.deni.gov.uk/inspection_services
- Health and social care: Monitoring the health and personal social services is the duty of the four health and social service councils –

one for each board area. The councils advise the public about services. They also advise on how services might be improved. www.dhsspsni.gov.uk/hss/index.asp

Scotland
● Education; HM Inspectorate of Education www.hmie.gov.uk
● Health: NHS Quality Improvement Scotland www.nhshealthquality.org
● Social services: Care Commission www.carecommission.com

Wales
● Health: Healthcare Inspectorate Wales www.hiw.wales.gov.uk
● Education: HM Inspectorate for Education and Training in Wales (Estyn) www.estyn.gov.uk
● Social Services: Care Standards Inspectorate for Wales www.csiw.wales.gov.uk

RCSLT
See Appendix 1 for a summary of speech and language therapy minimum service standards.

National clinical standards
National policy frameworks on service provision across the UK set out what individuals can expect to receive from the health service in major care areas or disease groups.

National clinical guidance and standards build on these frameworks and should form part of service development plans. Clinical guidance and standards are available from a number of sources:
● National Institute for Health and Clinical Excellence (NICE) www.nice.org.uk currently produces three kinds of guidance:
i. Technology appraisals – guidance on the use of new and existing medicines and treatments within the NHS in England and Wales.
ii. Clinical guidelines – guidance on the appropriate treatment and care of people with specific diseases and conditions within the NHS in England and Wales.
iii. Interventional procedures – guidance on whether interventional procedures used for diagnosis or treatment are safe enough and work well enough for routine use in England, Wales and Scotland
● Quality Improvement Scotland (QIS)

www.nhshealthquality.org/nhsqis/qis
● Provides advice and guidance to NHSScotland on effective clinical practice.
● Sets clinical and non-clinical standards of care to help improve performance.
● Scottish Intercollegiate Guidelines Network SIGN (Scotland) www.sign.ac.uk/guidelines develops evidence-based clinical guidelines for the NHS in Scotland.
● RCSLT produces clinical guidelines and position papers related specifically to speech and language therapy www.rcslt.org

9.1.3 Provision of services that comply with the standards

Consistent action is required locally in order to ensure that:
● national standards and guidance are reflected in the provision and development of local services
● local patient and public views become an integral part of reflection on and development of services to meet local needs
That action is guided by a system of governance and is backed up through lifelong learning by staff; through professional self-regulation and through external inspection.

What is governance?

Governance is a framework through which organisations are accountable for continuously safeguarding standards of service provision and for continuously improving the quality of services.

What is professional self-regulation?

Standards for individual professionals are set by the speech and language therapy regulatory body, the Health Professions Council (HPC) within its *Standards of Proficiency* (2003) and *Standards of conduct performance & ethics,* (2003) available at: www.hpc.org and by the RCSLT in chapter 1, Professional Framework.
Support practitioners are not currently (2006) regulated but should be guided by the code of ethics contained within the Professional Framework chapter.

9.1.4 Service monitoring and improvement

Standards will be assured through:
● external monitoring

● an internal system of governance covering all service functions

External monitoring

Inspectorates across the four countries use differing frameworks to monitor the quality of service provision. However, there is a general trend towards emphasising outputs and outcomes rather than structure and process.

For further information visit the websites referenced in National Service Standards section above.

Internal monitoring

Services will wish to monitor service performance in line with the requirements of external monitoring systems and service governance.

Performance across quality domains may be evidenced through:
● a range of clinical and service data, with an increasing emphasis on outputs and outcomes
● detailing of policies and procedures across a range of domains

Services should have available relevant, easily accessible and comprehensible information in order to support decision-making at service and commissioning levels.

Audit and service improvement

Continuous service audit allows for incremental changes to be implemented as part of ongoing service improvement.

Examples of information that services may wish to audit to evidence quality and quality improvements over time:

● **Accessibility:**
● waiting list figures for assessment and therapy
● proximity of specialist services and usage
● burden of travel for users
● compliance with Disability Discrimination Act (DDA)
● where individuals are seen.

● **Equity:**
● availability of level of expertise appropriate to the conditions being treated
● accessing of interpreters
● profiling of service users including ethnicity and languages spoken.

- **Effectiveness:**
- outcomes of intervention
- records of any negative effects that might be attributed to speech and language therapy intervention
- performance in relation to predetermined service goals and objectives
- number of complaints
- number of praises
- age/stage/frequency/intensity/style of therapeutic intervention in relation to outcomes.
- **Relevance:**
- range of services available
- individual/carer satisfaction.
- **Efficiency:**
- numbers of appointments offered and taken up by individuals or by specific cohorts of individuals in a given time period
- keeping of case notes
- length of waiting times.
- **Responsiveness:**
- user satisfaction.
- **Safety:**
- number of near misses or instances of harm being done
- **Appropriateness of resources, services and information**
- **Skilled staff in sufficient numbers**:
- numbers of staff and skill mix in relation to population
- caseload per member of staff
- workload per member of staff
- recruitment and retention figures
- each member of staff has a personal development plan
- CPD activity.
- **Networks across services and agencies**
- number of referrals from and to other agencies
- co-working figures
- number of second opinions sought.
- **Information systems collecting and providing relevant information:**
- information readily accessible and available.
- **Governance:**
- systems, policies and procedures in place in relation to all of the above

● clarity in relation to responsibilities and where accountability for given aspects of service decision-making lies.

Speech and language therapy practitioners should be aware of the criteria by which the therapy they provide will be examined. They will need to know about the policies and procedures, standards and performance measures set at national and local levels and in use within their working context.

9.2 Monitoring Clinical Effectiveness: Assessing the Impact and Outcomes of Clinical Services

Purpose of monitoring clinical effectiveness

● To provide a means of quality assurance.

● To identify both highly effective and less effective aspects of service practice.

● To identify efficient/effective speech and language therapy practice through comparison with other similar services.

● To monitor and improve service delivery.

● To provide information about service activity.

● To aid business case preparation and bids for service development.

● To enable the value of speech and language therapy to be communicated to stakeholders.

● To contribute to the speech and language therapy evidence base.

● To help focus practitioners on shared professional purpose through provision of framework for assessing the benefits of speech and language therapy.

● To clarify intended purpose of intervention.

● To enhance record keeping.

● To identify areas for change.

● To identify scope and boundaries of practice, eg skill mix, second opinions.

● To support decisions related to resource allocation.

● To manage clinical risk.

● As a basis for reflection.

In line with the current trend towards evidencing outcomes, the primary focus here is on clinical effectiveness, and evidencing the results of intervention with clients (whether individual or population).

Methods for collecting and analysing the health, educational and psychosocial benefits and outcomes for clients receiving speech and language therapy are likely to be influenced locally by commissioning requirements and the systems set up by managers to report on effectiveness.

Methods for assessing the impact of speech and language therapy need to be set within a model of working that emphasises the need for reflection and that holds the notion of health benefits and outcomes as an integral part of practice.

Figure 1 sets out a model of working which has quality improvement for the individual or at-risk group at its heart and embodies the notion of reflective practice that all practitioners are familiar with (RCSLT, 2005).

Plan: make a judgement about what the situation entails and how to best meet the needs identified.

Do: carry out the plan of action and document the results.

Check (study): evaluate the results.

Act: put the learning to good use by making any changes to practice that are indicated. Use the learning to inform the next stage of planning.

As can be seen, the model is relevant to four levels of working:
● the individual practitioner
● the team
● the service
● the commissioner.

Each level is informed and enhanced by information from the other levels. The model therefore describes a complex interdependency of action and reflection around meeting the needs of the individual or at-risk group and improving services.

Clinical effectiveness and multidisciplinary/multi-agency working

Speech and language therapy services are placing increasing emphasis on multidisciplinary/multi-agency working and multidisciplinary/multi-agency performance measures. For example, in the field of cleft lip and palate, surgical or 'team' outcomes are the norm, as opposed to speech and language therapy specific outcomes.

Services may find that their contribution is increasingly assessed by

Figure 1: Cycle of speech and language therapy intervention

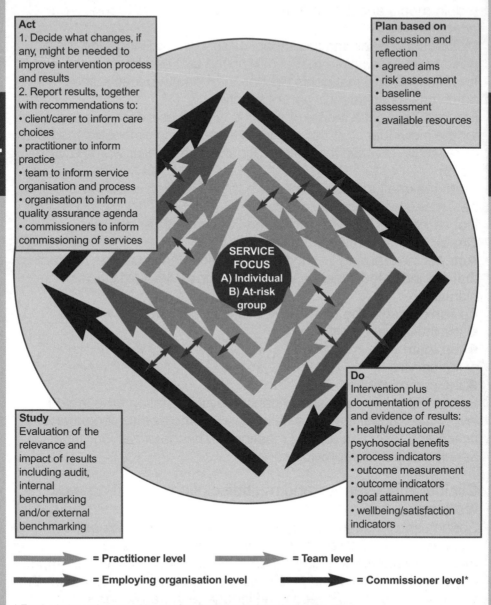

Act
1. Decide what changes, if any, might be needed to improve intervention process and results
2. Report results, together with recommendations to:
• client/carer to inform care choices
• practitioner to inform practice
• team to inform service organisation and process
• organisation to inform quality assurance agenda
• commissioners to inform commissioning of services

Plan based on
• discussion and reflection
• agreed aims
• risk assessment
• baseline assessment
• available resources

SERVICE FOCUS
A) Individual
B) At-risk group

Do
Intervention plus documentation of process and evidence of results:
• health/educational/psychosocial benefits
• process indicators
• outcome measurement
• outcome indicators
• goal attainment
• wellbeing/satisfaction indicators

Study
Evaluation of the relevance and impact of results including audit, internal benchmarking and/or external benchmarking

= Practitioner level   = Team level

= Employing organisation level   = Commissioner level*

* For the independent practitioner, often the commissioner is also the client.
* In some contexts, the employing organisation may also hold the commissioning role. In other contexts, the commissioning role is located externally.

broad team performance indicators, for example, an individual pupil's attendance and performance in an educational context.

Clinical effectiveness and evidence-based practice
Service standard 56: Clinical care standards are linked to the published research evidence base and consensus views on best practice
See section 5.3.6 on Evidence-based practice: research utilisation.

9.2.1 Health, educational and psychosocial benefits
The full range of health, educational and psychosocial benefits is best assured by services that offer a range of services targeting the needs of at-risk groups as well as the needs of referred individuals.

Health, educational and psychosocial benefits of speech and language therapy are as follows:
- improvement in general health and wellbeing
- increased independence
- improved participation in family, social, occupational and educational activities
- improved social and family relationships
- increased literacy skills
- reduction in the negative effects of communication disability and the harm or distress this may cause to the individual and others
- reduced risk of poor nutrition and invasive procedures such as surgical intervention in the case of individuals with swallowing disorders
- reduced health risks and length of hospital stay through the prevention of respiratory problems associated with swallowing difficulties
- reduced risk of surgical intervention by maintaining healthy voice mechanisms
- reduced risk of inappropriate prescribing of medication, for example, through diagnosis of autistic spectrum disorder as opposed to psychosis
- reduced risk of educational failure
- reduction in challenging behaviours including anti-social or crime-related activity

● reduced risk of social isolation
● prevention of certain speech, language and communication disorders
● increased participation in society.

Accruing benefits

Health, educational and psychosocial benefits are described from the perspective of the individual, but can be used to extrapolate benefits for the immediate family, for the local community and for broader society.

For example, an improvement in individual communication abilities can lead to:
● increased independence
● increased self esteem
● increased sense of citizenship
● improved relationships
● a decrease in anti-social behaviours
● a decreased risk of educational failure.

All of which will benefit the family and broader society and ultimately be of economical benefit.

9.2.2. Speech and language therapy outcomes

● diagnosis of communication and/or swallowing disorders
● maintenance of optimal communication and/or swallowing abilities
● improvement in the communication abilities of an individual in whatever language is appropriate to that person
● facilitating use of existing function
● facilitating optimal function following oral surgery, (eg cleft palate, tongue reduction, laryngectomy)
● reduction of communication anxiety and avoidance
● decreased impact of the speech, language and communication disorder (SLCD) on the individual's functioning
● provision and use of alternative or augmentative communication where oral communication is limited or precluded by a physical or psychological condition
● improvement in interaction and effective social communication
● increased awareness of others about communication and/or swallowing disorders, intervention and management
● improved communication environment

- greater opportunities for communication
- improvement in the individual's understanding of the nature and implications of a communication and/or swallowing disorder
- improvement in parenting skills.

9.2.3. Evidencing outcomes

1. Outcome indicators

Indicators are specific items of data that are tracked to give an indication of how intervention is having an impact. An indicator, or set of indicators, represents a concept that is related to the hoped for effects.

Concept	Indicator
Participation	Accessing of family, social, community, vocational and educational opportunities Exclusions from class, school, further education colleges or day services School attendance
Physical Health	Number of hospital admissions Child's weight and growth
Psychosocial health	Number of emergency assessment and treatment admissions due to placement breakdowns Number of incidents where an individual challenges supporting staff or relatives/carers Use of PRN medication or physical intervention
School readiness	Baseline measurements at school entry

By monitoring trends using indicators, services may gain evidence of a likely outcome for an individual or at-risk group.
Indicators are a useful adjunct to measurement systems, especially when change is not readily amenable to measurement. This is

typically the case when the main focus of intervention is to provide information and support, to modify/adapt regimes, or to prevent further health, education or psychosocial difficulties. In the latter circumstances, the use of peer-reviewed goals, health status measures, self-rating scales, questionnaires and analogue scales are also ways of reflecting on outcomes and providing information on the value added by speech and language therapy.

Goal attainment as outcome

As with other indicators, goal-based indicators detailing the number and percentage of clients who achieve/partially achieve/do not achieve their goals, are a useful adjunct to measurement. However, in order to be considered as an appropriate, quality indicator of effective intervention, goals need to conform to certain criteria.

Goal setting principles

Goals may relate to communication behaviour, skills, knowledge, attitudes, values, emotional state and medical condition of the referred individual.

Goals may also relate to the communication behaviour, skills and attitudes of those within the individual's environment

Goals should be:

● ethical
● relevant to the client, carers and context
● needs based
● evidence based (where evidence is available)
● focused on functional, participative aspects of life wherever possible
● formulated in conjunction with client/carer
● formulated in conjunction with other members of the team where appropriate
● specific, measurable, achievable, relevant and timed (SMART)
● defined in agreed terms, ie using shared terminology. This may involve using the client's opinion, in words or in another form of communication
● jargon-free
● take into account the skills and knowledge of the agent of change
● regularly reviewed
● discussed, agreed and evaluated with clients and, where appropriate, with carers.

Goal setting should be subject to periodic peer-review. **It should be noted that, because of the subjectivity and variability around goal setting, goal-achievement data cannot be aggregated and used as a benchmark for services.**

Goal setting when working within a multidisciplinary team setting
Within all agencies in the UK, there is an increasing emphasis on multidisciplinary working and joint goal setting.
Although goals in certain settings (for example, independent practice) or for certain individuals (for example, adults with dysfluent speech or pre-school children who are not accessing day care) may be uni-disciplinary, therapists may often need to link with other agencies or professions in setting goals.
There is currently no law covering joint team accountability. This means that each professional carries individual accountability for their actions carried out (or not carried out) within the team.
Where joint working is undertaken and where appropriate, any speech and language therapy-specific outcomes should link to those of other professionals.
Where achieving such outcomes is dependent on other professionals, the respective roles and contributions of personnel should be specified.

2. Measurement of outcomes

a) Qualitative measures
Wellbeing/satisfaction
Client/carer reports on changes in health and wellbeing following a period of intervention is a further way of evidencing the effectiveness of speech and language therapy. Health status measures, self-rating scales and questionnaires are all useful ways of capturing change.

b) Quantitative measures
Measurement involves the use of standardised, reliable and validated tools to record baseline and end-of-episode or discharge status. Measurements are particularly important for comparing results across services and establishing benchmarks. Thus they will support and promote service evaluation and multi-centre audit/research.
As part of individual profiling, standardised assessments or the use of instrumental tools, (eg acoustic computerised analysis and

videofluoroscopy) may be appropriate to measure baselines and change within specified aspects of functioning. However, the results of standardised assessments do not necessarily equate to outcomes that are, in turn, associated with health, educational and psychosocial benefits. Measures should be appropriate to the setting and to the aims and scope of the intervention. Therapists need to be clear what parameters they are measuring and that these are the relevant ones.

Example 1

Assessing the effects of speech and language therapy intervention in relation to children referred with eating/drinking difficulties

Possible outcomes of speech and language therapy intervention:
● resolution of difficulties
● avoidance of further risk through use of appropriate feeding strategies
● enhanced oral/pharyngeal function through a programme which modifies feeds or uses compensatory strategies
● modified/adapted regime through facilitation of adequate nutrition using non-oral methods, supported by appropriate non-nutritive programmes to sustain oral-motor function
● reduction of feeding anxiety and avoidance by supporting and reassuring carers.

Possible health, education and psychosocial benefits of speech and language therapy intervention:
● improvements in the child's health
● reduction in the number of hospital admissions
● improved participation in family mealtimes
● improved social and family relationships
● reduction in the negative effects of feeding difficulties and the harm or distress this may cause to the child and the family
● reduced risk of educational failure.

Outcome indicators to be tracked
● child's weight and growth
● hospital admissions due to right lobe aspiration infection
● school attendance
● goal achievement:
● jointly evaluated progress against specific goals at regular intervals
● implemented changes in the child's feeding regime which enhance oral/pharyngeal function.

Outcome measurement
A) Qualitative:

- questionnaire completion by parents/carers pre- and post-intervention
- diary of nutritional intake
- personal evaluations by children and young adults of any changes.
- reported changes in parents/carers management of feeding strategies which can improve the experience of mealtimes for the child.

B) Quantitative:
- re-assessment of skills using the same assessments, for example, videofluoroscopy, POSP, SOMA and so on.

Example 2
Assessing the effects of speech and language therapy intervention in relation a targeted at-risk group: Talking tots playgroup

Possible outcomes of speech and language therapy intervention:
- improved play skills
- improved communication skills
- improved parent/child interaction
- improved attention skills
- improved awareness of self as one of a group
- improved conformity within a group.

Possible health, education and psychosocial benefits of speech and language therapy intervention:
- increased access to school curriculum at school entry
- reduced risk of educational difficulties
- increased social participation
- improve parenting skills
- timely access to tier 3 services as appropriate
- improved social and family relationships.

Outcome indicators to be tracked:
- attendance/participation in group
- accessing of toy library by families
- proportion of children in sure start area with increased performance on school foundation measures
- goal achievement:
- jointly (parent and therapist) evaluated progress against specific goals at regular intervals.

Outcome Measurement
A) Qualitative:
- parent report on own confidence in parenting

● parent report on changes in child behaviour.

B) Quantitative:

● language assessment using Sure Start language measure (SSLM) pre and post group

● observational ratings related to child attention, concentration and interaction

● pre and post group measures of, eg number of opportunities parent provides for child to play and communicate; number of times the parent allows the child to take the lead; the number of times the parent provides good models of language.

For further information on outcomes see:

Squires, A J (Ed). *Rehabilitation of older people: a handbook for the multidisciplinary team,* Chapman Hall. 1996 (2nd Edition)

Frattali, C (Ed) *Measuring outcomes in speech-language pathology.* Thieme, 1998.

Enderby, P. "Making speech pathology practice evidence based: Is this enough?" in *Advances in Speech and Language Pathology,* 2004: 6.2; pp125-126.

9.3 The Relationship between Service Audit, Evaluation and Research

What is service audit?

A service audit cycle includes the following steps:

● observing current practice

● setting standards of care

● comparing practice to standards and implementing change.

This is a continuous process.

It has been suggested that audit is similar to research. The main difference is that whilst research aims to influence clinical practice in its totality, audit aims to influence activity on a local level.

Audit is useful when the need is not to understand practice in detail, but simply to look at outcome data.

What is service evaluation?

An evaluation is applied research for a purpose. It is a structured process concerned with making an assessment, judging an activity or a service against a set of criteria.

Evaluation is useful for looking in detail at service practice in order to see, for example:

● whether the service is meeting the needs of service users
● whether the service can be improved
● what happens to individuals after an intervention is finished
● whether resources are being used to the best advantage by providing care in a particular way
● whether the service should continue.

For further information see 9.4 Service Improvement and Development.

What is service research?

Research is designed to provide generalisable knowledge. The results of research are not just about specific programmes or areas, they have the likelihood of being applicable to similar services elsewhere. Many of the methods of research are those used in evaluation, but the focus is different, the scale of resources required is likely to be different, along with the level of skills and knowledge.

Is audit, evaluation or research to be chosen?

Services should be clear about the questions they are seeking to answer in order to ascertain whether audit, evaluation or research is required.

Consideration should also be given as to whether a mix of approaches is appropriate, for example, a local audit added to existing research findings will avoid the onus of a full scale evaluation but still provide some local data and greater credibility.

For further information see the: *Trent focus service evaluation* toolkit, available at the Department of Health's website, at:
www.dh.gov.uk/assetRoot/04/09/81/83/04098183.doc
www.dh.gov.uk/assetRoot/04/09/82/63/04098263.doc

9.4 Service Improvement and Development

9.4.1 Service improvement

Continuous service audit allows for incremental changes to be implemented as part of ongoing service improvement.
Service evaluation is designed to have a greater degree of impact

and may involve radical changes to service provision.

Some changes to service provision may be implemented within current resources whilst other, larger-scale changes may be classed as service development and require additional resources in order to be implemented.

9.4.2 Service development

Commissioning context

With all service development issues it is important to understand the process and context in which the development is taking place at local, regional and national levels.

The central themes across the UK across health and social care are:

● For patient care – the move from a professional to patient/service user centred focus, an increase in self-care and health promotion with the premise of the patient as an expert. An increase in focus on patient choice.

● For workforce issues – a move to an adaptable workforce that can meet the changing health and social care needs of the population as the demographic changes in the UK affect both health needs and the available workforce.

The need to demonstrate the quality and impact of care in terms of health, educational and psychosocial benefits is discussed in detail within 9.1 Quality Framework for Clinical Services and 9.2 Monitoring Clinical Effectiveness.

Drivers within health and social care for the four countries include: the *AHP Career Framework*, the *Knowledge and Skills Framework, Skills for Health and Lifelong Learning* as well as the priority areas/frameworks for each country based around children, cancer, coronary heart disease, diabetes, living with long term conditions, mental health, and older people, and changing directions for the allied health professions.

The governments are looking for a flexible workforce engaged in lifelong learning, with the skills to provide the right intervention and care, and the ability to change roles in response to the needs of the local community. Allied health professionals are being asked to express their shared knowledge and skills together with a statement about the specific nature of their expertise so that services can be provided more flexibly.

In each of the four countries structures have been set up with groups at national, regional and local levels to assess current service provision, future training places and future service provision. There are also workforce groups looking at care pathways and the relevant abilities and skills required of staff to provide quality care. There is increasing involvement in workforce planning from the government departments who take the lead for education and children's services in looking at the future workforce for children.

As a result there is a move towards the planning for new and developing established services in a multi-agency manner, looking at the:

● *needs* (what are the local health and social care needs of the population)

● *functions* (what are the functions required to meet those needs)

● *competencies* (what do the staff need to be able to do in order to fulfil those functions) required of the workforce in general and not of one service in isolation.

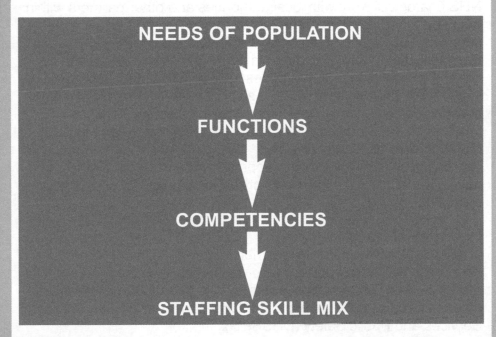

Planning cycles
Planning cycles and processes differ in the four UK countries in relation to their drivers, policies, and commissioners.

In England

As a result of new policy drivers including *Commissioning a Patient-led NHS* and the upcoming White Paper on the *Future of services: closer to home,* major changes are taking place in the commissioning and provision of services in England.

As yet it is unclear what the new planning cycles will be and it is important for those involved in planning services to:

● keep up to date with national policy drivers and priorities including payment by results. www.dh.gov.uk

● identify who the key stakeholders are at a local level that need to be influenced

● be actively engaged in the process of local implementation to inform decisions

● be informed of the planning cycle process in order to be proactive and make a timely and effective contribution.

In Scotland

NHS boards will work with local authorities and other partners within the community planning partnerships to develop joint local health improvement plans for each local authority area.

Each local NHS board will draw up a single local health plan for its area. The local health plan includes NHS action points from the joint local health improvement plans. It also includes the healthcare plans covering primary, community, secondary and tertiary services provided by NHS bodies in the board area. Priority areas can be found at: www.show.scot.nhs.uk

Any business case for new development within a service must be developed within the parameters of the local health plan in order to succeed.

In Northern Ireland

When the Northern Ireland Assembly resumes, funding for all public services in Northern Ireland will come directly from the Parliament to the Assembly. The Assembly will then delegate the budget to the different departments, including the Department of Health, Social Services and Public Safety (DHSSPS).

The DHSSPS then funds each of the health and services boards who, in turn, provide funding to local health and social care groups and the local health and social care trusts.

The priorities for funding are driven by the Northern Ireland Assembly but within the overall framework of the NHS (UK-wide). There are also specific priorities set by the UK Government and by the Northern Ireland Assembly. Each board, local health and social care group and trust will have its own priorities in line with the above. The funding allocation follows a similar timeframe to that in England. Each health and social services board has a health and wellbeing investment plan (HWIP) and each trust must have a service delivery plan to meet this investment plan.

In Wales
The Welsh Assembly Government is responsible for policy direction and for allocating funds to the NHS in Wales. The Assembly's NHS Wales Department currently allocates funds annually to the five existing regional health authorities.
The authorities buy health services from professionals in primary care, such as family doctors, dentists and opticians, and from the NHS trusts that provide secondary and community care.
Improving Health in Wales was launched in February 2001, setting out the long-term strategy for the NHS in Wales.
The new system aims to ensure that health services are designed and delivered locally. In order to achieve this, there will be a local health board in every area, building on existing local health groups. They will serve their own localities and decide what services are needed for local people, (eg family health, community health and hospital services).
Local health boards involve local doctors, nurses and other health professionals, representatives from the council (including elected members), voluntary organisations and the public. In the new system, local government, local health boards and the voluntary sector will work together more closely, so that there is a better coordination of services (particularly health and social services).
Information on the structures referred to in this section can be found on the Health of Wales Information Service (HOWIS) website, at: www.wales.nhs.uk

Assessing the need for local service development for a given client or population group
In assessing the need for service development there are several

processes that can be employed. These include:

a. consulting with commissioners, service users, referral agents and co-providers of services to assess levels of satisfaction

b. analysing current service provision in terms of activity, models of service delivery and outcomes

c. estimating current unmet need using epidemiological and demographic information

d. predicting future demands by consideration of local and national strategies and priorities.

a. Consultation process

Service standard 57: Service evaluation as the basis of a service development bid involves consultation with commissioners, service users, referral agents, and other services or agencies who are co-providers of services.

Consultation with commissioners

As bids for service development need to tie in with local planning processes and priorities, it is advisable to alert commissioners to the need for in-depth service evaluation at an early stage.

Consultation with co-providers

As most speech and language therapy services are not provided in professional isolation, the majority of plans for service development require the involvement and cooperation of others. The ability to demonstrate such cooperation may increase the likelihood of a successful development bid.

Consultation with other service leaders should include discussion related to the roles, functions and skills of the current staff and those required of the future workforce

Consultation with service users

User consultation and feedback is a main plank of government policy. Ethics and/or approval within the clinical governance arrangements of the organisation may be necessary for some methods of user consultation.

Different approaches to service user consultation may be used including:

● focus groups

- surveys

This will help identify:

- shortfall in current service delivery
- need for service improvement, perhaps involving a change in the model of service provision
- need for service growth.

Where an individual is asked to attend and contribute at formal meetings, appropriate consideration must be given to providing support in their preparation for, and during, the meetings as well as possible assistance in attending.

Consultation with local clinical leaders will be important when:

- reviewing a service for a specific client group
- seeking support with service change or development
- bid proposals that may be put forward.

b. Analysing activity and outcome data

Commissioners of services and workforce planners are interested not just in patient related activity, but in outcomes of interventions and likely impact both of therapy being available or not available. Linking benefits and activity data to the targets and priorities of local agencies will assist with development bids.

Information on local targets and priority areas is available from a variety of sources such as national policies and local agency improvement plans.

c. Estimating the current unmet need

An estimate of the unmet need of a client group or population group can be made by comparing actual referral rates with predicted referral rates (based on incidence/prevalence figures related to population figures).

Care should be exercised in using some information as for example, waiting list numbers and numbers of new referrals may simply reflect local patterns due to the presence or absence of specialists, multi disciplinary teams, or a particular model of service. Additionally the incidence or prevalence rates do not indicate the numbers of people who may benefit from or want speech and language therapy input.

For information on prevalence and incidence see chapter 8 Working with Specific Client Groups.

Statistical information on the local population can be found on several websites such as the national statistics and regional public health observatories.

Where an analysis of unmet need reveals that the safety of individuals is being put at risk or the efficacy of therapeutic input is seriously compromised, consideration must be given by the speech and language therapy manager to redesigning the model of service delivery, capping the caseload or withdrawing a service until further support can be achieved.

d. Predicting future demand

● **Nationally and local drivers** Relevant information can be found on regional council and local council websites and from other sources such as the government websites and public health observatories.

● **Local socio-economic influences**

Statistical information is available on the deprivation index and on age distribution. These help inform the analysis of present and future demand such as possible access issues or the likelihood of long-term and age related conditions.

See websites such as the national statistics and regional public health observatories:

www.statistics.gov.uk

www.pho.org.uk

● **National trends**

Examples include:

● an increasing number of adults and children/babies surviving with disabilities due to technological and medical advances

● use of technology to provide remote access to impairment therapy

● increasingly affordable and flexible technology to assist individuals with their communication.

Designing service options

Having identified the need for service development and having clarified the desired the outcomes and benefits of such a development, a range of service provision options should be explored.

Managers are advised to use best clinical-practice guidance in designing service options and to show how the predicted benefits and outcomes from the service change will be evidenced. These should be agreed with the commissioning agents. This process will usually continue to be undertaken in the context of a multidisciplinary or multi-agency forum.

For each option, the following issues are key:

- What model of service provision is to be adopted?
- What are the identified functions (eg assessment, therapy, training, enabling, care support) that will need to be carried out within the stated model of provision?
- What are the competencies associated with those functions (ie the detail of what staff will need to do)?
- What might the staffing skill mix look like based on the above?
- What are the other resources required to implement the stated service option?
- What are the cost implications (initial set-up costs and on-going costs)?

Role and service redesign is increasingly being promoted as a way of modernising or improving services as well as tackling the concerns over workforce recruitment and development in the coming years.

Information may be obtained from the Web Information Sharing Environment (WISE) on the NHS web portal at: www.wise.nhs.uk, as well as from the NHS Scotland website: www.show.scot.nhs.uk/workforcedevelopment, the National Leadership and Innovation Agency for Healthcare (NLIAH), via the Health of Wales Information Health website: www.wales.nhs.uk and the Northern Ireland Department of Health, Social Services and Public Safety www.dhsspsni.gov.uk, on the Workforce Development Unit section.

Resource implications of proposed service developments:
a) staffing
b) accommodation and other physical resources

a) Assessing Staffing levels required:
- skill-mix
- numbers of staff at differing levels of skill.

Skill mix

One aim of skill mix is to free staff to use their skills and knowledge to maximum effect.

Skill mix can have a positive affect on both staff recruitment and staff retention.

The *NHS Knowledge and Skills Framework* and *Skills for Health* (UK-wide) provide guidance on skills and competencies for staff functions.

In relation to a given context, an appropriate skill mix may reflect:

● a range of professionals
● different grades and specialties of SLTs
● bilingual therapists and or support workers
● support practitioners
● technicians
● generic workers
● administrative and clerical support.

Managers and commissioners should be aware of the range of influences on local skill mix requirements. See the diagram below.

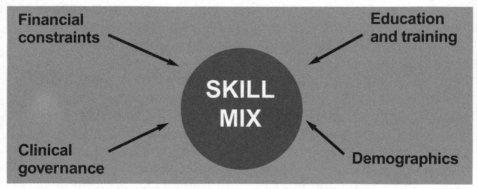

Financial constraints: it is helpful to gain some indication from commissioners of any financial constraints applying to service development bids

Clinical governance: a prime consideration should be the need to provide safe and effective services to individuals. This includes having staff who are competent in the required tasks and who are adequately supported by supervision processes.

There must be sufficient senior staff with designated time to supervise and support less experienced therapists and support practitioners in their clinical work.

Education and training: the types and levels of knowledge, skill and expertise required to meet the needs of the target group. This may include the need for highly specialised expertise.

Demographics (including geography, population, age groupings, health needs, socio-economic profile, deprivation and ethnic diversity).

Example 1. Diversity: the workforce should reflect the ethnic and socio-economic diversity of the local community. The workforce may need to include bilingual practitioners.

Example 2. Geography: services within a very rural context are likely to require staff to be have high levels of expertise across a range of functions; with access to very highly specialist services outwith the service. Services within an urban context are likely to be better placed to have staff with very high degrees of specialism within their skill mix.

Estimating numbers of speech and language therapist staff required at each level of skill within a given model of service provision
There has been much debate around assessing required staffing levels on the basis of nationally agreed notional caseloads. Guidance from workforce planners and the RCSLT *Workforce Planning Guidelines* (2006), is that notional caseloads on their own are insufficient for calculating staffing levels. This is because of the number of other variables that impact on working practice and what constitutes a manageable practitioner caseload. Variables include:

- chosen model of working
- local geography and accessibility
- range and number of local co-providers
- risk management issues
- grading of practitioner
- ratio of clinical: non-clinical practitioner time available.

For example, the competence, knowledge and skills expected of therapists varies according to grading. This will affect the clinical input expected and in turn may affect the numbers of people that they are able to see, eg a consultant therapist will be required to see people with complex issues who may require larger amounts of time than people with more straightforward issues. The consultant SLT may see less people in the clinical time available than a practitioner on a lower banding. In addition, the clinical time itself may be less as the consultant may have a range of other responsibilities in relation to research and development, providing practice-based learning opportunities and supervising other practitioners.

However, a notional caseload may be arrived at locally in relation to a given client group by taking all the variables into account. See figure below.

Figure 2: Influences on estimating notional caseload

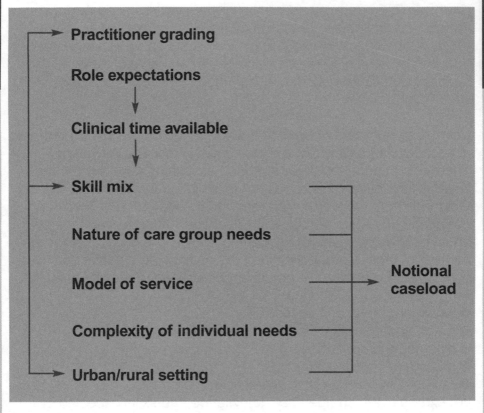

Further information on workload can be found in section 5.4.3 on Workload Management in Chapter 5.

Accommodation and other resource requirements

Non-staff costings involved in setting up the proposed service should be provided. This will include costings for accommodation, furnishings, equipment, and published assessments.

Recurrent costs should be estimated and set out separately (e.g. training and travel).

Accommodation should comply with the Disability Discrimination Act and incorporate the creation of communication-friendly environments.

Further information on the minimum standards of accommodation and equipment can be found in 5.4.1 on Accommodation.

It is important to ensure that staff have access to the most recently revised editions of assessments to ensure best practice.

Costings for training and travel needs may be estimated based on current levels of expenditure and the anticipated model of working.

9.4.3 Service development plans

Service development plans are required when any significant development of existing services or the creation of a new service is being considered. This may be as a result of:

● the development of extended scopes of practice/consultant posts
● a change in local demographics such as a large new housing estate or settlement of large numbers of refugees in an area
● redesign of a service to a care group
● developing service delivery into new areas
● a service failing to meet RCSLT standards and guidelines.

A service development plan is a process rather than just a document and may form the basis for performance management. These plans should be developed within the manager's local service and updated annually. Different organisations may have different terms for service/business plans and may hold them at a level other than the speech and language therapy service level. It is important for speech and language therapy services to be able to contribute to these plans. The planning process can provide a positive opportunity to engage staff within the service in both reviewing and planning service delivery. As procedures associated with service development planning will vary between organisations, managers should seek advice on the local process.. Information may be available from the business functions within organisations, eg corporate or performance directorates.

Information that could be included in a service plan includes:

● current service structure (eg skill mix, workforce profile, vacancies)

● details of service performance (eg ability to meet RCSLT minimum service standards, clinical audit, service outcomes)
● details of unmet clinical need
● broad details of the nature of the service development required to meet local health and social care needs
● how this links with national and local development priorities
● risk factors that may affect how the plan can be implemented
● costed service options including details of functions and competencies
● suggested performance indicators.

For information on national priorities see national policy documents available on the four government websites.

For information on local priorities, see local public health, health and local authority websites.

9.5 Development of Research Capacity within Services

Research capacity is a dimension of service organisation that many services currently need to develop.

What is research capacity?

Research capacity is a term that describes, "a process of individual and institutional development which leads to higher levels of skills and greater ability to perform useful research." (Trostle, 1992).

Whilst the traditional measures of research capacity building have tended to be outputs such as publications, funding applications and qualifications, other outputs might impact on professional outcomes including job satisfaction and confidence.

Professional research capacity is addressed at two service levels:
● individual
● organisation.

9.5.1 Individual responsibilities

Individuals need to:
● Document practice – especially interventions – that are well-designed, well-conducted and well-reported, to contribute to building our professional evidence base.
● Develop an awareness of research governance policy and local

protocols regarding conduct of research in NHS trusts.
- Collaborate with other speech and language therapy colleagues in both clinical and academic posts who have relevant experience and expertise in leading and in disseminating clinical research.
- Develop advanced skills in project management and contract management.
- Develop advanced skills in dissemination of results.
- Publish work to develop a track record for future funding applications.

9.5.2 Organisation responsibilities
Organisations need to:
- welcome local EBP/audit/research initiatives
- differentiate between audit, service evaluation and research (see section 9.3)
- be pro-active in support for national research projects, such as providing access to research participants
- promote and facilitate research and research culture within the department
- encourage local funding for research and appropriate locum cover
- identify priority areas for research relevant to the profession and service delivery
- provide appropriate levels of support for staff undertaking research
- raise awareness of service commissioners about the importance of research
- establish working protocols with researchers
- ensure that any employer requirements are met, (eg registration, research indemnity, research governance.

The NHS *Research and Development Research management and governance toolkit* provides advice, guidance and document templates: www.rdforum.nhs.uk/toolkit.htm
- meet regularly with any staff member undertaking research to be kept informed of progress and any problems encountered
- help the researcher to find solutions to any problems
- have a designated coordinator, preferably one who is already research-active, who participates in any employer-wide research networks, and who keeps abreast of available support for local research initiatives and acts as knowledge broker/pathfinder for

members of staff, (eg writing bids, how ethics committees work etc)
- have designated staff links to national AHP quality/EBP/research networks
- establish links with research-active staff in higher education institution/s
- provide for study leave for members of staff undertaking post-graduate education or for flexible terms of employment for research-active staff, to allow for splits between NHS employment and employment on funded research projects
- have a system to encourage SLTs to engage in research – write up their work to enhance the evidence base. Reduce barriers to involvement in research
- recognise that individuals in an organisation will have different levels of skill and knowledge about research and that the opportunities for training, development and support need to reflect this
- provide training for managers on the benefits of research
- facilitate dialogue between managers, academics and practitioners to ensure research meets organisational objectives.

Managers and SLTs should refer to national policy and guidance via websites for the government departments of the four countries of the UK.

9.5.3 Resources

RDInfo consists of three services providing access to details of research funding, training and advice:

1) *RDFunding* provides information on health-related research funding opportunities: www.rdfunding.org.uk

2) *RDLearning* provides information on learning opportunities: www.rdlearning.org.uk

3) *RDDirect* is a signposting service for researchers: www.rddirect.org.uk

RCSLT research group www.rcslt.org/resources/research

RCSLT Research Strategy.

RCSLT Position Paper *Approaching Research in Speech and Language Therapy,* 2003. www.rcslt.org.uk

PCT Competencies: Education, Training and Research, National Primary and Care Trust development programme, 2005. www.natpact.nhs.uk

9.6 Services Responding to Imposed Structural Change

The following is a set of general principles for speech and language therapy managers that can be applied to any situation where structural change is occurring.

9.6.1 Context of change

● Identify why the change is being proposed – what is the policy context for the change?
● What are the intended outcomes/benefits being proposed to service delivery?
● Establish who relevant colleagues are and work with them, eg AHP colleagues. This will help to achieve a critical mass of professionals working together and will provide mutual support eg working with physiotherapy and occupational therapy colleagues within children's services.
● Determine whether the change is going to affect only the internal organisation or whether there are also implications for other agencies, eg education, social services. How does the proposed change affect:
● the financial budget
● structures
● systems
● processes
● care pathways
● workforce and skill mix.
● If the implications of the change are far reaching the issues should be raised and addressed with key stakeholders in the relevant agencies. Ensure that there is a sound evidence base for issues to be raised.
● Determine whether the proposed change has implications for the speech and language therapy profession as a whole.

9.6.2 Implications for service users

● Look at the change from the point of view of service users. Consider what the benefits are to service users if the change occurs.
● Assess whether the change is going to affect prioritisation and/or distribution of resources. It *should not* affect your clinical prioritisation but may affect how your resources are distributed.

● Map the service user's journey/care pathway currently and within the new structure. Assess any difference in the distribution and/or availability of resources. Raise awareness that SLTs have a duty of care that will often go beyond limited, prescribed packages, and encourage a whole systems approach to be taken, eg long-term management of a dysphasic client.

9.6.3 Clinical governance

● Services should assess whether they can still meet the agreed minimum RCSLT professional standards within the new structure.
● Provide explicit and, wherever possible, evidence-based clinical guidelines and care pathways that are currently used to provide services to your local population. If these are not currently used within the service, urgently develop them. It should still be possible to provide the service based on these within the new structure.
● Encourage a culture of openness and good communication. This is the key to supporting staff through the change process. It is essential that there is effective communication throughout the speech and language therapy department concerned, and that there are mechanisms in place to facilitate dialogue in both directions, i.e. from top down and vice versa. This may include the following discussions:
● making the strategic objectives clear to staff
● building a shared vision of the better future. Compare this with the current one, and identify the work that has to be done to move from one to the other
● providing leadership to help individuals move forward and regularly review progress.
● Analyse and then specify the risks to the service user that may arise from these changes, and identify strategies to minimise these risks, eg provision of continuous care from acute into community settings.
● Engage service users in debate about the impact of the change, eg Sure Start debates, local stroke clubs. Use this information to influence decision makers.
● Ensure systems for profession specific CPD and clinical supervision are going to be maintained. In addition, opportunities for multidisciplinary/inter-professional CPD and supervision should be enhanced.
● Be proactive within the local network to ensure the ability to

influence both the strategic leads within the organisation, eg members of the board, and the strategic leads in other organisations, eg the local education authority.

● Ensure systems for managing staff effectively are going to be maintained. There should be clarity around staff accountability and management authority. If an SLT is not going to be managing the service, the interface between professional leadership and service management should be made explicit, e.g. input to the appraisal process, managing staff performance, skill mix within the service, identification of training needs.

● Ensure there are systems in place for the professional lead to contribute to local implementation of national strategy across health, education and social services agendas.

● Check if the changes may have any effect on speech and language therapy ethical/professional issues and highlight these if appropriate.

9.6.4 Resources

● Lewin's three phase model: unfreezing, moving, re-freezing. Lewin's force field analysis tool which assumes that in any change situation there are two forces – those driving the change and those opposing or restraining it. Completion of the force field analysis may lead to an onset of realism (Lewin, 1947).

● Nadler and Tushman provide a diagnostic model of change, which can be used to help understand the current situation and the way it might respond to intervention. It helps individuals decide on their own method of intervention to facilitate change, and act proactively (Nadler & Tushman, 1997).

● *Understanding Organisations* by Charles Handy (1993) has chapters on managing change in organisations, and is used in the Open University course that links with the Institute of Health Services managers' course on *Managing Health Services*.

● NHS leadership programmes include modules on project planning, risk management, problem solving, organisational development, information technology, networking, presentation and assertiveness.

References

Department of Health. *The new NHS: modern, dependable*, 1997. www.dh.org.uk

Huycke, L & All, AC. Quality in health care and ethical principles in

Journal of Advanced Nursing, 2000:32(3); pp562-571.

Lewin, K. Frontiers in group dynamics in *Human Relations*, 1947:1 pp5-41.

Maxwell, RJ. Quality assessment in health in *British Medical Journal,* 1984:288; pp1470-72.

Nadler, DA & Tushman, ML. *Competing by design: The power of organizational architecture.* Oxford University Press, 1997.

Ovretveit, J. *Evaluating Health Interventions.* Open University Press, 1998.

Trostle, J. Research Capacity building & international health: Definitions, evaluations & strategies for success in *Soc.sci.med*, 1992:35(11); pp1321-1324.

RCSLT. CQ3 Quality Assurance Expert Group, 2005. (Diagram based on the *Deming Plan, Do, Study, Act* (PDSA) Cycle).

Appendix 1
Summary of minimum service standards for service organisation and provision

Service standard 1: The service audits its performance against the RCSLT minimum service standards as part of a regular process of service review. (Section 5.2)

Service standard 2: Policies are reviewed at least once every three years. (Section 5.2)

Service standard 3: The service has a system for monitoring SLT's HPC registration status. (Section 5.3.1)

Service standard 4: Exit interviews are conducted with all staff leaving the service. (Section 5.3.2)

Service standard 5: All staff have a clear and up-to-date contract of employment. (Section 5.3.3)

Service standard 6: All staff have a clear and up-to-date job description. (Section 5.3.3)

Service standard 7: The service has a system for monitoring staff absence. (Section 5.3.3)

Service standard 8: The service provides a planned orientation, induction and support programme for all new staff, including locum staff, and returners to practice. (Section 5.3.3)

Service standard 9: The service has an up-to-date organisation and service profile showing clear lines of responsibility and accountability within the organisation. (Section 5.3.3)

Service standard 10: All staff have an annual performance review supported by a systematic approach to training and development including a PDP and appropriate CPD opportunities. (Section 5.3.3)

Service standard 11: The service has a system for reviewing the requirements of a post in terms of knowledge and skills. (Section 5.3.3)

Service standard 12: The service has agreed mechanisms in place to support practitioners working within external agencies. (Section 5.3.3)

Service standard 13: The service has an up-to-date policy and system of clinical supervision for all clinical staff. (Section 5.3.3)

Service standard 14: All SLTs access an appropriate form of clinical supervision at least once every 12 weeks. (Section 5.3.3)

Service standard 15: The service has a system for accessing clinical advice or second opinions. (Section 5.3.3)

Service standard 16: The service uses the competency based framework to structure the learning of the newly-qualified practitioner during the initial twelve month period and as evidence of readiness to transfer to full RCSLT membership. (Section 5.3.4)

Service standard 17: The service supports the monitoring of clinical practice through managerial and clinical supervision, staff development review and personal development plans. (Section 5.3.5)

Service standard 18: The service has a clear and up-to-date policy for dealing with staff concerns about clinical care, including a confidential procedure for staff to follow. (Section 5.3.5)

Service standard 19: As appropriate, service managers are involved in influencing and defining the objectives of the wider organisation. (Section 5.3.5)

Service standard 20: All staff have the opportunity to participate in the planning, decision making and formulating of policies that affect service provision. (Section 5.3.5)

Service standard 21: The service has clear and up-to-date administrative policies that relate to speech and language therapy working practices. These are written by or in consultation with a registered SLT. (Section 5.3.5)

Service standard 22: RCSLT's professional standards and

guidelines inform the development of policy and practice. (Section 5.3.5)

Service standard 23: The service has a strategic and systematic approach within each clinical team to establish an evidence-based resource as the basis for provision of clinical care, organisation of services and service development. (Section 5.3.6)

Service standard 24: The service has a system to collect information for service management purposes and to meet contractual obligations. Information is collected on a consistent and regular basis. (Section 5.3.7)

Service standard 25: The design of service documents includes a code to allow for audit trails and identification of source. (Section 5.3.7)

Service standard 26: All staff maintain personal learning portfolios and reflect on learning gained through practice, both individually and in teams. (Section 5.3.9)

Service standard 27: All staff have access to a personal development review at least once every twelve months. (Section 5.3.9)

Service standard 28: The service has a clear and up-to-date staff training and development policy. (Section 5.3.9)

Service standard 29: The service has sufficient and appropriate resources to support the principal functions of the service. (Section 5.4)

Service standard 30: The financial resources of the service are planned, managed and controlled. (Section 5.4)

Service standard 31: Equipment used in therapy is non-hazardous to the client and conforms with health and safety standards. This includes regular cleaning of equipment in accordance with infection control guidance. (Section 5.4)

Service standard 32: The service has a range of relevant and up-to-date literature available to support the client and/or carer in understanding the nature and extent of any given swallowing or communication disorder. (Section 5.4)

Service standard 33: The service has a written statement of philosophy, core purpose and operational policy. (Section 5.4)

Service standard 34: All staff (including those in remote areas) are aware of available resources and are able to access them as appropriate. (Section 5.4.3)

Service standard 35: The service has a mechanism for ongoing monitoring of staff workloads. (Section 5.4.3)

Service standard 36: The urgency or priority of referrals is determined in a systematic and equitable manner. Prioritisation systems are evidence-based as far as possible and clearly documented. (Section 5.4.3)

Service standard 37: Written records are kept of each individual's care. (Section 5.5.3)

Service standard 38: The service has clear standards of record keeping in line with Data Protection Act (1998) principles and RCSLT guidance that are reviewed and audited on a regular, at least annual, basis. (Section 5.5.3)

Service standard 39: The service has a clear and up-to-date policy on the confidentiality, use, security and disclosure of health information. (Section 5.5.4)

Service standard 40: The service has a clear and up-to-date policy detailing the process through which individuals (or their advocates) have access to their records in line with the Data Protection Act (1998). (Section 5.5.4)

Service standard 41: The service has a clear and up-to-date policy relating to the length of retention and ultimate disposal of clinical records which complies with legislation and RCSLT guidance. (Section 5.5.4)

Service standard 42: The service has a clear and up-to-date policy relating to storage and disposal of audio and visual recordings. (Section 5.5.4)

Service standard 43: The service has clear and up-to-date risk-management policy and guidelines. (Section 5.6.1)

Service standard 44: The service a clear and up-to-date local policy and procedures for handling complaints. (Section 5.6.2)

Service standard 45: The service has a clear and up-to-date policy related to health, safety and protection of staff and clients. (Section 5.6.4)

Service standard 46: The service involves service users in the evaluation and development of services. (Section 5.7)

Service standard 47: The service has a clear and up-to-date policy for dealing with media enquiries. (Section 5.8)

Service standard 48: The service has a clear and up-to-date policy on the management of student placements. (Section 5.9.3)

Service standard 49: Where the service head is not a qualified speech and language therapist, there is a system of professional representation to the service manager on matters relating to clinical issues. (Section 5.9.4)

Service Standard 50: Where there are gaps or shortfalls against standards in the service, there is clear evidence that the service is taking steps to develop and improve the service. (Section 6.2.3)

Service standard 51: The service has a strategy in relation to health inequalities and is able to demonstrate actions taken to reduce these inequalities. (Section 6.2.3)

Service Standard 52: There are clear and up-to-date written policies on admission to and discharge from speech and language therapy services for referred individuals (level 3 services). (Section 6.2.4)

Service standard 53:The service has links with voluntary organisations vocational/employment agencies, and local support groups to complement the work of the service. (Section 6.2.4)

Service standard 54: There are clear written care pathways for each speech and language therapy care group that reflect and anticipate the needs of clients, many of whom have enduring, complex and multiple health and social needs. (Section 6.3.1)

Service standard 55: Where specialist services are not available within the immediate service or local district there is a pathway and clear procedures for individuals to access these outwith the region. (Section 6.3.1)

Service standard 56: Clinical care standards are linked to the published research evidence-base and consensus views on best practice. (Section 9.2)

Service standard 57: Service evaluation as the basis of a service development bid involves consultation with commissioners, service users, referral agents, and other services or agencies that are co-providers of services. (Section 9.4.3)

Notes on terminology:

Clear is used to denote text that is, as far as possible, free from ambiguity.

Up-to-date is used to denote policy content that has been reviewed and revised to reflect the current context and thinking and that the review has occurred within the last three years.

Appendix 2

Sources of further support and information for individuals, their families and professionals

The following list of organisations is not intended to be exhaustive, but to provide a starting point for people seeking further information in relation to communication and swallowing disorders.

Every reasonable effort has been made to ensure that the information was accurate at the time of publication.

ACE Centre Advisory Trust
www.ace-centre.org.uk provides assessment, advice and training in the use of technology for young people with physical and communication difficulties.

A C T Aid for Children with Tracheostomies
www.actfortrachykids.com provides information and support for families who have children with tracheostomies

ACT www.act.org.uk works to improve care and services for all children in the UK with life-threatening or terminal conditions and their families.

fasic www.afasic.org.uk provides information and support for children and young people with speech and language impairments and their families.

Alcoholics Anonymous www.alcoholics-anonymous.org.uk is a fellowship of men and women who share their experience, strength and hope with each other that they may solve their common problem and help others to recover from alcoholism.

Alzheimers Organisation www.alzheimers.org.uk is a care and research charity for people with dementia, their families and carers.

Aphasia help www.aphasiahelp.org provides information for people with aphasia, including a penpal service.

ARCOS (Association for the rehabilitation of Communication skills) www.arcos.org.uk provides information and support for people who have acquired communication problems.

ASH Scotland is the leading voluntary organisation campaigning for effective tobacco control legislation and providing an expert information service. www.ashscotland.org.uk

ASLTIP www.helpwithtalking.com provides support for SLTs in independent practice. ASLTIP holds a list of independent practitioners that may be contacted.

Ataxia UK www.ataxia.org.uk supports people affected by ataxia with research, information, welfare grants, campaigning and the opportunity to meet and help others in a similar position.

Becta (British Educational Communications & Technology Agency) www.becta.org.uk contains online version of the journal *Deafblind Perspectives.*

Ben Walton Trust www.benwaltontrust.org is a charity that offers direct patient support and advice and information on oral cancers.

BILD (British Institute for Learning Disabilities) www.bild.org.uk provides information and support in relation to learning disability.

BDA (British Deaf Association) www.signcommunity.org.uk provides information and support for the Deaf.

Birth Defects Foundation www.bdfcharity.co.uk is a UK charity that provides information and support and nurse advice for all birth defects.

BLISS www.bliss.org.uk provides support for parents and families of newborn babies requiring special care.

British Aphasiology Society www.bas.org.uk is a national interest group formed to foster the development of the study of aphasia

British Association for Counselling and Psychotherapy www.bacp.co.uk provides information on counselling and psychotherapy. Holds a list of registered psychotherapists.

British Psychoanalytic Council www.bcp.org.uk provides information on psychoanalytic psychotherapy. Holds a list of registered psychotherapists.

British Dental Health Foundation offers free expert advice on oral health problems including mouth cancer. Provides an information leaflet *Tell me about mouth cancer* which has information on the causes, diagnosis and treatments of mouth cancer. www.mouthcancer.org.uk

British Dyslexia Association www.bda-dyslexia.org.uk offers advice, information and help to families, professionals and individuals with dyslexia. Committed to raising awareness and understanding of dyslexia.

British Cochlear Implant Group www.bcig.co.uk provides information on cochlear implants.

British Dietetics Association www.bda.uk.com provides advice on diet, nutrition and lifestyle, offering essential information from authorities in the field of diet and food information. List of registered dietitians held.

British Stammering Association www.stammering.org provides information and support on stammering.

British Voice Association www.british-voice-association.com provides information on healthy voice use and care and prevention of voice problems.

CancerBACUP www.cancerbacup.org.uk is a free one-to-one service that provides counselling and emotional support for people with cancer and their families and friends.

Cancer Help UK www.cancerhelp.org.uk is a free information service about cancer and cancer care for people with cancer and their families.

Cancer in Scotland www.show.scot.nhs.uk/sehd/cancerinscotland identifies the wide range of activities necessary to prevent, detect and improve treatment and care for people with cancer in Scotland.

Cancer Laryngectomee Trust www.cancerlt.org offers free help to sufferers of cancer of the larynx, people who have had a laryngectomy and their carers.

CALL Centre (Communication Aids for Language and Learning)

w.callcentre.education.ed.ac.uk provides specialist expertise in chnology for children who have speech, communication and/or writing difficulties.

Changing Faces www.changingfaces.org.uk supports and represents people who have disfigurements of the face or body from any cause.

CBIT (Child Brain Injury Trust) www.cbituk.org aims to improve the quality of life for all children and young people who have an acquired brain injury.

CLAPA (Cleft lip and Palate Association) www.clapa.com provides information on services and advice on cleft lip and palate.

CommunicAbility – The James Powell (UK) Trust www.communicability.smartchange.org provides advice on simple communication aid equipment

Communication Matters www.communicationmatters.org.uk is a national voluntary organisation of members concerned with augmentative and alternative communications.

Connect see UK Connect.

Contact a Family www.cafamily.org.uk is a UK charity for families with disabled children offering information on specific conditions and rare disorders.

Council for Disabled Children www.ncb.org.uk/cdc deals with policy and practice issues for disabled children and young people and those with special educational needs.

Deafblind UK (The Association of Deafblind and Dual Sensory Impaired People) www.deafblind.org.uk provides information and support for individuals who are deafblind.

Different Strokes www.differentstrokes.co.uk specialises in the support of young stroke survivors and their carers.

DIPex (Database of Individual Experiences) www.dipex.org is a website that reports on a wide variety of personal experiences of health and illness. People can watch, listen to or read interviews, find reliable information on treatment choices and where to find support. The site covers heart disease, epilepsy, screening programmes and cancers.

Down's Syndrome Association www.downs-syndrome.org.uk provides information, counselling and support for people with Down's syndrome, their families and carers, as well as for professionals.

Dyspraxia Foundation www.dyspraxiafoundation.org.uk supports individuals and families affected by developmental dyspraxia.

EQUIP Electronic Quality Information for Patients
www.equip.nhs.uk is a gateway to quality health and social care
information for UK patients, their families and carers. Provides
information about risks, symptoms and treatment options as well as
where to seek support and advice (in UK).

Foundation for people with learning disabilities
www.learningdisabilities.org.uk provides information about issues
affecting the lives of people with learning disabilities.

Fragile X Society www.fragilex.org.uk provides information and
support related to Fragile X.

Headlines www.headlines.org.uk provides information on conditions
associated with Craniosynostosis.

Headway www.headway.org.uk provides information and promotes
understanding of all aspects of brain injury.

Healthyliving www.healthyliving.gov.uk promotes Scotland's healthy
living programme and is designed to help people attain a healthier
diet and a more active lifestyle by providing resources, advice and
support on healthy eating and physical activity.

Home Farm Trust www.hft.org.uk provides a range of services
including supported living, registered care homes, advocacy,
supported employment, short-term breaks (respite) and day services
for individuals with learning disability.

Hospice Information Service www.hospiceinformation.info

Huntingtons Disease Association www.hda.org.uk provides health
care information and details of medical research into curing
Huntington's Disease.

I CAN www.ican.org.uk provides a combination of specialist therapy
and education for children with the most severe and complex
disabilities, information for parents and training and advice for
teachers and other professionals.

Learning Disabilities UK www.learningdisabilitiesUK.org.uk
provides information and support for people with learning disability.

Let's Face It (Head and Neck Cancer Support Group)
www.lets-face-it.org.uk offers one to one support and befriending,
telephone communication and letter writing. Provides literature
information and resources for recovery.

Long Term Medical Conditions Alliance www.lmca.org.uk is the
umbrella body for national voluntary organisations working to meet
the needs of people with long-term health conditions.

MacMillan Cancer Relief www.macmillan.org.uk supports people with cancer and their families with specialist information, treatment and care.

Maggie's Centres Scotland www.maggiescentres.org aims to help people with cancer to be as healthy in mind and body as possible and enable them to make their own contribution to their medical treatment and recovery.

Marie Curie Cancer Care www.mariecurie.org.uk is a comprehensive cancer care charity, providing practical nursing care at home and specialist multidisciplinary care through its ten Marie Curie centres.

MaxAppeal www.maxappeal.org.uk provides information and support in relation to velo-cardial facial syndrome (VCFS).

Mencap www.mencap.org.uk campaigns for equal rights for children and adults with a learning disability and offers a variety of services to them and their families.

Mental Health Foundation www.mentalhealth.org.uk aims to help people survive, recover from and prevent mental health problems.

MIND (National Association for Mental Health) www.mind.org.uk provides information on all aspects of mental health.

Motor Neurone Disease Association www.mndassociation.org provides information and support in relation to MND.

Mouth Cancer Foundation (MCF) www.rdoc.org.uk aims to help patients, carers and health professionals find free information on mouth cancers easily. It provides direct links to the relevant sections of existing cancer sites and includes patient experiences as well as an online support group.

Multiple Sclerosis Society www.mssociety.org.uk provides information and support in relation to MS.

Muscular Dystrophy Campaign www.muscular-dystrophy.org provides information and support in relation to MD.

NAPLIC (National Association of Professionals concerned with Language) www.naplic.org.uk exists to promote and increase the awareness and understanding of language impairment in children.

NASEN www.nasen.org.uk is an organisation for the education, training, development and support of all those working within the field of special and additional support needs.

National Cochlear Implant Users Association www.nciua.demon.co.uk

The National Association of Deafened People www.nadp.org.uk a UK organisation representing deafened people, providing information and support to enable them to regain their independence and quality of life.

National Association of Laryngectomee Clubs (NALC) www.nalc.ik.com provides information and support for those living with laryngectomy.

National Autistic Society www.nas.org.uk

National Deaf Children's Society www.ndcs.org.uk

National Parent Partnership Network www.parentpartnership.org.uk is a national organisation supporting and enabling parents and carers of children with special educational needs.

Neurological Alliance www.neural.org.uk provides details of organisations that can offer help and assistance to people with a neurological condition.

OAASIS (Office for Advice, Assistance, Support and Information on Special needs) www.oaasis.co.uk provides support for parents of children with special needs.

Pain Association www.painassociation.com provides support for all cancer patients suffering from pain. Offers the opportunity for patients and their carers to join support groups.

Parkinson's Disease Society www.parkinsons.org.uk provides support, advice and information to people with Parkinson's in the UK, their carers, families and friends.

PSP Association www.pspeur.org provides information and support for those with Progressive Supranuclear Palsy.

Rehab UK www.rehabuk.org works in the area of brain injury and brain injury services.

Rethink www.rethink.org provides information and support for those affected by severe mental illness.

Royal National Institute for the Blind www.rnib.org.uk provides education and information services.

Royal National Institute for Deaf People www.rnid.org.uk provides education and information services

Samaritans www.samaritans.org.uk is available 24 hours a day to provide confidential emotional support for people who are experiencing feelings of distress or despair, including those which may lead to suicide.

Smoking and Tobacco unwrapped www.hebs.org/topics/smoking/index.htm provides advice and support on giving up smoking.

The Sarah Matheson Trust www.msaweb.co.uk offers support, information and services to people living with Multiple System Atrophy.

SCOPE www.scope.org.uk is a UK disability organisation whose focus is people with cerebral palsy.

Scottish Association for Mental Health www.samh.org.uk operates a range of services across Scotland for people with mental health problems.

Sense www.sense.org.uk supports people of all ages who are deafblind or have associated disabilities.

The Shaftesbury Society www.shaftesburysociety.org works with disabled people and local communities to achieve social inclusion, empowerment and justice.

Speakability www.speakability.org.uk dedicated to helping aphasic individuals rebuild communication through information services, self-help groups and education.

The Stroke Association www.stroke.org.uk provides information and support for people living with the effects of stroke.

Talking point www.talkingpoint.org.uk provides information and resources about children with speech, language and communication difficulties.

UK Connect www.ukconnect.org is a national charity working collaboratively with people with aphasia.

UK Council for Psychotherapy www.psychotherapy.org.uk promotes the profession of psychotherapy. Holds a register of psychotherapists.

Voice Care Network UK www.voicecare.org.uk provides information about the care, development and use of the speaking voice.

Index

Page numbers in italic refer to figures or tables.

Fair Employment and Treatment (Northern Ireland) Order, 1998 70-1
feeding difficulties 321-4
   in cleft palate 322
   in craniofacial anomalies 301, 323
FEES *see* Fibre Optic Endoscopic Evaluation of Swallowing
fees for SLT services, guidelines 11
Fibre Optic Endoscopic Evaluation of Swallowing (FEES)
   managing risks 328
   RCSLT policy statement 91, 94
financial issues *see* resource management
focus groups 432
Folia Phoniatrica 45
foreign SLTs
   EU nationals 41-2
   non-EU nationals 43-4
foster parents, and consent to care 19
framing 33
Freedom of Information Act, 2000 62, 141
Friedreich's ataxia
   prevalence 357
   see also neurological disorders
frontal lobe head injuries 281
Fulfilling Lives Rehabilitation in Palliative Care (NCHSPCS 2000) 349

gastro-oesophageal reflux (GOR)
   in adults with learning difficulties 330
   in children 322
gifts and hospitality 11
Glasgow Coma Scale 272
'glue ear' 310-11
goal attainment measures 422-3
goal setting 208-9, 422-3
   examples 424-6
governance 415-16
   definitions 413
   see also clinical governance
Government
   defined 52
   functions of Parliament 52

invasive procedures, RCSLT guidelines 334
IPR 105
INVOLVE (engagement in research) 167

job descriptions 102
joint commissioning arrangements 432
    see also commissioning for service development; partnership
    working
Joint Inspection of Children's Services and Inspection of Social Work
    Services (Scotland) Bill (Nov 2005) 68
journals, RCSLT 90-1

KSF (Knowledge and Skills Framework) 124

language competence 41
language impairments *see* specific language impairment
laryngeal cancer 335-6
    see also head and neck cancers
laryngectomy, risk factors 338
learning disabilities *see* adult learning disability; consent issues
learning organisations 114-16
learning problems, and language impairment 368
legal frameworks 13-30
    accountability levels 13-15, *16-17*
    Acts of Parliament 38, 52, 59-72, 81-2
    consent issues 15, 21-2
    professional judgements 35
legal statements 236-7
legal/medical reports 237-9
levels of service provision 184, *185*
Lewin's Force Field Analysis tool 445
liability, indemnity insurance 8-9, 85-6
lifestyle initiatives 73-4
light sensitivity 376
line management 104-5
litigation, NHS funding schemes 157-8

mainstream schools 224-5
management of treatments *see* interventions management

Notes

Notes

Notes

Notes

Notes

Notes